Public Health Consequences of Social Isolation and Loneliness

Public Health Consequences of Social Isolation and Loneliness

Guest Editors

Ami Rokach

David Berman

MDPI

Basel • Beijing • Wuhan • Barcelona • Belgrade • Novi Sad • Cluj • Manchester

Guest Editors
Ami Rokach
Department of Psychology
York University
Toronto
Canada

David Berman
Department of Psychology
York University
Toronto
Canada

Editorial Office
MDPI AG
Grosspeteranlage 5
4052 Basel, Switzerland

This is a reprint of the Special Issue, published open access by the journal *International Journal of Environmental Research and Public Health* (ISSN 1660-4601), freely accessible at: https://www.mdpi.com/journal/ijerph/special_issues/0MS48NL974.

For citation purposes, cite each article independently as indicated on the article page online and as indicated below:

Lastname, A.A.; Lastname, B.B. Article Title. *Journal Name* **Year**, *Volume Number*, Page Range.

ISBN 978-3-7258-5859-0 (Hbk)
ISBN 978-3-7258-5860-6 (PDF)
https://doi.org/10.3390/books978-3-7258-5860-6

Contents

About the Editors

Ami Rokach

Ami Rokach, Ph.D., is a member of the psychology department at York University in Toronto Canada, and is a clinical psychologist who has been researching and teaching about loneliness, human sexuality, and psychotherapy for the past 40 years. Ami is the Editor-in-Chief of the *Journal of Psychology: Interdisciplinary and Applied.*

David Berman

David Berman, is a Ph.D. Student at York University's Historical, Theoretical, and Critical Studies of Psychology program. His research interests have included the history of emotions and constructs, including boredom, love, willpower, and anxiety, with additional focus on neoliberal subjectivity, long-term care, and suicide. David is an associate editor of the *Journal of Psychology: Interdisciplinary and Applied.*

International Journal of
Environmental Research and Public Health

MDPI

Editorial

Loneliness: An Existential and Public Health Issue

Ami Rokach * and David Berman

Department of Psychology, Faculty of Health, York University, Toronto, ON M3J 1P3, Canada; davideb.htc@yorku.ca
* Correspondence: rokach@yorku.ca

1. Loneliness, a Universal Issue

Interpersonal relationships are a fundamental human need [1]. Indeed, having strong social and personal relationships contributes to multiple forms of physical and mental health and well-being [2,3]. Loneliness is part of life. Whether frequently or rarely, all humans know the deep and passing pangs of loneliness, of feeling dejected, unimportant, forgotten, and alone [4]. The results of recent studies have revealed an increase in the number of people who state that they have nobody to confide in, demonstrating a significant loss of social contacts compared to past generations [5]. Loneliness may be reactive, when it is experienced as a reaction to a life event, or essential, when it is interwoven into one's personality [6]. There are several variables that are associated with loneliness, such as living alone, being unmarried, not participating in social groups, and having fewer friends to turn to in times of need [7]. Additionally, lack of social support, be it from a close family or friends, may further exacerbate the experience of loneliness [8].

McCullough [9] observed that when one does not feel related to others, feels that one does not matter to them, the feeling of loneliness tends to increase. In the study by A. Flett et al. [10], the authors examined the relationship between belief in mattering to others and loneliness in a sample of 232 undergraduate students. Their results revealed a robust and significant correlation between feeling that one does not matter to others and experiencing loneliness.

Although some may be more vulnerable to the effects of loneliness, it would appear that all are bound to experience this feeling [11]. But who are the lonely? In a study in which lonely people were asked about their experiences, responses such as feeling detached, distanced, and isolated were highlighted. The lonely reported that they feel unimportant, that they do not matter to others, that they are, sometimes, even unnoticed by those around them, and that while they may be surrounded by caring people, they *feel* that no one cares [6].

In addition, the public health implications of loneliness are considerable, given its far-reaching impact on both quality of life and overall health. The results of numerous studies have established clear links between loneliness and adverse health outcomes, including worse cardiovascular and cognitive health [12], a risk factor for dementia and Alzheimer's disease [13], greater likelihood of stroke [14], increased risk of depression [15], and elevated mortality [16].

The present Special Issue includes a variety of articles and studies, the results of which highlight the richness of the experience of loneliness and capture its effects across different age groups and life journeys. This Special Issue is divided into five conceptual sections:

2. Part 1: Defining and Assessing Loneliness

Mills et al. (Contribution 1) focused, in their study, on loneliness in adults with opioid use disorder. They highlighted the psychological correlates of loneliness and its effects on those struggling with addiction.

Rokach et al. (Contribution 2) describe, in their article, the development and validation of a scale aimed at assessing how loneliness is expressed and experienced in intimate relationships. They review the Loneliness in Intimate Relationships Scale (LIRS) in their article.

3. Part 2: Loneliness and Physical and Mental Disorders

Vallee (Contribution 3) highlights the association between loneliness and cardiac problems. Indeed, as the current literature indicates, in general, a positive correlation between loneliness and atherosclerotic cardiovascular disease was found.

Einav & Margalit (Contribution 4) investigated the feeling of loneliness before and after the COVID-19 pandemic, as many individuals experienced loneliness and social alienation during this particular period. They found lower levels of loneliness and a sense of coherence among those questioned before the COVID-19 pandemic compared to those measured after the pandemic.

Patrono et al. (Contribution 5) also sought to determine the impact that COVID-19 had on young adults living in Italy. They found an alarming positive correlation between the length of experienced loneliness and youth rule-breaking behaviour.

Goldberg et al. (Contribution 6) address the isolation and related stigma of family members who live with and care for those with mental health problems. Their results indicated that those living with a mentally ill relative experienced comparatively higher levels of stigma by association compared with those who did not live with such a relative. The authors reported that both groups experienced moderate levels of loneliness and noted that the cohabiting relatives perceived themselves as lacking support from friends and other family members.

4. Part 3: Loneliness in Various Age Groups

Wright & Silard (Contribution 7) examined loneliness in young adult workers in Western Europe. Their results indicated that workers feel invisible at work, have a thwarted sense of belonging to their employers, and consequently experience regular relational deficiencies due to automation and individualisation of work practices.

Ezeokonkwo et al. (Contribution 8) focused their study on older adults and examined the relationship between their interpersonal goals and loneliness. Their results showed that interpersonal goals were significantly negatively associated with loneliness. In other words, those with higher compassion and self-image goals experienced less loneliness.

Ramírez López (Contribution 9) examined the role of functional deficits, depression, and cognitive symptoms in Mexican older adults on their perceived loneliness. Loneliness was found to be associated with depression and low levels of instrumental activities of daily living but not with cognitive impairment.

5. Part 4: Loneliness and Destructive Behaviours

Herczyk et al. (Contribution 10) focused on a sample of individuals with substance abuse disorder and explored the association between loneliness and mindfulness in this particular population. They found that rates of loneliness, depression, and anxiety did not differ between those who continued treatment and those who did not. They noted that rates of mindfulness, which was associated with effective treatment in preliminary findings, were significantly lower among those not retained versus those retained.

Rokach & Chan (Contribution 11) focus on love and the devastating effects of infidelity. It is acknowledged that infidelity, and its negative effects, is relatively prevalent among Western societies. In this particular study, infidelity was associated with loneliness, which may be the cause as well as the result of infidelity, in addition to the association between infidelity and stress and heartache. Infidelity can damage a loving, romantic relationship to the point of its demise.

Yong, R.K.F. (Contribution 12) explored the effects of unemployment and living alone on loneliness and suicidality in Japan. Their results indicated that unemployment and living alone each elevated the risk of suicidality, with the highest rate among unemployed men aged 40–59 living alone. Among women, interaction was most evident for those aged 40–59 and 25 and sub-additive at $\geq$60.

6. Part 5: Addressing Loneliness

Matthaeus et al. (Contribution 13) conducted a study on online dyadic socio-emotional vs. mindfulness-based training. They found that a mental training approach, based on a 12-min novel online practice routine conducted with a partner, was quite effective in reducing pain and could potentially help address the increasing problem of loneliness in our society.

Bjørnøy Urke et al. (Contribution 14) compared the efficacy of a single-tiered vs. multi-tiered approach at preventing loneliness in students from upper secondary schools in Norway. The results highlighted that a multi-tier intervention reduced the feeling of loneliness in the second year of upper secondary school and did so by utilizing a caring school approach during the students' first year. In contrast, the single-tier intervention was associated with increased loneliness due to a decrease in the perception of a caring school climate.

Johnsrud et al. (Contribution 15) sought to explore the effect of outdoor activities on an individual's health and loneliness. They examined the impact of garden installations at inexpensive summer cottages, where dwellers tended and cared for various plants. They found that maintaining such a garden positively impacts self-perceived well-being and physical health through exercise and outdoor activities. They also noted that the allotment garden, which individuals tended to, strongly impacts perceived health, well-being, and sense of coherence for the individuals, by promoting outdoor activities and social interaction while preventing feelings of loneliness and isolation.

Cattaneo et al. (Contribution 16) explored how Nature-Based Social Prescription (NBSPs)-guided group activities could assist people experiencing social isolation and loneliness. They uncovered a holistic health paradigm linking nature, community, and well-being, in addition to stark ecological inequities with limited green-space access in deprived districts, and discovered work challenges that rose as a result of the urgent needs of individuals facing significant socio-economic challenges in demanding contexts. NBSP appears to be a promising approach to addressing loneliness.

Dwyer (Contribution 17) views digital interventions, such as artificial intelligence companions, as methods for fostering connection and mitigating individual negative experiences of loneliness. Based on communication studies and behavioural information design, the author found that loneliness is understood both as an emotional or interpersonal state and as a logical consequence of hegemonic digital and technological design paradigms. The author proposes a model for evaluating and designing digital public health interventions that resist behavioural enclosure and support autonomy, relational depth, systemic accountability, and structural transparency.

* *

The impact of loneliness can be devastating and long-lasting. Mijuskovic [17] poignantly described our social milieu as becoming increasingly contaminated and ironically claimed separation is becoming one of the only things we share. Although responsibility and commitment toward one another are the true salvation of our communities, collaboration has dwindled and been replaced by competition (see also Surkalim et al., [18]).

While these structural causes of loneliness are persistent, the experience of loneliness can be brief, where bouts of the experience have been termed transient loneliness. Loneliness may be experienced occasionally and may not be associated with long-term negative effects [19]. However, experiencing loneliness on a regular or chronic basis may induce a host of emotional, behavioural, and cognitive implications [20,21].

Through this Special Issue, we have not only attempted to highlight the destructive effects of loneliness but also indicate that loneliness need not be a constant companion. Loneliness can, indeed, be addressed, controlled, and need not rule our lives. It has been repeatedly demonstrated that the first step in addressing loneliness is what we have attempted to achieve herein: admit—to ourselves—that we are lonely, recognize and address the learned helplessness which prevents many individuals from actively improving their lot in life, explore the reasons that we experience such isolation, and earnestly attempt to control the loneliness we experience.

Concluding Comments

This Special Issue highlights the multifaceted nature of loneliness, its profound impact on individuals and communities, and what its alarming rise reveals about our present age. To this end, this Special Issue includes diverse investigations into the causes and correlates of loneliness amidst persistent political, technological, economic, and global health challenges. These studies include works that underscore the troubling links between loneliness and issues such as anxiety, depression, and substance abuse (Contributions 1 and 10), all of which appear to be intractable issues plaguing Western societies.

This Special Issue also explores innovative approaches to understanding loneliness within intimate relationships. While such relationships are often viewed as a safeguard against loneliness, this research highlights how they can instead contribute to this issue, particularly when confronted with conflict and infidelity (Contribution 11). Developments in this area of study are further supported by the introduction of a new Loneliness in Intimate Relationships Scale (Contribution 2).

Other contributions examine the impact of the COVID-19 pandemic, wherein the social isolation experienced during lockdowns was linked to heightened levels of loneliness thereafter (Contribution 4). Additionally, this research shows that male youths who lived through the lockdowns exhibited increased rates of rule-breaking behaviours (Contribution 5). While extensive research will be required to fully contextualize the long-term psychological effects of this global disruption on millions of individuals, it is already clear that societies will be grappling with its consequences for many years to come.

Addressing the complex nature of loneliness, this Special Issue also examines its associations with both physical and psychological disorders, whereby Vallée (Contribution 3) draws attention to how loneliness is a risk factor for cardiovascular disease in men, while Goldberg et al. (Contribution 6) explore the stigmatization faced not only by individuals with mental illness but also by their families. This stigma is linked to a lack of compassion, relationships, and understanding and elevated levels of loneliness.

In the included articles, loneliness was acknowledged as a pervasive issue across all age groups. Younger workers, for instance, often experience loneliness during work hours, struggling to build meaningful connections with coworkers in modern workplaces that prioritize competition over collaboration (Contribution 7). Similarly, Urke et al. (Contribution 14) investigated various approaches to reduce student loneliness. In contrast, López et al. (Contribution 9) and Ezeokonkwo et al. (Contribution 8) examined the close relationship between loneliness and older adults, highlighting how a decline in interpersonal goals and instrumental activities can leave individuals increasingly vulnerable in later life.

These research efforts also included practical approaches to understanding and addressing loneliness, such as how mindfulness can help mitigate substance abuse disorder and loneliness (Contribution 10). Similarly, Urke et al. (Contribution 14) showed that a multi-tier intervention of mindfulness effectively reduced loneliness in students. Another study in this Special Issue examined the positive impact of gardening on loneliness, showing how an improved sense of coherence and increased physical activity can provide meaningful benefits (Contribution 15).

The 17 included papers reveal the complexities surrounding the manifestation and experience of loneliness. They underscore the need for remediation efforts that extend beyond individual-level interventions to include social and workplace considerations. The apparent surge in loneliness in modern life has been linked to a raft of social issues, including the lack of community [7], the decline of "third spaces" [22], and the pervasive influence of social media and related technologies [23]. Addressing these challenges will require a herculean effort that includes collective and community-driven contributions.

With the inevitability of future global pandemics and growing concerns about bird flu [24,25], it is crucial to prioritize efforts to understand and mitigate loneliness, particularly in the context of the reintroduction of government-mandated social restrictions. It is also worth reevaluating the heavy reliance on technological solutions for combating loneliness and fostering sociability. Such approaches have often proven to be of limited efficacy and, in some instances, may have exacerbated the problem [26,27]. The need to investigate the associated harms of these technologies is only made more pressing with the introduction of AI tools and AI-integrated humanoid robotics to explicitly provide "companionship" and address loneliness [28]. Much like social media, governments appear intent on allowing these technologies to proliferate without any serious consideration of the harm they might cause. Because of these existing concerns and developments, emphasizing authentic human interactions and community-building efforts seems more important than ever. While these technologies hold the promise of keeping people connected, especially during times of government-mandated social restrictions, they should be integrated into methods that enhance and support existing social connections and practices rather than allowing them to further encroach on how we interact and connect with one another.

Despite the above concerns, research efforts like those presented in this Special issue offer hope—a powerful confound to loneliness—along with the connections fostered as academics unite to address this pressing issue. These efforts can inform policy approaches that emphasize public and professional education programs aimed at raising awareness and reducing stigma, while ensuring that the negative health consequences of loneliness are not only recognized but addressed through innovative prevention strategies, comprehensive assessment frameworks, and targeted treatment approaches. In this spirit, Ami and I extend our deepest gratitude to the authors of these papers, the diligent reviewers whose contributions are integral to the journal's output, the readers who engage with these works, the wider editorial staff, who made it all possible, and the journal managers for their thoughtful oversight.

Our greatest hope is that these efforts will inspire future research and foster connections within the academic community, empowering us to address loneliness in our work and personal lives.

Author Contributions: Conceptualization, A.R. and D.B.; resources, A.R. and D.B.; writing—original draft preparation, A.R. and D.B.; writing—review and editing, A.R. and D.B. All authors have read and agreed to the published version of the manuscript.

Funding: This research received no external funding.

Conflicts of Interest: The authors declare no conflict of interest.

List of Contributions:

1. Mills, R.; Zullig, K.J.; Theeke, L.A.; Lander, L.R.; Hobbs, G.R.; Herczyk, J.; Davis, S.M. Assessing Loneliness among Adults Receiving Outpatient Treatment with Medication for Opioid Use Disorder (MOUD). *Int. J. Environ. Res. Public Health* **2022**, *19*, 13481. https://doi.org/10.3390/ijerph192013481.
2. Rokach, A.; Sha'ked, A.; Ben-Artzi, E. Loneliness in Intimate Relationships Scale (LIRS): Development and Validation. *Int. J. Environ. Res. Public Health* **2022**, *19*, 12970. https://doi.org/10.3390/ijerph191912970.
3. Vallée, A. Association between Social Isolation and Loneliness with Estimated Atherosclerotic Cardiovascular Disease Risk in a UK Biobank Population-Based Study. *Int. J. Environ. Res. Public Health* **2023**, *20*, 2869. https://doi.org/10.3390/ijerph20042869.
4. Einav, M.; Margalit, M. Loneliness before and after COVID-19: Sense of Coherence and Hope as Coping Mechanisms. *Int. J. Environ. Res. Public Health* **2023**, *20*, 5840. https://doi.org/10.3390/ijerph20105840.
5. Patrono, A.; Invernizzi, A.; Placidi, D.; Cagna, G.; Calza, S.; Oppini, M.; Rechtman, E.; Papazaharias, D.M.; Reichenberg, A.; Lucchini, R.G.; et al. Impact of COVID-19-Related Social Isolation on Behavioral Outcomes in Young Adults Residing in Northern Italy. *Int. J. Environ. Res. Public Health* **2022**, *19*, 16496. https://doi.org/10.3390/ijerph192416496.
6. Goldberg, J.O.; McKeag, S.A.; Rose, A.L.; Lumsden-Ruegg, H.; Flett, G.L. Too Close for Comfort: Stigma by Association in Family Members Who Live with Relatives with Mental Illness. *Int. J. Environ. Res. Public Health* **2023**, *20*, 5209. https://doi.org/10.3390/ijerph20065209.
7. Wright, S.L.; Silard, A.G. Loneliness in Young Adult Workers. *Int. J. Environ. Res. Public Health* **2022**, *19*, 14462. https://doi.org/10.3390/ijerph192114462.
8. Ezeokonkwo, F.C.; Sekula, K.L.; Stokes, J.E.; Theeke, L.A.; Zoucha, R.; Troutman-Jordan, M.; Sharma, D. Relationships between Interpersonal Goals and Loneliness in Older Adults: A Cross-Sectional Study. *Int. J. Environ. Res. Public Health* **2023**, *20*, 1914. https://doi.org/10.3390/ijerph20031914.
9. López, A.B.R.; Rodríguez-Agudelo, Y.; Paz-Rodríguez, F.; Tafoya, S.A.; López, B.G.; Olavarrieta, C.D. The Role of Functional Deficits, Depression, and Cognitive Symptoms in the Perceived Loneliness of Older Adults in Mexico City. *Int. J. Environ. Res. Public Health* **2024**, *21*, 977. https://doi.org/10.3390/ijerph21080977.
10. Herczyk, J.M.; Zullig, K.J.; Davis, S.M.; Mallow, J.; Hobbs, G.R.; Davidov, D.M.; Lander, L.R.; Theeke, L. Association of Loneliness and Mindfulness in Substance Use Treatment Retention. *Int. J. Environ. Res. Public Health* **2023**, *20*, 6571. https://doi.org/10.3390/ijerph20166571.
11. Rokach, A.; Chan, S.H. Love and Infidelity: Causes and Consequences. *Int. J. Environ. Res. Public Health* **2023**, *20*, 3904. https://doi.org/10.3390/ijerph20053904.
12. Yong, R. The Double Burden of Isolation and Unemployment: Suicide Risk in Structurally Vulnerable Populations in Japan—A Case Study of Akita Prefecture (2018–2022). *Int. J. Environ. Res. Public Health* **2025**, *22*, 1447. https://doi.org/10.3390/ijerph22091447.
13. Matthaeus, H.; Godara, M.; Silveira, S.; Hecht, M.; Voelkle, M.; Singer, T. Reducing Loneliness through the Power of Practicing Together: A Randomized Controlled Trial of Online Dyadic

Socio-Emotional vs. Mindfulness-Based Training. *Int. J. Environ. Res. Public Health* **2024**, *21*, 570. https://doi.org/10.3390/ijerph21050570.

14. Urke, H.B.; Larsen, T.B.; Kristensen, S.M.E. Preventing Loneliness and Reducing Dropout: Results from the COMPLETE Intervention Study in Upper Secondary Schools in Norway. *Int. J. Environ. Res. Public Health* **2023**, *20*, 6299. https://doi.org/10.3390/ijerph20136299.
15. Johnsrud, M.; Goth, U.S.; Skjerve, H. The Impact of Urban Allotment Gardens on Physical and Mental Health in Norway. *Int. J. Environ. Res. Public Health* **2024**, *21*, 720. https://doi.org/10.3390/ijerph21060720.
16. Cattaneo, L.; Daguzan, A.; Vélez, G.G.; Gentile, S. Conceptualising a Community-Based Response to Loneliness: The Representational Anchoring of Nature-Based Social Prescription by Professionals in Marseille, Insights from the RECETAS Project. *Int. J. Environ. Res. Public Health* **2025**, *22*, 1400. https://doi.org/10.3390/ijerph22091400.
17. Dwyer, L. Loneliness by Design: The Structural Logic of Isolation in Engagement-Driven Systems. *Int. J. Environ. Res. Public Health* **2025**, *22*, 1394. https://doi.org/10.3390/ijerph22091394.

References

1. Allen, K.-A.; Gray, D.L.; Baumeister, R.F.; Leary, M.R. The need to belong: A deep dive into the origins, implications, and future of a foundational construct. *Educ. Psychol. Rev.* **2022**, *34*, 1133–1156. [CrossRef]
2. Floyd, K. *Affectionate Communication in Close Relationships*; Cambridge University Press: Cambridge, UK, 2019. [CrossRef]
3. Holt-Lunstad, J. Why social relationships are important for physical health: A systems approach to understanding and modifying risk and protection. *Annu. Rev. Psychol.* **2018**, *69*, 437–458. [CrossRef]
4. McComb, S.E.; Goldberg, J.O.; Flett, G.L.; Rose, A.L. The double jeopardy of feeling lonely and unimportant: State and trait loneliness and feelings and fears of not mattering. *Front. Psychol.* **2020**, *11*, 563420. [CrossRef]
5. Cacioppo, J.T.; Cacioppo, S. Older adults reporting social isolation or loneliness show poorer cognitive function 4 years later. *Evid. Based Nurs.* **2014**, *17*, 59–60. [CrossRef] [PubMed]
6. Rokach, A. *The Psychological Journey to and From Loneliness: Development, Causes, and Effects of Social and Emotional Isolation*; Academic Press: Cambridge, MA, USA, 2019.
7. Holt-Lunstad, J.; Smith, T.B.; Layton, J.B. Social relationships and mortality risk: A meta-analytic review. *PLoS Med.* **2010**, *7*, e1000316. [CrossRef] [PubMed]
8. Chang, E.C.; Chang, O.D.; Martos, T.; Sallay, V.; Lee, J.; Stam, K.R.; Batterbee, C.N.H.; Yu, T. Family support as a moderator of the relationship between loneliness and suicide risk in college students: Having a supportive family matters! *Fam. J.* **2017**, *25*, 257–263. [CrossRef]
9. McCullough, M.E.; Larson, D.B. Religion and depression: A review of the literature. *Twin Res.* **1981**, *2*, 126–136. [CrossRef]
10. Flett, G.L.; Goldstein, A.L.; Pechenkov, I.G.; Nepon, T.; Wekerle, C. Antecedents, correlates, and consequences of feeling like you don't matter: Associations with maltreatment, loneliness, social anxiety, and the five-factor model. *Personal. Individ. Differ.* **2016**, *92*, 52–56. [CrossRef]
11. Cacioppo, J.T.; Cacioppo, S.; Cole, S.W.; Capitanio, J.P.; Goossens, L.; Boomsma, D.I. Loneliness across phylogeny and a call for animal models. *Perspect. Psychol. Sci.* **2015**, *10*, 202–212. [CrossRef]
12. Cené, C.W.; Beckie, T.M.; Sims, M.; Suglia, S.F.; Aggarwal, B.; Moise, N.; Jiménez, M.C.; Gaye, B.; McCullough, L.D. Effects of objective and perceived social isolation on cardiovascular and brain health: A scientific statement from the American Heart Association. *J. Am. Heart Assoc.* **2022**, *11*, e026493. [CrossRef]
13. Akhter-Khan, S.C.; Tao, Q.; Ang, T.F.A.; Itchapurapu, I.S.; Alosco, M.L.; Mez, J.; Piers, R.J.; Steffens, D.C.; Au, R.; Qiu, W.Q. Associations of loneliness with risk of Alzheimer's disease dementia in the Framingham Heart Study. *Alzheimer's Dement.* **2021**, *17*, 1619–1627. [CrossRef]
14. Soh, Y.; Kawachi, I.; Kubzansky, L.D.; Berkman, L.F.; Tiemeier, H. Chronic loneliness and the risk of incident stroke in middle and late adulthood: A longitudinal cohort study of US older adults. *EClinicalMedicine* **2024**, *73*, 102639. [CrossRef]
15. Loades, M.E.; Chatburn, E.; Higson-Sweeney, N.; Reynolds, S.; Shafran, R.; Brigden, A.; Linney, C.; McManus, M.N.; Borwick, C.; Crawley, E. Rapid systematic review: The impact of social isolation and loneliness on the mental health of children and adolescents in the context of COVID-19. *J. Am. Acad. Child Adolesc. Psychiatry* **2020**, *59*, 1218–1239. [CrossRef]
16. Holt-Lunstad, J.; Smith, T.B.; Baker, M.; Harris, T.; Stephenson, D. Loneliness and social isolation as risk factors for mortality: A meta-analytic review. *Perspect. Psychol. Sci.* **2015**, *10*, 227–237. [CrossRef]
17. Mijuskovic, B.L. *Loneliness in Philosophy, Psychology, and Literature*; iUniverse: Bloomington, IN, USA, 2012.

18. Surkalim, D.L.; Luo, M.; Eres, R.; Gebel, K.; van Buskirk, J.; Bauman, A.; Ding, D. The prevalence of loneliness across 113 countries: Systematic review and meta-analysis. *Br. Med. J.* **2022**, *376*, e067068. [CrossRef] [PubMed]
19. DiTomasso, E.; Fizzel, S.R.; Robinson, B.A. Chronic loneliness within an attachment framework: Process and interventions. In *Addressing Loneliness: Coping, Prevention and Clinical Interventions*; Sha'ked, A., Rokach, A., Eds.; Routledge: New York, NY, USA, 2015.
20. Hawkley, L.C.; Cacioppo, J.T. Loneliness matters: A theoretical and empirical review of consequences and mechanisms. *Ann. Behav. Med.* **2010**, *40*, 218–227. [CrossRef] [PubMed]
21. Stickley, A.; Koyanagi, A. Loneliness, common mental disorders and suicidal behavior: Findings from a general population survey. *J. Affect. Disord.* **2016**, *197*, 81–87. [CrossRef] [PubMed]
22. Putnam, R.D. *Bowling Alone: The Collapse and Revival of American Community*; Simon Schuster: New York, NY, USA, 2000.
23. Hunt, M.G.; Marx, R.; Lipson, C.; Young, J. No more FOMO: Limiting social media decreases loneliness and depression. *J. Soc. Clin. Psychol.* **2018**, *37*, 751–768. [CrossRef]
24. Kniss, K.; Sumner, K.M.; Tastad, K.J.; Lewis, N.M.; Jansen, L.; Julian, D.; Reh, M.; Carlson, E.; Williams, R.; Koirala, S.; et al. Risk for infection in humans after exposure to birds infected with highly pathogenic avian influenza A (H5N1) virus, United States, 2022. *Emerg. Infect. Dis.* **2023**, *29*, 1215. [CrossRef]
25. Webby, R.J.; Uyeki, T.M. An update on highly pathogenic avian influenza A (H5N1) virus, clade 2.3. 4.4 b. *J. Infect. Dis.* **2024**, *230*, 533–542. [CrossRef]
26. Primack, B.A.; Shensa, A.; Sidani, J.E.; Whaite, E.O.; Lin, L.Y.; Rosen, D.; Colditz, J.B.; Radovic, A.M.; Miller, E. Social media use and perceived social isolation among young adults in the US. *Am. J. Prev. Med.* **2017**, *53*, 1–8. [CrossRef] [PubMed]
27. Sharabi, L.L.; Von Feldt, P.A.; Ha, T. Burnt out and still single: Susceptibility to dating app burnout over time. *New Media Soc.* **2024**. [CrossRef]
28. Business Wire. Realbotix Unveils New Robotic Technology at CES 2025. *Business Wire*. Available online: https://www.businesswire.com/news/home/20250107953617/en/Realbotix-Unveils-New-Robotic-Technology-At-CES-2025?utm_source=chatgpt.com (accessed on 7 January 2025).

International Journal of
Environmental Research and Public Health

MDPI

Article

Assessing Loneliness among Adults Receiving Outpatient Treatment with Medication for Opioid Use Disorder (MOUD)

Rosalina Mills [1], Keith J. Zullig [1,*], Laurie A. Theeke [2], Laura R. Lander [3], Gerry R. Hobbs [4], Johnathan Herczyk [1] and Stephen M. Davis [5]

1 Department of Social and Behavioral Sciences, School of Public Health, West Virginia University, Morgantown, WV 26506, USA
2 School of Nursing, George Washington University, Washington, DC 20052, USA
3 Department of Behavioral Medicine and Psychiatry, Rockefeller Neurosciences Institute, School of Medicine, West Virginia University, Morgantown, WV 26506, USA
4 Department of Statistics, West Virginia University, Morgantown, WV 26506, USA
5 Department of Health Policy, Management, & Leadership, School of Public Health, West Virginia University, Morgantown, WV 26506, USA
* Correspondence: kzullig@hsc.wvu.edu; Tel.: +1-304-293-1091; Fax: +1-304-293-6685

Abstract: Loneliness is a significant risk factor for substance use, however, impacts of treatments on loneliness are relatively unexplored. Living in a rural location is a greater risk factor for loneliness. This study examined data from a quasi-experimental study in rural Appalachia, comparing the effectiveness of Mindfulness-Based Relapse Prevention (MBRP) versus Treatment as Usual (TAU) among adults receiving MOUD in outpatient therapy. Our objective was to determine whether observed reductions in self-reported craving, anxiety, depression, and increased perceived mindfulness would also improve loneliness reports. Eighty participants (n = 35 MBRP; n = 45 TAU) were included in the analysis from a group-based Comprehensive Opioid Addiction Treatment program. Outcomes tracked included craving, anxiety, depression, mindfulness, and loneliness as measured by the Revised UCLA Loneliness Scale (R-UCLA). A linear mixed model ANOVA determined the significance of the treatments on changes in loneliness scores at baseline, 12 weeks, 24 weeks, and 36 weeks post-recruitment. Both groups reported significantly reduced loneliness over the course of the study ($F = 16.07$, $p < 0.01$), however there were no significant differences between groups. Loneliness was also significantly positively ($p < 0.01$) correlated with anxiety (0.66), depression (0.59), and craving (0.38), and significantly ($p < 0.01$) inversely correlated (-0.52) with mindfulness. Results suggest that participation in MOUD group-based outpatient therapy has the potential to diminish loneliness and associated poor psychological outcomes. Thus, it is possible that a more targeted intervention for loneliness would further diminish loneliness, which is important as loneliness is linked to risk for relapse.

Keywords: medication for opioid use disorder outpatient therapy; treatment; intervention; loneliness; R-UCLA

1. Introduction

Substance use disorder (SUD) is prevalent in the United States and is defined as problematic and disordered use of substances such as alcohol, cannabis, cocaine, heroin, hallucinogens, inhalants, prescription opioids, sedatives, stimulants, and/or other drugs, according to the Diagnostic and Statistical Manual of Mental Disorders, Fifth Edition (DSM-5) criteria [1,2]. It is currently estimated that 20 million people aged 12 and older struggle with substance use disorders in the United States [3]. Furthermore, the use of opioids has become a national health crisis with over 80,000 Americans dying from opioid-related overdoses in 2021 [4]. Hence, there is a continuing need for research and treatments targeting potential risk factors for opioid use disorder (OUD), which is defined by DSM-5 diagnostic criteria as the disordered use of a prescription opioid, heroin, or both [5].

Existing literature has shown that Americans with psychological problems or psychiatric diagnoses are more likely to develop SUD and use opioids than Americans without these illnesses [6–8]. Loneliness is a significant stressor that has been consistently linked to negative physical, social, and psychological health outcomes [9–11]; including depression and anxiety, as well as with the use of alcohol, cigarettes and other substances [12–15]. Although loneliness prevalence varies by country and age group, it is typically highest among adults [16]. The national prevalence of loneliness in the United States is estimated to be between 11–22% for adults [17,18], and 35% for adults aged 45 and older [19]. One U.S. study found that 76% of sampled community-dwelling adults reported moderate or high levels of loneliness [20].

It is important to distinguish loneliness from social isolation. Social isolation is the lack of social contact and regular human interaction, while loneliness is the distressing feeling associated with being alone or isolated [21]. It is possible for people to be socially isolated and not lonely; contrarily, it is also possible to feel lonely while in the company of others. Loneliness and social isolation have both been associated with negative outcomes, such as mortality and mood and anxiety disorders [19,22,23]. While literature studying the relationship between social isolation and loneliness is sparse, an increase in social isolation, or a reduction in social networks, is a predictor of loneliness [24].

Loneliness has already been identified as a risk factor for opioid use [25–27]; and associated with relapse in people with OUD, women with depression and in treatment for OUD, and for people who use methamphetamine [26,28,29]. Thus, it may be critical to assess for and address loneliness as part of SUD treatment, yet this is not part of routine care for people with SUD [26,30]. Although mental health treatments that target loneliness have been developed [31,32], a recent systematic review identified only nine longitudinal studies that investigated loneliness in SUD treatment [13], and even fewer highlighted a need to investigate interventions for loneliness during OUD treatment [13]. Given the limited studies on loneliness, mindfulness and SUD treatment, there is a continuing need to study loneliness and its impact on recovery among those receiving treatment for OUD. In addition, these prior studies were predominantly conducted in urban areas, leaving a significant gap in the literature when seeking to understand the impact of loneliness on people who live in rural areas like Appalachia, a known area of extreme disparity in SUD.

Rurality, Loneliness, and SUD

Appalachia is a rural region of the United States spanning 205,000 square miles, from New York State to Mississippi [33]. Appalachia has also been disproportionately affected by opioid overdoses and overdose death rates compared to the rest of the United States [33]. West Virginia, in particular, has the highest drug overdose deaths per capita, with rates peaking at 52.8 per 100,000 people in 2019 [34]. The highest proportion of these overdose deaths was from opioid misuse [34]. COVID-19 has reversed any effects of overdose reduction; recent estimates show overdose death increased from 2019 to 2020 by 45% in West Virginia [35].

West Virginia's rural characteristics may also play a role in barriers to adequate healthcare. Nearly half of West Virginia's counties do not provide waivers to prescribe buprenorphine, an evidence-based treatment for OUD [36]. Living in a rural location is also a substantially greater risk factor for social isolation and loneliness [37,38]. Despite these facts, there is a dearth of research on loneliness in substance-using, rural populations, and especially Appalachian populations.

The current study is a secondary analysis of data examining loneliness levels among adults receiving Medication for Opioid Use Disorder (MOUD) in outpatient therapy in a rural Appalachian state as part of an intervention testing the effectiveness of Mindfulness-Based Relapse Prevention (MBRP). Conducted over a period of 36 weeks, the intervention from which these data are derived demonstrated significantly reduced self-reported craving, anxiety, and depression as perceived mindfulness increased among MBRP/MOUD participants when compared to treatment as usual (TAU) cognitive behavioral therapy MOUD participants [39]. The intervention was not designed with the intent to address loneliness among participants, nor has there been any empirical investigation into an intervention's potential impact on loneliness. However, there is a clear theoretical premise for such an investigation given previous research connecting loneliness to SUD.

Examining depression and anxiety is also important for the purposes of this study, given that these factors have been found to be prevalent in rural populations [40], and are also associated with loneliness and OUD [22,41]. Mood disorders often co-occur with SUD [41], therefore the results from the current study are more robust by also measuring depression and anxiety in addition to loneliness.

Existing evidence suggests that craving may also potentially influence substance use, specifically in OUD treatment populations [42]. Craving symptoms have been found to be associated with depression, anxiety, and negative social exchanges [42]. The importance of social support in the context of OUD treatment is highlighted by evidence demonstrating that daily positive social exchanges, that is, social support and positive interactions with others, helped reduce cravings experienced by patients in OUD treatment [42], providing additional evidence to study loneliness during OUD treatment. Thus, craving was included in the study as an indicator of future substance use, and as a factor that may be influenced by loneliness.

Mindfulness is also an important factor to consider when examining loneliness and OUD treatment. Mindfulness interventions specific to SUD address the relapse cycle by cultivating the awareness of triggers, attending mindfully to the discomforts the triggers elicited, and teaching targeted skills to cope with craving, thus facilitating the recovery process [43,44].

Systemic reviews, as well as individual randomized controlled trials, have shown that mindfulness-based interventions can significantly reduce loneliness [45–48]. Mindfulness training has been demonstrated to reduce loneliness in participants throughout the course of 6 to 8-week interventions [47]. However, when examined in the context of MOUD treatment, recent research suggests loneliness and other indicators of mental health (e.g., depression, anxiety, etc.) and well-being were not significantly reduced by MOUD alone after the first 6 months of treatment [49]. This research highlights a clear need for behavioral therapy and support in tandem with MOUD during treatment, such as mindfulness.

Thus, our study objective was to determine whether loneliness levels would improve among adults in MOUD outpatient treatment also receiving behavioral therapy. Our overall hypothesis was that over the course of the study, as participants engaged in the recovery process addressing psychological processes associated with OUD (e.g., anxiety, depression, and craving), reports of loneliness would also decrease. Anxiety, depression, and craving were included in the study owing to their relationship to loneliness in the literature. However, given the preliminary nature of the study, no hypotheses were made regarding between-group differences in loneliness reports.

2. Materials and Methods

Data were derived from a study conducted from September 2017–December 2019 that included participants recruited during the intermediate stage of treatment (patients with at least 90 consecutive days substance free) from a large, Mid-Atlantic university's Comprehensive Opioid Addiction Treatment (COAT) program. Project investigators met with interested and eligible participants to describe the study, administer consent, and conduct baseline data assessments. Participants were then given the option to enroll in MBRP plus MOUD or remain in TAU MOUD. MBRP/MOUD group participants were assigned to attend bi-weekly 60-min group therapy sessions for 24 weeks. For a full description of the intervention, see Zullig et al. [39]. The referent university's Institutional Review Board approved this study.

All analyses were conducted in SAS version 9.4. Descriptive statistics were first calculated followed by a linear mixed model ANOVA where fixed effects are reported in the results. For this analysis, we were specifically interested in determining whether loneliness levels would improve among intervention participants. Linear mixed models (also called multilevel models) are a method for analyzing data that are non-independent, multilevel/hierarchical, and longitudinal, which allowed us to explore the difference between effects within and between groups. Linear mixed models effectively use all of the available data to estimate change over time and is a preferred method to last value carried forward methods often used in intent-to-treat analyses. The analysis controlled for the demographic variables age, sex, marital status, education levels, employment status, and insurance specified a priori. We also used ANOVA to examine the correlations between the changes in loneliness at 36 weeks for the baseline demographic variables. Cohen's d was used to calculate effect sizes to determine the magnitude of statistically significant findings. Lastly, we performed a series of correlations at baseline to assess the strength of the association between perceived loneliness and negative psychological health outcomes [9–11] including depression and anxiety. An alpha level of 0.05 was used to determine the statistical significance of all analyses.

Measures

Study outcomes were participants' self-reported craving, depression, and anxiety levels; mindfulness; and loneliness. All measures were administered at baseline, after 12 weeks, post-intervention (24 weeks), and again 36 weeks post-intervention to MBRP/MOUD and TAU/MOUD study participants.

Craving symptoms. Craving symptoms were measured by the 14-item Desire for Drugs Questionnaire (DDQ). Response options are (a) strongly disagree, (b) disagree, (c) undecided, (d) agree, and (e) strongly agree with values from 1 (strongly disagree) to 5 (strongly agree) assigned. The sum of the response values (range 14–70) was the outcome of interest with higher values indicative of greater cravings. The DDQ has previously demonstrated acceptable validity and internal consistency reliability with estimates above 0.80 [50]. The baseline internal consistency estimate for the DDQ in this study was 0.78.

Depression. Depression was assessed using the 5-item Overall Depression Severity and Impairment Scale (ODSIS). Each item has 4 response options that are summed (range 0–20) with a total score of 8 or higher used to determine a depression diagnosis (correctly classifies over 80%). The scale has demonstrated acceptable validity and internal consistency reliability with estimates exceeding 0.91 [51]. The baseline internal consistency estimate for the ODSIS in this study was 0.89.

Anxiety. Anxiety was assessed using the 5-item Overall Anxiety Severity and Impairment Scale (OASIS). Each OASIS item has 4 response options that are summed (range 0–20) with a total score of 8 or higher used to determine an anxiety diagnosis (correctly classifies over 80%). The scale has demonstrated acceptable validity and internal consistency reliability with estimates exceeding 0.80 [52,53]. The baseline internal consistency estimate for the OASIS in this study was 0.92.

Mindfulness. Mindfulness was measured with the 39-item self-report 5-Facet Mindfulness Questionnaire (FFMQ). Response options are (a) never or very rarely true, (b) rarely true, (c) sometimes true, (d) often true, and (e) very often or always true with values from 1 (never or very rarely true) to 5 (very often or always true). For this study, the sum of the responses for the total scale were divided by 5 (range 1–5) with higher values indicating greater mindfulness. The FFMQ has demonstrated adequate validity and internal consistency with estimates ranging from 0.75 to 0.91 for the five subscales in prior research [54]. The baseline internal consistency estimate for the FFMQ total scale in this study was 0.89.

Loneliness. Loneliness was assessed using the 20-item Revised-UCLA Loneliness Scale (R-UCLA) [55]. This scale is a self-report Likert scale, with 4 answer options for each item: (1) never, (2) sometimes, (3) often, and (4) always. Nine of these 20 items are reverse-scored; the minimum score for this scale is 20, while the maximum is 80, with lower values indicating improved perceptions of loneliness. The R-UCLA scale is considered the gold standard for measuring loneliness given (1) its ease of administration, (2) acceptable reliability and validity [56], and (3) ability to measure change over time [56,57]. The prevalence of loneliness in many studies using the R-UCLA indicate feeling lonely "at least some of the time" [58], with a threshold of 44 or greater for the full 20-item UCLA scale [59]. Therefore, it is the scale most often used in studies of loneliness, particularly as those pertaining to SUD [13]. The baseline internal consistency estimate for the R-UCLA in this study was 0.92.

3. Results

A total of 80 participants were included in the analysis (MBRP/MOUD, n = 35; TAU/MOUD, n = 45). The intervention flow chart is provided in Figure 1 and group baseline demographics are located in Table 1. The overall sample mean age was 36.3 (SD = 8.7).

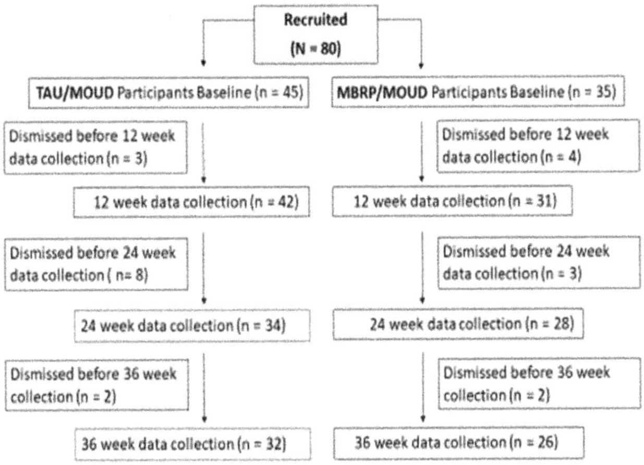

Figure 1. Intervention flowchart.

Table 1. MBRP Intervention Demographic Data by Group and Total (N = 80).

Demographic	TAU (n = 45)	MBRP (n = 35)	Total	*p*-Value
Marital Status				0.63
Single	28 (60.9%)	18 (39.1%)	46	
Married	8 (50.0%)	8 (50.0%)	16	
Divorced or Separating	9 (50.0%)	9 (50.0%)	18	
Sex				0.12
Male	24 (64.9%)	13 (35.1%)	37	
Female	21 (51.2%)	20 (48.9%)	41	
Other	0 (0.0%)	2 (100.0%)	2	
Race				n/a
White	45 (56.3%)	35 (43.8%)	80	
Employment				0.95
Full Time	18 (58.1%)	13 (41.9%)	31	
Part Time	8 (53.3%)	7 (46.7%)	15	
Unemployed	19 (55.9%)	15 (44.1%)	34	
Education				0.10
Did Not Finish High School	3 (37.5%)	5 (62.5%)	8	
High School Graduate/GED	30 (66.7%)	15 (33/3%)	45	
Some College or Greater	11 (40.1%)	16 (59.3%)	27	
Insurance				0.59
Medicaid	34 (52.3%)	31 (47.8%)	65	
Medicare	3 (0.6%)	2 (0.4%)	5	
Private	7 (70.0%)	3 (30.0%)	10	

TAU = Treatment as Usual; MBRP = Mindfulness Based Relapse Prevention (Intervention).

For categorical characteristics in Table 1, no significant differences were detected at baseline between MBRP/MOUD and TAU/MOUD participants within marital status ($p = 0.63$), sex ($p = 0.12$), employment ($p = 0.95$), education ($p = 0.10$), or insurance ($p = 0.59$). A t-test comparing groups in age revealed MBRP/MOUD group participants were statistically significantly ($p = 0.02$) younger (M = 34.9, SD = 6.9) than TAU group participants (M = 37.3, SD = 10.3). However, the effect size for this difference was small (Cohen's d = 0.21), suggesting this difference was not practically important.

Results of the regression analysis are located in Figure 2. Results suggest both MBRP/MOUD and TAU/MOUD groups reported significantly reduced loneliness over the course of the study ($F = 16.07$, $p < 0.0001$, Cohen's d = 0.20) even after controlling for the covariates. However, no significant differences in loneliness reports were detected in the interaction between weeks and groups over the 36-week time period ($F = 0.88$, $p = 0.35$).

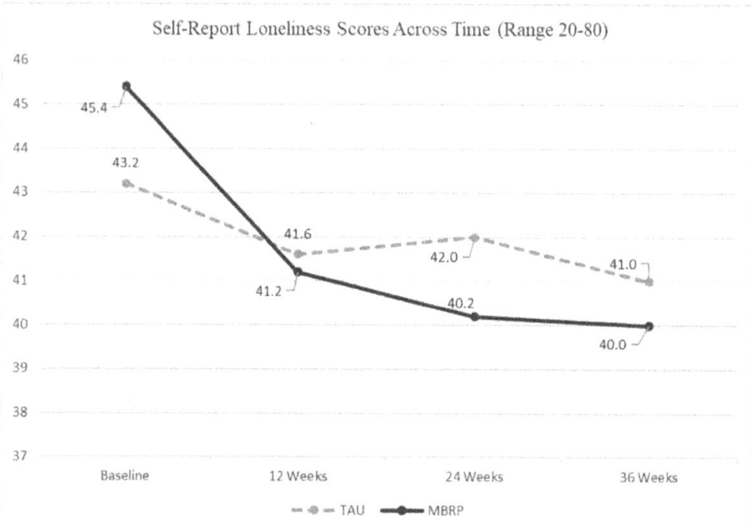

Figure 2. Self-Report Loneliness Scores by Group across the 36 Week Intervention from the Linear Mixed Model.

Nevertheless, given the sharper reductions in reported loneliness scores observed among MBRP/MOUD participants in comparison to the TAU/MOUD participants between the baseline and 12-week data, we investigated the decline in loneliness across time in the MBRP/MOUD group and found significance ($F = 13.83$, $p < 0.001$). This exploratory result suggests loneliness decreased in the MBRP/MOUD group more than the TAU/MOUD group from baseline to 12 weeks.

ANOVA results examining the correlations between the changes in loneliness at 36 weeks for the baseline demographic variables yielded no statistically significant findings. The p-values for these analyses were 0.85 for age, 0.79 for sex, 0.09 employment, 0.48 for education, and 0.34 for insurance.

Loneliness was significantly positively ($p < 0.01$) correlated with anxiety, depression, and craving. Specifically, baseline correlation coefficients between loneliness and anxiety, depression, and craving were 0.66, 0.59, and 0.38, respectively. Loneliness and mindfulness were also significantly ($p < 0.01$) inversely correlated at baseline $r = -0.52$. However, when separated by intervention condition (i.e., MBRP/MOUD and TAU/MOUD), the associations between mindfulness and loneliness were stronger for individuals in the MBRP/MOUD group. For instance, the baseline correlation coefficient between loneliness and mindfulness in the MBRP/MOUD group was -0.59 ($p < 0.01$) in comparison to the TAU/MOUD group $r = -0.39$ ($p < 0.05$).

4. Discussion

Although loneliness has been identified as a possible risk factor for SUD or OUD [26,27] in cross-sectional studies and as a possible reason for relapse [25] in qualitative research, limited research has explored the longitudinal association between loneliness and its correlates among those receiving MOUD in outpatient treatment [13]. Moreover, we were able to locate only two longitudinal studies on outpatient OUD treatment. The first was conducted with urban adults receiving buprenorphine treatment and suggests that very lonely adults with substance use disorder may have more difficulty with cessation [60]. For instance, participants in their study with the highest levels of loneliness were most likely to have non-prescribed opioids present in their oral fluid or urine during drug testing [60]. The second was also conducted with participants in a large metropolitan city receiving MOUDs and no behavioral therapy and found loneliness was not significantly reduced after six months treatment [49].

Findings from the current study suggest both TAU/MOUD and MBRP/MOUD groups reported statistically significantly reduced perceptions of loneliness over the course of the intervention, however the effect was "small". It is worth underlining that although the effect size was small, these results were found despite the fact that neither TAU/MOUD nor MBRP/MOUD were specifically designed with the intent of addressing loneliness among participants.

In addition, no significant differences in loneliness reports were detected in the interaction between weeks and groups. Nevertheless, additional exploratory analysis detected a significant intervention effect where loneliness decreased in the MBRP/MOUD group more sharply when compared to the TAU/MOUD group over the first 12 weeks. However, analyses examining the correlations between the changes in loneliness at 36 weeks for the baseline demographic variables yielded no statistically significant findings. The results suggest age, sex, employment status, education levels, and insurance status were not important confounders.

This is not the first study to postulate that a mindfulness intervention has potential to help with loneliness. A recent systematic review with meta-analysis on mindfulness as a treatment for loneliness concluded that mindfulness intervention was useful in relieving loneliness among participants with no mental health conditions [47]. In addition, Creswell and colleagues reported that mindfulness based programs can help with loneliness and isolation in adults [45]. However, the current study may be the first to document that loneliness can be diminished in people with OUD with concurrent psychological problems where between 43% to 49% of the sample (depending on group) reported anxiety above the clinical threshold and between 38% to 65% of the sample reported depression above the clinical threshold [39].

The higher initial levels of reported loneliness in this population are congruent with prior scientific literature indicating that people with substance use disorder experience loneliness [28]. This knowledge paired with the findings of statistically significantly lower levels of loneliness at 36-weeks post recruitment is consistent with the research suggesting that engaging in social changes during the early phase of OUD treatment may lead to loneliness [13,60,61].

This study presents new information about loneliness and its relation to healing in people with OUD. The information begins to fill a critical need for knowledge and could be used to inform designs for more precise interventions among individuals who experience loneliness and have SUD. Current treatment programs often encourage patients to avoid previous friendships or associations in order to avoid substance use triggers or opportunities [60]. This is a needed lifestyle change for successful recovery but programs do not always offer ways to combat the loneliness and isolation that can ensue when a person enters treatment. Acknowledging loneliness as a potential real problem that occurs when people with SUD try to heal will mean incorporating strategies that target loneliness and isolation into treatment programs.

It is also key to avoid conflating social isolation with loneliness when treating OUD. The unique constructs of isolation and loneliness require different treatment, plans to rebuild a supportive network and frequent contacts, and plans to address the maladaptive thinking that often accompanies loneliness. Recent research has shown that mindfulness training may be effective at reducing loneliness and increasing social contact for adults [46]. Therefore, although speculative, the reduction in perceived loneliness within both groups over the 36-week intervention may, in part, be attributed to the fostering of new social groups and increased social support that were created throughout the course of treatment. Loneliness may have improved over time in both groups due to the sharing of common experiences which fosters social supports in treatment groups. Group therapy has been recognized as the treatment of choice for SUD for decades owing to addiction being associated with depression, anxiety, isolation, denial, shame, and the need for social skills building [62].

The correlational findings are not surprising given that loneliness has been positively associated with both depression and anxiety in previous research, and is a known precursor to a variety of mental illnesses [63,64]. The correlations from the current study support the current narrative identifying loneliness as a predictor for anxiety and depression. As perceptions of loneliness decreased, so did reports of depression and anxiety. The inverse association between loneliness and mindfulness is also consistent with the expectation that increased perceived mindfulness would be associated with decreased, or improved, perceptions of loneliness in the present study, regardless of treatment [46].

This study is one of the first to offer information about the relationship between loneliness and drug craving. Prior studies have reported loneliness and drug cravings as independently associated with depression and anxiety [65]. In fact, loneliness and drug craving have typically been coupled together and studied as a combined effect on substance use, depression, and anxiety [65]. While there is a direct relationship between loneliness and substance use itself [13,30,65], the relationship between loneliness and drug craving alone is understudied. Future studies should include measures of loneliness, social connectedness, and social isolation in order to better understand the influence of each on use and relapse, as well as to further understand how the psychological construct of loneliness influences cravings. This is important since cravings are both psychological and physiological.

Limitations

The study employed a quasi-experimental study design, and therefore, selection bias and confounding cannot be ruled out given that participants were not randomized to groups. A statistically significant difference between groups at baseline was detected for age, however age was not a significant predictor in the analysis. No other significant demographic differences were detected between groups at baseline. We also cannot definitively conclude that the OUD treatments caused the positive reductions in loneliness reports given the study design. Future randomized controlled trials are necessary to fully understand the effect of interventions targeting loneliness in this population. Our study sample also identified primarily as white, which while representative of the Appalachian region, it does limit generalizability to other populations. It is also possible that our sample size may have left the study somewhat underpowered. Quantitatively, MBRP/MOUD participants experienced approximately 2.5 times more improvement in loneliness from baseline to 12 weeks than TAU/MOUD participants and consistently better loneliness levels throughout the intervention. Studies with larger samples may have different conclusions [39].

5. Conclusions

Study results provide additional support to the literature suggesting that loneliness may be an important construct to address for individuals in MOUD treatment. The prevalence of loneliness in this study and in existing research [13] coupled with the dearth of empirical studies conducted in the context of MOUD treatment make it critical to continue this work. Novel interventions are needed for people with OUD so that they are implementable on a large scale. While interventions for loneliness in populations who use substances are sparse, some intervention studies have demonstrated success in diminishing loneliness in other populations. For example, interactive workshops and the LISTEN intervention demonstrated effectiveness in an elderly Appalachian population [31]. Other potential strategies include mindfulness training, social support interventions and social cognitive training [32,46]. Results from the current study suggest that testing the potential transferability of these successful strategies to populations who use substances offers future researchers potential avenues to explore. In addition, full consideration will be given on how these findings could inform the design of telehealth-based interventions. Future qualitative studies could provide additional insights into understanding what mattered most to people with OUD who experience loneliness.

Recognizing loneliness as a unique health risk worthy of assessment and intervention in this population and others will be key to treating people who experience loneliness. The current study was conducted pre-pandemic but it is important to note that there may be even a greater need to include loneliness when studying addiction due to increases in both addiction and loneliness reported during the COVID-19 pandemic [12,57,66].

Author Contributions: Conceptualization, K.J.Z. and L.A.T.; methodology, K.J.Z. and G.R.H.; software, K.J.Z. and G.R.H.; validation, K.J.Z. and G.R.H.; formal analysis, G.R.H., K.J.Z.; investigation, K.J.Z., L.R.L. and L.A.T.; resources, K.J.Z. and L.R.L.; data curation, K.J.Z., L.R.L. and G.R.H.; writing—original draft preparation, R.M., K.J.Z.; writing—review and editing, K.J.Z., R.M., L.A.T., L.R.L., J.H. and S.M.D.; visualization, K.J.Z. and L.A.T.; supervision, K.J.Z.; project administration, K.J.Z. and L.R.L.; funding acquisition, K.J.Z. and L.R.L. All authors have read and agreed to the published version of the manuscript.

Funding: This research was supported in part by Grant Number, 6R49CE002109-05-06, funded by the US Centers for Disease Control and Prevention. Its contents are solely the responsibility of the authors and do not necessarily represent the official views of the Centers for Disease Control and Prevention or the Department of Health and Human Services.

Institutional Review Board Statement: The study was conducted in accordance with the Declaration of Helsinki, and approved by the Institutional Review Board of West Virginia University (Protocol # 1708720058, approved on 26 August 2017.

Informed Consent Statement: Informed consent was obtained from all subjects involved in the study from which these data were obtained for secondary analysis.

Data Availability Statement: The datasets used and/or analyzed during the current study are available from the corresponding author on reasonable request.

Conflicts of Interest: The authors declare no conflict of interest.

References

1. Grant, B.F.; Saha, T.D.; Ruan, W.J.; Goldstein, R.B.; Chou, S.P.; Jung, J.; Hasin, D.S. Epidemiology of DSM-5 drug use disorder: Results from the National Epidemiologic Survey on Alcohol and Related Conditions—III. *JAMA Psychiatry* **2016**, *73*, 39–47. [CrossRef] [PubMed]
2. McCabe, S.E.; West, B.T.; Jutkiewicz, E.M.; Boyd, C.J. Multiple DSM-5 substance use disorders: A national study of US adults. *Hum. Psychopharmacol. Clin. Experimental* **2017**, *32*, e2625. [CrossRef] [PubMed]
3. National Center for Drug Abuse Statistics. Drug Abuse Statistics. 2022. Available online: https://drugabusestatistics.org/ (accessed on 29 May 2022).
4. National Center for Health Statistics. U.S. Overdose Deaths in 2021 Increased Half as Much as in 2020—But Are Still Up 15%. 2022. Available online: https://www.cdc.gov/nchs/pressroom/nchs_press_releases/2022/202205.htm (accessed on 29 May 2022).
5. Jones, C.M.; McCance-Katz, E.F. Co-occurring substance use and mental disorders among adults with opioid use disorder. *Drug Alcohol Depend.* **2019**, *197*, 78–82. [CrossRef] [PubMed]
6. Davis, M.A.; Lin, L.A.; Liu, H.; Sites, B.D. Prescription opioid use among adults with mental health disorders in the United States. *J. Am. Board Fam. Med.* **2017**, *30*, 407–417. [CrossRef]
7. Kelly, T.M.; Daley, D.C. Integrated treatment of substance use and psychiatric disorders. *Soc. Work Public Health* **2013**, *28*, 388–406. [CrossRef] [PubMed]
8. Ross, S.; Peselow, E. Co-Occurring Psychotic and Addictive Disorders. *Clin. Neuropharmacol.* **2012**, *35*, 235–243. [CrossRef]

9. Kelly, D.; Steiner, A.; Mazzei, M.; Baker, R. Filling a void? The role of social enterprise in addressing social isolation and loneliness in rural communities. *J. Rural. Stud.* **2019**, *70*, 225–236. [CrossRef]
10. Luo, Y.; Hawkley, L.C.; Waite, L.J.; Cacioppo, J.T. Loneliness, health, and mortality in old age: A national longitudinal study. *Soc. Sci. Med.* **2012**, *74*, 907–914. [CrossRef]
11. Tremeau, F.; Antonius, D.; Malaspina, D.; Goff, D.C.; Javitt, D.C. Loneliness in schizophrenia and its possible correlates. An exploratory study. *Psychiatry Res.* **2016**, *246*, 211–217. [CrossRef]
12. Horigian, V.E.; Schmidt, R.D.; Feaster, D.J. Loneliness, Mental Health, and Substance Use among US Young Adults during COVID-19. *J. Psychoact. Drugs* **2020**, *53*, 1–9. [CrossRef]
13. Ingram, I.; Kelly, P.J.; Deane, F.P.; Baker, A.L.; Goh, M.C.W.; Raftery, D.K.; Dingle, G.A. Loneliness among people with substance use problems: A narrative systematic review. *Drug Alcohol. Rev.* **2020**, *39*, 447–483. [CrossRef]
14. Stickley, A.; Koyanagi, A.; Koposov, R.; Schwab-Stone, M.; Ruchkin, V. Loneliness and health risk behaviours among Russian and U.S. adolescents: A cross-sectional study. *BMC Public Health* **2014**, *14*, 366. [CrossRef]
15. Wootton, R.E.; Greenstone, H.S.R.; Abdellaoui, A.; Denys, D.; Verweij, K.J.H.; Munafò, M.R.; Treur, J.L. Bidirectional effects between loneliness, smoking and alcohol use: Evidence from a Mendelian randomization study. *Addiction* **2021**, *116*, 400–406. [CrossRef] [PubMed]
16. Surkalim, D.L.; Luo, M.; Eres, R.; Gebel, K.; van Buskirk, J.; Bauman, A.; Ding, D. The prevalence of loneliness across 113 countries: Systematic review and meta-analysis. *BMJ* **2022**, *376*, e067068. [CrossRef]
17. DiJulio, B.L.; Hamel, L.; Munana, C.; Brodie, M. *Loneliness and Social Isolation in the United States, the United Kingdom, and Japan: An International Survey*; Kaiser Family Foundation: San Francisco, CA, USA, 2018. Available online: https://files.kff.org/attachment/Report-Loneliness-and-Social-Isolation-in-the-United-States-the-United-Kingdom-and-Japan-An-International-Survey (accessed on 20 November 2019).
18. Kaiser Family Foundation; The Economist. Survey on Loneliness and Social Isolation in the United States, the United Kingdom, and Japan. 2018. Available online: http://files.kff.org/attachment/Topline-Kaiser-Family-Foundation-The-Economist-Survey-on-Loneliness-and-Social-Isolation-in-the-United-States-the-United-Kingdom-and-Japan (accessed on 30 May 2022).
19. National Academies of Sciences, Engineering, and Medicine. *Social Isolation and Loneliness in Older Adults: Opportunities for the Health Care System*; The National Academies Press: Washington, DC, USA, 2020. [CrossRef]
20. Lee, E.E.; Depp, C.; Palmer, B.W.; Glorioso, D.; Daly, R.; Liu, J.; Jeste, D.V. High prevalence and adverse health effects of loneliness in community-dwelling adults across the lifespan: Role of wisdom as a protective factor. *Int. Psychogeriatr.* **2019**, *31*, 1447–1462. [CrossRef] [PubMed]
21. NIH National Institutes on Aging. Loneliness and Social Isolation—Tips for Staying Connected. National Institutes of Health. 2021. Available online: https://www.nia.nih.gov/health/loneliness-and-social-isolation-tips-staying-connected#:~{}:text=Loneliness%20is%20the%20distressing%20feeling,while%20being%20with%20other%20people (accessed on 15 May 2021).
22. Barg, F.K.; Huss-Ashmore, R.; Wittink, M.N.; Murray, G.F.; Bogner, H.R.; Gallo, J.J. A mixed methods approach to understanding loneliness and depression in older adults. *J. Gerontol. Ser. B* **2006**, *61*, S329–S339. [CrossRef] [PubMed]
23. Theeke, L.A.; Mallow, J. Loneliness and quality of life in chronically ill rural older adults. *Am. J. Nurs.* **2013**, *113*, 28–37. [CrossRef] [PubMed]
24. Petersen, J.; Kaye, J.; Jacobs, P.G.; Quinones, A.; Dodge, H.; Arnold, A.; Thielke, S. Longitudinal relationship between loneliness and social isolation in older adults: Results from the cardiovascular health study. *J. Aging Health* **2016**, *28*, 775–795. [CrossRef] [PubMed]
25. Laudet, A.B.; Magura, S.; Vogel, H.S.; Knight, E.L. Perceived reasons for substance misuse among persons with a psychiatric disorder. *Am. J. Orthopsychiatry* **2004**, *74*, 365–375. [CrossRef]
26. Polenick, C.A.; Cotton, B.P.; Bryson, W.C.; Birditt, K.S. Loneliness and Illicit Opioid Use Among Methadone Maintenance Treatment Patients. *Subst. Use Misuse* **2019**, *54*, 2089–2098. [CrossRef]
27. Vyas, M.V.; Watt, J.A.; Yu, A.Y.; Straus, S.E.; Kapral, M.K. The association between loneliness and medication use in older adults. *Age Ageing* **2021**, *50*, 587–591. [CrossRef] [PubMed]
28. Johnson, J.E.; Schonbrun, Y.C.; Nargiso, J.E.; Kuo, C.C.; Shefner, R.T.; Williams, C.A.; Zlotnick, C. "I know if I drink I won't feel anything": Substance use relapse among depressed women leaving prison. *Int. J. Prison. Health* **2013**, *9*, 169–186. [CrossRef] [PubMed]
29. Newton, T.F.; De La Garza, R., 2nd; Kalechstein, A.D.; Tziortzis, D.; Jacobsen, C.A. Theories of addiction: Methamphetamine users' explanations for continuing drug use and relapse. *Am. J. Addict.* **2009**, *18*, 294–300. [CrossRef] [PubMed]
30. Hosseinbor, M.; Yassini Ardekani, S.M.; Bakhshani, S.; Bakhshani, S. Emotional and social loneliness in individuals with and without substance dependence disorder. *Int. J. High Risk Behav. Addict.* **2014**, *3*, e22688. [CrossRef]
31. Theeke, L.A.; Mallow, J.A.; Moore, J.; McBurney, A.; Rellick, S.; VanGilder, R. Effectiveness of LISTEN on loneliness, neuroimmunological stress response, psychosocial functioning, quality of life, and physical health measures of chronic illness. *Int. J. Nurs. Sci.* **2016**, *3*, 242–251. [CrossRef]
32. Veronese, N.; Galvano, D.; D'Antiga, F. Interventions for reducing loneliness: An umbrella review of intervention studies. *Health Soc. Care Community* **2021**, *29*, e89–e96. [CrossRef]
33. Meit, M.; Heffernan, M.; Tanenbaum, E. Investigating the impact of the diseases of despair in Appalachia. *J. Appalach. Health* **2019**, *1*, 7–18. [CrossRef]

34. Centers for Disease Control and Prevention (CDC). Drug Overdose Mortality by State. 2021. Available online: https://www.cdc.gov/nchs/pressroom/sosmap/drug_poisoning_mortality/drug_poisoning.htm (accessed on 17 September 2021).
35. Department of Health and Human Resources (DHHR). West Virginia Experiences Increase in Overdose Deaths; Health Officials Emphasize Resources. 2020. Available online: https://dhhr.wv.gov/News/2021/Pages/West-Virginia-Experiences-Increase-in-Overdose-Deaths;-Health-Officials-Emphasize-Resources.aspx (accessed on 17 September 2021).
36. Andrilla, C.H.A.; Moore, T.E.; Patterson, D.G.; Larson, E.H. Geographic distribution of providers with a DEA waiver to prescribe buprenorphine for the treatment of opioid use disorder: A 5-year update. *J. Rural. Health* **2019**, *35*, 108–112. [CrossRef]
37. Henning-Smith, C.; Ecklund, A.; Lahr, M.; Evenson, A.; Moscovice, I.; Kozhimannil, K. Key Informant Perspectives on Rural Social Isolation and Loneliness. University of Minnesota Rural Health Research Center. 2018. Available online: http://rhrc.umn.edu/wp-content/uploads/2019/01/1539002382UMNpolicybriefKeyInformantPerspectivesonRuralSocialIsolationandLoneliness.pdf (accessed on 5 March 2021).
38. Savikko, N.; Routasalo, P.; Tilvis, R.S.; Strandberg, T.E.; Pitkälä, K.H. Predictors and subjective causes of loneliness in an aged population. *Arch. Gerontol. Geriatr.* **2005**, *41*, 223–233. [CrossRef]
39. Zullig, K.J.; Lander, L.R.; Tuscano, M.; Garland, M.; Hobbs, G.R.; Faulkenberry, L. Testing Mindfulness-Based Relapse Prevention with medications for opioid use disorder among adults in outpatient therapy: A quasi-experimental study. *Mindfulness* **2021**, *12*, 3036–3046. [CrossRef]
40. Friedman, B.; Conwell, Y.; Delavan, R.L. Correlates of late-life major depression: A comparison of urban and rural primary care patients. *Am. J. Geriatr. Psychiatry* **2007**, *15*, 28–41. [CrossRef] [PubMed]
41. Nkyi, A.K.; Ninnoni, J.P.K. Depression, Purpose in Life, Loneliness and Anxiety Among Patients with Substance Use Disorders in Ankaful Psychiatric Hospital in Ghana. *J. Psychosoc. Rehabil. Ment. Health* **2020**, *7*, 263–271. [CrossRef]
42. Knapp, K.S.; Bunce, S.C.; Brick, T.R.; Deneke, E.; Cleveland, H.H. Daily associations among craving, affect, and social interactions in the lives of patients during residential opioid use disorder treatment. *Psychol. Addict. Behav.* **2020**. Advance online publication. [CrossRef] [PubMed]
43. Bowen, S.; Witkiewitz, K.; Dillworth, T.M.; Chawla, N.; Simpson, T.L.; Ostafin, B.; Larimer, M.E.; Blume, A.W.; Parks, G.A.; Marlatt, G.A. Mindfulness meditation and substance use in an incarcerated population. *Psychol. Addict. Behav.* **2006**, *20*, 343–347. [CrossRef] [PubMed]
44. Bowen, S.; Witkiewitz, K.; Clifasefi, S.L.; Grow, G.; Chawla, N.; Hsu, S.H.; Carroll, H.A.; Harrop, E.; Collins, S.E.; Lustyk, M.K.; et al. Relative efficacy of mindfulness-based relapse prevention, standard relapse prevention, and treatment as usual for substance use disorders: A randomized clinical trial. *JAMA Psychiatry* **2014**, *71*, 547–556. [CrossRef]
45. Creswell, J.D.; Irwin, M.R.; Burklund, L.J.; Lieberman, M.D.; Arevalo, J.M.; Ma, J.; Cole, S.W. Mindfulness-based stress reduction training reduces loneliness and pro-inflammatory gene expression in older adults: A small randomized controlled trial. *Brain Behav. Immun.* **2012**, *26*, 1095–1101. [CrossRef]
46. Lindsay, E.K.; Young, S.; Brown, K.W.; Smyth, J.M.; Creswell, J.D. Mindfulness training reduces loneliness and increases social contact in a randomized controlled trial. *Proc. Natl. Acad. Sci. USA* **2019**, *116*, 3488–3493. [CrossRef]
47. Teoh, S.L.; Letchumanan, V.; Lee, L.H. Can mindfulness help to alleviate loneliness? A systematic review and meta-analysis. *Front. Psychol.* **2021**, *12*, 402. [CrossRef]
48. Zhang, N.; Fan, F.M.; Huang, S.Y.; Rodriguez, M.A. Mindfulness training for loneliness among Chinese college students: A pilot randomized controlled trial. *Int. J. Psychol.* **2018**, *53*, 373–378. [CrossRef]
49. Hooker, S.A.; Lonergan-Cullum, M.; Levy, R.; Nissly, T.; Sherman, M.D. Longitudinal assessment of mental health and well-being in patients being treated with medications for opioid use disorder in primary care. *Addict. Behav. Rep.* **2021**, *13*, 100348. [CrossRef]
50. Franken, I.H.A.; Hendriks, V.M.; van den Brink, W. Initial validation of two opiate craving questionnaires: The Obsessive Compulsive Drug Use Scale and the Desires for Drug Questionnaire. *Addict. Behav.* **2002**, *27*, 675–685. [CrossRef]
51. Bentley, K.H.; Gallagher, M.W.; Carl, J.R.; Barlow, D.H. Development and validation of the Overall Depression Severity and Impairment Scale. *Psychol. Assess.* **2014**, *26*, 815–830. [CrossRef] [PubMed]
52. Campbell-Sills, L.; Norman, S.B.; Craske, M.G.; Sullivan, G.; Lang, A.J.; Chavira, D.A.; Bystritsky, A.; Sherbourne, C.; Roy-Byrne, P.; Stein, M.B. Validation of a brief measure of anxiety-related severity and impairment: The Overall Anxiety Severity and Impairment Scale (OASIS). *J. Affect. Disord.* **2009**, *112*, 92–101. [CrossRef]
53. Norman, S.B.; Hami Cissell, S.; Means-Christensen, A.J.; Stein, M.B. Development and validation of an overall anxiety severity and impairment scale (OASIS). *Depress. Anxiety* **2006**, *23*, 245–249. [CrossRef] [PubMed]
54. Baer, R.A.; Smith, G.T.; Hopkins, J.; Krietemeyer, J.; Toney, L. Using self-report assessment methods to explore facets of mindfulness. *Assessment* **2006**, *13*, 27–45. [CrossRef] [PubMed]
55. Russell, D. UCLA Loneliness Scale (Version 3): Reliability, validity, and factor structure. *J. Personal. Assess.* **1996**, *66*, 20–40. [CrossRef]
56. Russell, D.W.; Peplau, L.A.; Cutrona, C.E. The revised UCLA Loneliness Scale: Concurrent and discriminant validity evidence. *J. Personal. Soc. Psychol.* **1980**, *39*, 472–480. [CrossRef]
57. Groarke, J.M.; Berry, E.; Graham-Wisener, L.; McKenna-Plumley, P.E.; McGlinchey, E.; Armour, C. Loneliness in the UK during the COVID-19 pandemic: Cross-sectional results from the COVID-19 Psychological Wellbeing Study. *PLoS ONE* **2020**, *15*, e0239698. [CrossRef]

58. Kuwert, P.; Knaevelsrud, C.; Pietrzak, R.H. Loneliness among older veterans in the United States: Results from the National Health and Resilience in Veterans Study. *Am. J. Geriatr. Psychiatry* **2014**, *22*, 564–569. [CrossRef]
59. Wilson, C.; Moulton, B. *Loneliness among Older Adults: A National Survey of Adults 45+. Knowledge Networks and Insight Policy Research*; AARP: Washington, DC, USA, 2010; Available online: https://assets.aarp.org/rgcenter/general/loneliness_2010.pdf (accessed on 22 March 2022).
60. McDonagh, J.; Williams, C.B.; Oldfield, B.J.; Cruz-Jose, D.; Olson, D.P. The Association of Loneliness and Non-prescribed Opioid Use in Patients With Opioid Use Disorder. *J. Addict. Med.* **2020**, *14*, 489–493. [CrossRef]
61. Ingram, I.; Kelly, P.J.; Deane, F.P.; Baker, A.L.; Dingle, G.A. Perceptions of loneliness among people accessing treatment for substance use disorders. *Drug Alcohol Rev.* **2020**, *39*, 484–494. [CrossRef] [PubMed]
62. Center for Substance Abuse Treatment (CSAT). *Substance Abuse Treatment: Group Therapy*; (Treatment Improvement Protocol (TIP) Series, No. 41) 1 Groups and Substance Abuse Treatment; Substance Abuse and Mental Health Services Administration: Rockville, MD, USA, 2005. Available online: https://www.ncbi.nlm.nih.gov/books/NBK64223/ (accessed on 26 November 2021).
63. Dziedzic, B.; Sarwa, P.; Kobos, E.; Sienkiewicz, Z.; Idzik, A.; Wysokiński, M.; Fidecki, W. Loneliness and Depression among Polish High-School Students. *Int. J. Environ. Res. Public Health* **2021**, *18*, 1706. [CrossRef] [PubMed]
64. Erzen, E.; Çikrikci, Ö. The effect of loneliness on depression: A meta-analysis. *Int. J. Soc. Psychiatry* **2018**, *64*, 427–435. [CrossRef] [PubMed]
65. Chen, X.; Qiu, N.; Zhai, L.; Ren, G. Anxiety, Loneliness, Drug Craving, and Depression Among Substance Abusers in Sichuan Province, China. *Front. Pharmacol.* **2021**, *12*, 623360. [CrossRef]
66. Volkow, N.D. Collision of the COVID-19 and addiction epidemics. *Ann. Intern. Med.* **2020**, *173*, 61–62. [CrossRef]

International Journal of
Environmental Research and Public Health

MDPI

Article

Loneliness in Intimate Relationships Scale (LIRS): Development and Validation

Ami Rokach [1,*], Ami Sha'ked [2] and Elisheva Ben-Artzi [2]

[1] Department of Psychology, York University, Toronto, ON M3J 1P3, Canada
[2] Academic Center for Law & Business, Ramat Gan 5224213, Israel
* Correspondence: rokach@yorku.ca

Abstract: Intimate relationships have been shown to be loneliness positively related to self-esteem. Happiness and well-being and have also been regarded as a buffer against loneliness. Nevertheless, substantive research indicates that intimate relationships and marriage can produce or result in loneliness and thus seriously affect the person's physical, emotional and spiritual well-being. Loneliness in intimate relationships may damage the relationship if it goes on, and thus, this newly developed scale has been introduced to aid clinicians and researchers in discovering loneliness in an intimate union so it can be addressed before it negatively affects the union. Since none of the measures of loneliness tap loneliness as experienced in intimate relationships, a new rating scale, the Loneliness in Intimate Relationships Scale (LIRS), was developed and tested psychometrically. The generation of items followed a qualitative approach based on a semi-structured questionnaire administered to 108 volunteers from the general Israeli population, theoretical and empirical literature, and assessments of expert psychologists. In a second study (N = 215), a self-report scale assessing loneliness in intimate relationships was developed. This was followed by psychometric and construct validity evaluations with a new sample of 306 participants. Analyses revealed that loneliness in intimate relationships is experienced mainly in terms of three aspects: detachment, hurt, and guilt. Exploratory and confirmatory factor analyses and validity tests indicate that the final 14-item Loneliness in Intimate Relationship Scale is a well-structured, reliable, and valid scale tapping emotional, behavioral, and cognitive manifestations of loneliness in intimate relationships.

Keywords: loneliness; intimacy; intimate relationships; marriage; assessment

1. Loneliness in Intimate Relationships Scale (LIRS): Development and Validation

Establishing and maintaining close intimate relationships with a significant other has been recognized as a fundamental human motivation [1,2]. Similarly, marriage is perceived as the most intimate officially sanctioned adult bonding, serving as a primary source of affection, love, support [3,4] and physical and emotional well-being [5].

In the US, approximately sixty percent of adults (60% of males and 57% of females) aged 18 and over are married, while overall, 72% have experienced marriage and may thus be married, divorced, or widowed. Marriage, or a long-term intimate commitment, is central in Western culture, and although they presently have smaller chances of succeeding, they are still, by and large, the preferred lifestyles adult [4]. Strong [4] suggested that intimate relationships buffer against loneliness, positively affect our self-esteem, and are shown to be related to happiness, contentment, and a sense of well-being [6]. In close relationships, intimacy has been rated as more important for relationship satisfaction than autonomy, individuality, freedom, agreement, or sexual satisfaction [7].

This, however, does not prevent the married from experiencing loneliness. For example, Tornstam [8] found that 40% of married people in Sweden experienced more loneliness than unmarried people. It may intuitively seem paradoxical that a person can be both married and lonely. However, when marriages lose their vitality, spouses become prone to loneliness [9]. There is a tendency to believe that marriage and intimate relations tend to fend off loneliness because a companion is always around. However, Barbour [10] found that 20% of wives and 24% of husbands are significantly lonely, and as loneliness increases in the marriage or intimate relationship, so does depression.

Loneliness in marriage may be especially distressing because it is inconsistent with expectations about marriage and may have a significant effect on one's physical, emotional and spiritual well-being [11,12]. As indicated by Fincham and Rogge [13], there are two approaches that examine the construct of relationship quality. One focuses on the relationship, or the interpersonal exchange between the couple, namely their interaction, the manner in which they resolve conflicts, and their communication patterns. The other, the intrapersonal approach, which the present study took, focuses on subjective judgments of each partner and her or his evaluation of the marriage or intimate relationship.

Helping couples deal with conflicts, problematic issues, or dissatisfaction is what marital and couple therapists commonly do. However, in order to be effective, therapy needs to be clear as to what to focus on and address the specific aspects of the relationship that need the therapist's help and attention. There are a variety of assessment tools geared to examine couple relationships and problematic issues, including the Locke–Wallace Marital Adjustment Scale [14] the Quality of Relationship Inventory [15], the Brief Romantic Relationship Interaction Coding Scheme [16], the Kansas Marital Satisfaction Scale [17], and the Retired Spousal Intrusion Scale [18]. However, although important, valid and reliable instruments have been developed for assessing different aspects of relationships, none address the issue of loneliness, which can be highly disruptive and damaging to an intimate relation.

We, therefore, developed a new scale, the Loneliness in Intimate Relationships Scale [LIRS], which aims to fulfill this need. It is expected that there may be a moderate association between the present general loneliness scales and the one described herein since the one that we developed addresses relational issues that were not addressed in the existing loneliness questionnaires. The present manuscript does not check this assumption, and that will be addressed by our planned future research project. The present paper describes research aimed at developing a new scale for assessing loneliness in relationships for adults and testing its basic psychometric properties regarding reliability and validity. The development of the Loneliness in Intimate Relationships Scale followed the standard principles of a non-reactive methodology for questionnaire construction described in the *Standards for Educational and Psychological Testing* (APA, 2014). Such methodology ensures that the scale covers all aspects of the construct and meets the highest validity and reliability criteria. Table 1 presents the stages in the development of the Loneliness in Intimate Relationships Scale.

Table 1. Stages of the development of the loneliness in intimate relationships scale for adults.

Study 1		Qualitative study aimed to generate items for the Loneliness in Intimate Relationships Scale (LIRS)
	Phase I	Generation of items based on a semi-structured open-ended questionnaire and removal of overlapping items
	Phase II	Domains identification and initial classification of items into categories
	Phase III	Collection of items derived from different sources: (1) theoretical and empirical literature relevant to loneliness in intimate relationships, and (2) impressions, evaluations and assessments derived from the clinical practice of two expert psychologists, specialists in couples therapy
	Phase IV	Item evaluation with respect to clarity, ambiguousness and comprehensibility
	Phase V	Item reformulation based on the item evaluations
Study 2		Final scale development (N = 215)
Study 3		Structural evaluation (N = 306)
Study 4		Construct validity

2. Study 1

Generating items for the loneliness in intimate relationships scale.

Study 1 was designed to generate a large pool of items relevant to loneliness in intimate relationships, which would serve as the pool for developing the final scale. In the present study, the collection of items was based on both naive participants' descriptions and professional literature and therapists' input evaluations based on clinical practice relevant to loneliness in intimate relationships. Study 1 was therefore carried out as a qualitative exploration aimed at assessing items and domains of loneliness in relationships.

2.1. Method

2.1.1. Participants

A total of 108 participants from the general Israeli population (70 women) volunteered to participate in the study. The participants represented a broad range of demographic characteristics and were solicited from all walks of life. Age ranged between 19 and 59 years (M = 36.09, SD = 10.71). Education ranged between 10 and 18 years (M = 14.00, SD = 2.17). Seventy-nine (73%) of the participants were in a steady relationship at the time of the study. The study was approved by the Institutional Review Board of the Center for Academic Studies.

2.1.2. Semi-Structured Questionnaire

A semi-structured questionnaire was administered, in which the participants were asked to freely describe their reflections and feelings during an experience in which they felt lonely during a close/intimate relationship. The participants received the following instructions, "We are attempting to understand loneliness in intimate relationships by investigating how it is experienced. We would appreciate your reflections on an experience of loneliness in an intimate relationship. Please refer to a specific period or situation in which you felt lonely in an intimate relationship and describe what you felt or thought through the following five guiding aspects, as listed below. It is important that you to realize that there are no "right" or "wrong" responses to these aspects/questions. People are different, and we are interested in your personal experience."

The participants were then asked to freely refer to the following aspects of the situation: (1) "Describe, in a number of sentences, the situation/period in which you felt lonely"; (2) "Describe the thoughts you had about yourself and the relationship"; (3) "Describe the feelings you had about yourself and the relationship"; (4) "What did you want to happen to change the feeling of loneliness?"; and (5) "How did you deal with the situation?" The participants were not given a time limit for answering the questionnaire.

2.2. Results and Discussion

2.2.1. Listing and Categorization of the Data

A qualitative content analysis was performed on the 108 transcripts by two psychology students after having been trained by the researchers. Data were analyzed according to the following stages: (1) reduction of descriptions to precise terms; (2) identification of separate single-content statements; (3) removal of redundant items; (4) initial categorization of items into clusters. The descriptions reported by the participants yielded a wide range of statements. In the first stage of the analysis, two psychology students read all 108 protocols and recorded all the statements. Of the 108 transcripts, 533 separate single-content statements (verbatim) were identified (e.g., "I felt anger," "I thought our relationship was over"). Next, similarly worded statements were given a common label. For example, "I felt lonely" and "I sensed loneliness" were grouped together. Decisions on item grouping were carried out based on the two judges' full agreement. A list of 156 different items that were mentioned by at least one of the 108 participants was obtained.

The three authors then grouped the listed items into non-overlapping categories that they proposed. Items assessing similar issues were gathered to make up a subscale (category). The authors performed the categorization task separately. Inter-judge reliabilities were computed using a conservative method of percent agreement between judges for each category separately (i.e., the percentage of items that two judges grouped in the same category). The inter-judge agreement on all categories ranged between 0.80 and 0.90. Items for which there was no judge agreement were removed from the list. This stage resulted in a 138-item list.

2.2.2. Analysis of Existing Relevant Scales and Clinical Practice

Finally, we made a thorough analysis of existing relevant scales, as follows: Social and Emotional Loneliness Measure [19], de Jong Gierveld Loneliness Scale [20], Differential Loneliness Scale [21], Loneliness-Deprivation Scale [22], Loneliness and Social Dissatisfaction Questionnaire—Modified [23], Loneliness Questionnaire [24], Social and Emotional Loneliness Scale for Adults [25], Revised UCLA Loneliness Scale [26], Social and Emotional Loneliness Scale for Adults [27], and the Social and Emotional Loneliness Scale for Adults—Short Version [28]. Appraisals derived from the above-mentioned scales and clinical practice experience yielded an additional 28 items relevant to loneliness in intimate relationships. These items were added to the item list derived from the semi-structured questionnaires' content analysis, such that when an item was identified as belonging to one of the categories but did not appear in it, the judges added it to that category. When an item could not be grouped into any of the proposed categories, the judges created a new category for it. This procedure was carried out separately by three judges: two of the authors (E.B. & A.R.) and an additional psychology student. Inter-judge reliabilities were computed, yielding an inter-judge agreement on all categories ranging between 0.81 and 0.89. Items for which there was no full judge agreement were removed from the list. This procedure resulted in a list of 123 items grouped into 29 content categories.

Next, each item of the 123-item list was evaluated by two psychology students who worked separately regarding its clarity and comprehensibility. Items that did not meet these criteria were removed from the list or were rephrased based on an agreement by the three authors. This procedure resulted in a 66-item list which comprised the first version of the Loneliness in Intimate Relationship Scale. Table 2 presents the 29-category list derived from the content analysis of the semi-structured questionnaires, existing relevant scales and clinical practice. Each category consisted of 2–3 relevant items (e.g., "I felt sadness," "I felt that our love is fading").

Table 2. Categories derived from content analysis of the semi-structured questionnaires, relevant scales and clinical practice.

Category Name
Pain
Hopelessness
Emotional hurt
Anger
Frustration
Crying
Stress
Lacking partnership
Lack of intimacy
Misunderstanding
Lack of love
Sadness
Unavailability/lack of support
Emotional shut-off
Concerns about the fate of the relationship
Lack of appreciation
Helplessness
Insecurity
Self-blame

Table 2. *Cont.*

Category Name
Hope for change
Low self-esteem
Perceived partner's indifference to the relationship
Disengagement
Fear of end of relationship
Thoughts about suitability
Disrespect
Depression
Sense of failure
Self-pity

3. Study 2

Study 2 was designed to develop a self-report scale assessing loneliness in intimate relationships based on the results of the content analysis described in Study 1.

3.1. Method

3.1.1. Participants

A total of 215 participants from the general Israeli population (181 women) volunteered to participate in the study. Age ranged between 20 and 64 years (M = 33.95, SD = 10.49). Education ranged between 8 and 16 years (M = 12.10, SD = 0.96). Overall, 148 (69%) of the participants were in a steady relationship at the time of the study, while 65 (30%) were not. Two participants did not indicate their relationship status. A total of 43 (20%) participants reported feeling lonely at the time of the study, and 69 (32%) reported that when they experienced loneliness, it was "on a more or less continuous basis." The study was approved by the Institutional Review Board of the Center for Academic Studies.

3.1.2. Loneliness in Intimate Relationships Scale—Version 1

The first version of the Loneliness in Intimate Relationships Scale (LIRS) consisted of the 66 items derived from Study 1 (see Appendix A). The participants were given the following instructions: "We are attempting to understand loneliness in intimate relationships by investigating how it is experienced. We would appreciate your reflections on an experience in which you felt lonely during a close/intimate relationship. Please read each of the following statements and decide how much it describes what you felt or thought during a specific period or situation in which you felt lonely in a close relationship. Please respond according to the following 6-point scale ranging from 1 = totally not describes my experience to 6 = totally describes my experience. It is important for you to realize that there are no "right" or "wrong" answers to these questions. We are interested in how you felt. Please note that in this questionnaire, partner refers to a romantic 'partner' of either gender."

3.2. *Results and Discussion*

Exploratory Factor Analysis

The analysis was based on the responses of 215 participants, representing an adequate participants-per-item ratio (1:3.3) [29]. The ratings of the 66 items of the first version of the Loneliness in Intimate Relationship Scale were subjected to a principal components factor analysis with oblique factor rotation. Because rotated factors were only modestly correlated ($\bar{r}$ = 0.39), we reanalyzed the data using a varimax factor rotation. The number of factors to extract was determined by parallel analysis, which has been shown to provide more accurate estimates of the number of factors to retain than Kaiser's criterion of eigenvalues > 1 [30]. To establish the level for meaningful eigenvalues we conducted a principal-components factor analysis on random data ("Monte Carlo") generated from the raw data. We used O'Connor's SPSS software [31] to generate the random data set and to compute eigenvalues (and 95% CIs) on the random data set. Each parallel data set is based on column-wise random shufflings of the values in the raw data matrix using Castellan's (1992, BRMIC, 24, 72–77) algorithm. The distributions of the original raw variables are exactly preserved in the shuffled versions used in the parallel analyses. Permutations of the raw data set are thus. We computed 10,000 datasets, which is considered more than sufficient. Parallel analysis of the 66 items based on the mean eigenvalues and 95th eigenvalue obtained from random data indicated a four-factor solution accounting for 55.4% of the items' variance, with the first factor accounting for 41.6% of the total variance. However, several items had poor factor loadings on all the factors ($L < 0.40$) or had high factor loadings on more than one factor ($L \geq 0.40$) and were therefore removed from the list. The remaining 14 items were subjected to a principal components factor analysis with oblique factor rotation. Because rotated factors were only modestly correlated ($\bar{r} = 0.35$), we reanalyzed the data using a varimax factor rotation. Parallel analysis of the 14 items based on the mean eigenvalues and 95th eigenvalue obtained from random data indicated a three-factor solution, accounting for 61.8% of the items' variance, with the first factor accounting for 41% of the total variance. Factor 1 includes six items: 5, 8, 10, 11, 12, 13; factor 2 includes four items: 1, 2, 3, 4; and factor 3 also includes four items: 6, 7, 9, 14. Table 3 presents item loadings and factors' statistics. Inspection of item loadings in Table 3 indicates that all items have distinct loadings on the three factors. Analysis of item content suggests that factor 1 represents thoughts and feelings concerning detachment and separation, factor 2 represents feelings of hurt and pain, and factor 3 represents a sense of guilt and responsibility. The final 14-item version appears in Appendix A.

Table 3. Factor loadings and statistics of the loneliness in intimate relationships second 14-item version—Study 3.

Item	Factor		
	Detachment	Hurt	Guilt
13. I thought about ending our relationship	**0.78**	0.29	0.08
12. I wondered whether we are suitable	**0.74**	0.24	0.20
8. I invested in the relationship without getting back	**0.74**	0.21	0−.08
11. I felt that I could not continue like this	**0.73**	0.35	0.15
10. I felt that I was not important to him/her	**0.72**	0.26	0.12
5. My husband/partner had no time for me	**0.59**	0.08	0.19
2. I felt hurt	0.34	**0.86**	0.06
1. I felt a deep sense of pain	0.24	**0.83**	0.17
3. I felt insulted	0.23	**0.83**	0.15
4. I was very tense	0.36	**0.61**	0.15
6. I felt that I was not fulfilling my part in the relationship	−0.02	−0.02	**0.78**
7. I felt guilty for my misdeeds in the marriage/relationship	0.13	0.24	**0.74**
14. I thought that I was infantile	0.06	0.18	**0.61**
9. I felt that I was not worthy of his love	0.24	0.03	**0.56**
Mean	3.41	3.96	2.62
SD	1.38	1.41	1.12
% Explained Variance	**40.5%**	**11.7%**	**8.7%**

Note: Bold and underlined loadings indicate the item's affiliation to factors.

4. Study 3

Study 3 was designed to validate the structure pattern of the 14-item version of the LIRS that emerged in study 2 and to analyze its psychometric properties.

4.1. Method

4.1.1. Participants

A group of 306 participants from the general Israeli population (158 women) volunteered to participate in the study. They were recruited from all walks of life. Age ranged between 18 and 54 years (M = 26.99, SD = 6.95). Education ranged between 8 and 14 years (M = 11.99, SD = 0.44). A total of 135 (44%) of the participants were in a steady relationship at the time of the study, 169 (56%) were not. Two participants did not indicate their relationship status. Overall, 69 (23%) participants reported feeling lonely at the time of the study, and 87 (31%) reported that when they experienced loneliness, it was "on a more or less continuous basis." The study was approved by the Institutional Review Board of the Center for Academic Studies.

4.1.2. Loneliness in Intimate Relationships Scale—Version 2 (14 Items)

The 14-item LIRS version was used. The participants were given the instructions described in Study 2.

4.2. Results and Discussion

4.2.1. Exploratory Factor Analysis

In order to further ensure the structure validity of the LIRS, the goodness-of-fit to the data of the three-factor solution extracted from the exploratory factor analysis was compared to an equivalent random model using a structural equation modeling approach (AMOS, SPSS 21.0). The sample size (N = 306) was adequate for a confirmatory analysis (Kline, 2011). The equivalent random model was comprised of items 1, 5, 6, 7, 11, and 13 in factor 1, items 2, 3, 9, and 12 in factor 2, and items 4, 8, 10, and 14 in factor 3. The evaluated goodness-of-fit indicators included the overall χ^2. The evaluated descriptive indexes were the incremental fit index (IFI), the comparative fit index (CFI), and the root-mean-square error of approximation (RMSA), being complementary descriptive indexes (Schumacker & Lomax, 2012). The results of the confirmatory analyses comparing the goodness-of-fit to the data of the original and random three-factor models for the final 14-item version of the LIRS are presented in Table 4.

Table 4. Goodness-of-fit of the confirmatory analyses of the original and random models of the english version of the LIRS (14 items)—Study 3.

Model	χ^2	df	χ^2 Difference	p Difference	IFI	CFI	RMSA	p RMSA
Original	246.44 ***	74			0.91	0.91	0.09	<0.001
Random	619.04 ***	74	372.60	<0.001	0.72	0.71	0.16	<0.001

Note: *** $p < 0.001$.

As shown in Table 4, the original three-factor model fit the data well. Although the χ^2 was significant (which is expected with large samples), all the descriptive indexes indicated a satisfactory goodness-of-fit. Moreover, the χ^2 difference between the original and random models was significant, and all descriptive indexes of the random model indicated a poor fit to the data for the random model. Standardized factor coefficients are presented in Figure 1. Finally, as indicated in Figure 1, the three factors were moderately related.

Taken as a whole, the exploratory and confirmatory factor analyses indicate that the final 14-item version of the Loneliness in Intimate Relationship Scale (LIRS) is a well-structured and reliable scale depicting emotional, behavioral, and cognitive reactions and coping with loneliness in intimate relationships.

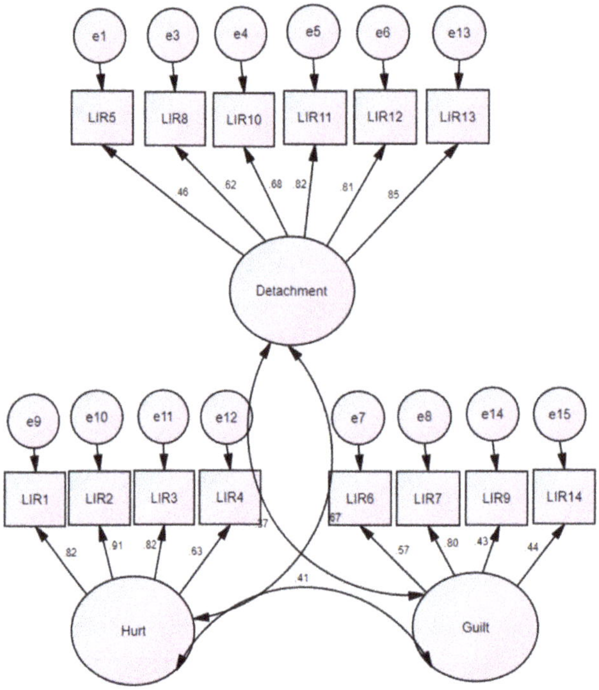

Figure 1. Standardized coefficients for the LIRS final version three-factor model—Study 3.

4.2.2. Confirmatory Factor Analysis

In order to further ensure the structure validity of the LIRS, the goodness-of-fit to the data of the three-factor solution extracted from the exploratory factor analysis was compared to an equivalent random model using a structural equation modeling approach (AMOS, SPSS 21.0). The sample size (N = 306) was adequate for a confirmatory analysis (Kline, 2011). The equivalent random model was comprised of items 1, 5, 6, 7, 11, and 13 in factor 1, items 2, 3, 9, and 12 in factor 2, and items 4, 8, 10, and 14 in factor 3. The evaluated goodness-of-fit indicators included the overall χ^2. The evaluated descriptive indexes were the incremental fit index (IFI), the comparative fit index (CFI), and the root-mean-square error of approximation (RMSA), being complementary descriptive indexes (Schumacker & Lomax, 2012). The results of the confirmatory analyses comparing the goodness-of-fit to the data of the original and random three-factor models for the final 14-item version of the LIRS are presented in Table 4.

As shown in Table 4, the original three-factor model fit the data well. Although the χ^2 was significant (which is expected with large samples), all the descriptive indexes indicated a satisfactory goodness-of-fit. Moreover, the χ^2 difference between the original and random models was significant, and all descriptive indexes of the random model indicated a poor fit to the data for the random model. Standardized factor coefficients are presented in Figure 1.

Taken as a whole, the exploratory and confirmatory factor analyses indicate that the final 14-item version of the Loneliness in Intimate Relationship Scale (LIRS) is a well-structured and reliable scale depicting emotional, behavioral, and cognitive reactions and coping with loneliness in intimate relationships.

5. Study 4

The purpose of this study was to assess the construct validity of the LIRS. Specifically, we performed two sets of concurrent validity tests. We tested the relationships between the subscales of the LIRS and other scales tapping close but different constructs, namely general loneliness, social loneliness, interpersonal needs, and depression. All these concepts were expected to be moderately positively associated with all LIRS subscales. We also compared the levels of loneliness in intimate relationships as established by the LIRS subscales for individuals who described their experience of loneliness in intimate relationships as continuous with those who described it as a specific state-related event. It was predicted that levels of loneliness in intimate relationships would be elevated for the former group. All of the above evidence would provide further support for the psychometric strength of the LIRS.

5.1. Method

5.1.1. Participants

The 306 individuals who participated in study 3 took part in the present study.

5.1.2. Measures

The 14-item version of the Loneliness in Intimate Relationships Scale (LIRS) developed in studies 1–3 was used. The participants were given the instructions described in study 3. This final version of the LIRS was comprised of three subscales: detachment (6 items), hurt (4 items), and guilt (4 items). The score for each subscale is computed by averaging the ratings of the relevant items, with higher scores reflecting greater feelings of detachment, hurt, and guilt. Study 4 revealed satisfactory internal reliabilities for all three subscales ($\alpha = 0.86, 0.87, 0.64$ for the detachment, hurt, and guilt subscales, respectively.

The Revised UCLA Loneliness Scale (UCLA-R) [32] is the most widely used self-report measure of loneliness for both adolescents and adults. The scale consists of 20 items, of which 10 are positive (e.g., "There are people I can talk to") and 10 are negative (e.g., "People are around me but not with me"). Respondents are asked to indicate how often (1 = never, 2 = rarely, 3 = sometimes, or 4 = often) they feel the way described in each item. Positive items (1, 4, 5, 6, 9, 10, 15, 16, 19 and 20) were reverse-coded prior to analysis. The total score is the sum of all 20 items, with higher scores reflecting greater feelings of loneliness. The UCLA-R scale has been found to have high internal consistency, with $\alpha = 96$ and test-retest reliability = 0.94 [26,33]. In the present study, the UCLA-R also had a high internal consistency ($\alpha = 0.91$).

The Social and Emotional Loneliness Scale for adults—short version (SELSA-S) is a 15-item questionnaire that measures loneliness as a multidimensional construct. The SELSA-S has three 5-item subscales: romantic loneliness, family loneliness, and social loneliness. In the present study, we used only the social loneliness subscale (e.g., "I feel part of a group of friends"). Items are rated on a 7-point Likert scale that ranges from 1 (strongly disagree) to 7 (strongly agree). Items 1, 2 and 4 were reverse-coded prior to analysis. The total score is the mean of all 5 items, with higher scores reflecting greater feelings of social loneliness. The SELSA-S has been shown to be a reliable and valid measure of adult loneliness [28]). In the present study, the social loneliness subscale had high internal reliability ($\alpha = 0.82$).

The Interpersonal Needs Questionnaire (INQ) [34,35] is a 15-item self-report measure of interpersonal needs tapping perceived burdensomeness (6 items) and thwarted belongingness (9 items). Respondents indicate the degree to which statements are true for them on a 7-point Likert-type scale that ranges from 1 ("not true for me at all") to 7 ("very true for me"). Items 7, 8, 10, 13, 14 and 15 were reverse-coded prior to analysis. The total scores are the mean of all the items in the relevant subscales, with higher scores reflecting greater feelings of perceived burdensomeness and thwarted belongingness. The INQ has shown evidence of high levels of validity (Van Orden et al., 2012). Internal consistencies of the INQ scales in the current study were high (INQ-TB $\alpha = 0.92$, INQ-PB $\alpha = 0.74$).

The Beck Depression Inventory (BDI) [36] is a questionnaire consisting of 21 groups of statements referring to different aspects of depression. Respondents are asked to endorse statements characterizing how they have been feeling throughout the past two weeks.

The maximum total score for all 21 items is 63. The BDI has shown evidence of high levels of validity and reliability [36,37].

All the scales were administered in a counter-balanced order in two forms. No order effect was found.

5.2. Results and Discussion

The means and standard deviations for the different measures are presented in Table 5. Pearson correlations among the LIRS subscales (see Table 6) suggest that detachment is highly associated with hurt (r = 0.63), whereas guilt has lower associations with both detachment (r = 0.28) and hurt (r = 0.34).

Table 5. Descriptive statistics of the study measures—Study 4.

Scale	M	SD	95% CI
LIRS			
Detachment	3.44	1.37	3.29–3.59
Hurt	3.97	1.40	3.81–4.14
Guilt	2.62	1.12	2.49–2.76
UCLA	38.41	11.25	37.25–39.60
SEISA (Social)	2.64	1.25	2.51–2.79
INQ			
Perceived burdensomeness	1.58	1.13	1.45–1.72
Thwarted belongingness	3.46	0.77	3.38–3.54
BDI	11.14	9.86	8.69–11.05

Table 6. Pearson correlations between the LIRS subscales and loneliness and depression measures.

	LIRS Subscales		
	Detachment	**Hurt**	**Guilt**
UCLA	0.20 ***	0.21 ***	0.34 ***
SELS-A (Social)	0.18 **	0.19 ***	0.27 ***
INQ			
Perceived burdensomeness	0.16	0.16	0.19 ***
Thwarted belongingness	0.24 ***	0.18 ***	0.24 ***
BDI	0.31 ***	0.31 ***	0.30 ***

Note: ** $p < 0.003$; *** $p < 0.001$.

The relationships between the LIRS three subscales and loneliness and depression measures were computed in order to assess the validity of the LIRS (see Table 6). Bonferroni's formula was used to adjust the α level from 0.05 to 0.05 divided by fifteen, or 0.003. Only values of $p \leq 0.003$ were considered to be significant. It was hypothesized that all three subscales of the LIRS would be positively but moderately associated with all other measures.

As indicated in Table 6, most of the correlations between the LIRS subscales and the criteria variables were in the expected positive direction, indicating that greater loneliness in intimate relationships is related to higher levels of reported general and social loneliness and greater interpersonal needs and depression. The non-significant associations between the detachment and hurt subscales of the LIRS and the perceived burdensomeness subscale of the INQ provide support for the discriminant validity of the LIRS, which refers to the distinctiveness of different constructs [38]. These results validate the LIRS as tapping loneliness and social detachment tendencies, yet measuring new and unique aspects of loneliness, namely loneliness in intimate relationships, which are not addressed by any other measure.

To further validate the LIRS as a measure of loneliness in intimate relationships, we compared the patterns of its subscales between individuals who reported that when they experienced loneliness, it was on a more or less continuous basis, with those reporting that it was related to a specific occasion. The results are presented in Table 7.

Table 7. Descriptive and Inferential Statistics of LIRS by Type of Loneliness.

	Type of Loneliness					
LIRS Subscales	**Continuous**		**Specific**		***F* (1, 280)**	η_p^2
	M	SD	M	SD		
Detachment	4.04	1.27	3.30	1.33	19.09 ***	0.06
Hurt	4.44	1.24	3.89	1.37	9.87 ***	0.03
Guilt	3.00	1.23	2.46	1.03	14.70 ***	0.05

Note: *** $p < 0.001$.

A multivariate analysis of variance (MANOVA) conducted on the three LIRS subscales means with the type of loneliness (continuous/specific) as IV revealed a significant multivariate effect of type of loneliness, F (3, 278) = 9.09, $p < 0.001$. As expected, univariate analyses (see Table 7) revealed that the level of loneliness in intimate relationships is greater for individuals who experienced loneliness in a relationship on a continuous, not state-related basis, compared with individuals whose loneliness experience was more specific and state-related. This pattern emerged for all three LIRS subscales.

Finally, despite not having preliminary hypotheses regarding gender differences in LIRS scales, we wished to explore them. The results are presented in Table 8. A multivariate analysis of variance (MANOVA) conducted on the three LIRS subscales means with gender as IV revealed a significant multivariate effect of gender, F (3, 299) = 9.14, $p < 0.001$. Univariate analyses revealed that women experience significantly higher levels of detachment and hurt, while men experience significantly higher levels of guilt.

Table 8. Descriptive and Inferential Statistics of LIRS by Gender.

LIRS Subscales	**Men**		**Women**		***F* (1, 301)**	η_p^2
	M	SD	M	SD		
Detachment	3.22	1.36	3.63	1.36	6.77 **	0.02
Hurt	3.65	1.38	4.24	1.38	13.55 ***	0.04
Guilt	2.76	1.19	2.50	1.06	4.16 *	0.01

Note: * $p < 0.05$, ** $p < 0.01$, *** $p < 0.001$.

Taken as a whole, the results of Study 4 provide support for the validity properties of the LIRS.

6. Conclusions

Various pitfalls, stumbling blocks, and hazards, such as hurt feelings, ostracism, jealousy, lying, and betrayal, may harm emotional relations and feelings of love [39]. We want and need to be loved by our intimate partners and hope that our relational value—the degree to which our partner considers our intimate relationship valuable, important, and close—is as high as we perceive it to be. It is painful to discover that our partner may perceive it as lower than we would like it to be perceived. A dissonance is thus created between what we envision it to be and what our partner apparently sees in it. Should relational devaluation occur, and we are no longer thought of as positively as before, we experience pain, anger, hurt, and loneliness [40,41] described ideal romantic love as a situation where the one I love loves me back since "Out of all the people she could love, she chooses to love me. That suggests that the reason why she loves me should be to do with the things that set me apart from others" (p. 163). When those feelings seem to change, when one stops feeling so valued and special to their partner, it may lead to their feeling neglected, unappreciated, and thus lonely. When one is not as important to one's lover as one knows one was in the past, it ushers in loneliness, sadness, and longing to recreate what was, what made one feel so good and special in the first place.

The newly created scale is expected to be valuable, not only for researchers in the areas of loneliness and marital relationships but for clinicians as well, who would be able to identify specific shortcomings in the relationships which contribute to loneliness and thus be able to more specifically address them.

7. Limitations

There are several scales in use for assessing relationships, couple's satisfaction, and loneliness. However, none addresses the specific issue of loneliness that may exist in intimate relations, which needs to be identified and measured. The present study was designed to integrate theoretical frameworks of loneliness in intimate relationships with empirical data, resulting in the development of a new scale, the Loneliness in Intimate Relationships Scale (LIRS). The preliminary versions of the LIRS were based on semi-structured questionnaires administered to a large heterogenic Israeli sample and on analyses of existing relevant scales. Exploratory and confirmatory factor analyses resulted in a well-structured 14-item scale depicting emotional, behavioral, and cognitive reactions and coping with loneliness in intimate relationships. The analyses revealed that the experience of loneliness in intimate relationships encompasses three main aspects: detachment, hurt, and guilt. Rokach and Brock [12] developed a scale to explore the qualitative aspects of loneliness in general. Their five-dimensional model included those very same factors: the hurt, which is a salient ingredient of loneliness, the hurt that follows feeling alone and unwanted, and the detachment that some people resort to in order to prevent further rejections, hurt, and pain. The LIRS evidenced excellent reliability levels with internal consistency estimates in the 90s. Furthermore, construct validity tests showed that, as expected, the LIRS subscales are positively related to higher levels of reported general and social loneliness and greater interpersonal needs and depression and are more prevalent among individuals who experienced loneliness in a relationship on a continuous, not state-related, basis.

Being connected is one of the most important human needs. It is so important that it affects not only emotional and physical well-being but is directly related to mortality rates. Studies have demonstrated a steep rise in mortality rates among socially isolated individuals [42]. However, being lonely does not necessarily reflect being unconnected with other human beings. The empirical and clinical literature conceptualizes loneliness as a two-dimensional construct, discriminating between objective loneliness, which reflects the quantity of one's social interactions, and subjective loneliness, which concerns the quality of those interactions and reflects dissatisfaction with one's social relationships, or as described by Weiss [43], as a "gnawing, chronic disease without redeeming features" (in [44], p. 446). Nevertheless, these two aspects of loneliness are not necessarily associated. According to Gottman's [44,45] Distance and Isolation Cascade model, deterioration of marital distress can eventually result in disengagement, isolation, and loneliness. Gottman depicts the process leading from emotional flooding within a relationship to the feeling that any attempt to discuss problems will be pointless and futile—an approach that will eventually lead to emotionally parallel lives. When a couple reaches this advanced stage of relational deterioration, there is a complete absence of expressions of love and affection, and the partners experience emotional isolation, disengagement, and loneliness. Partners then find themselves emotionally uninvolved with and unavailable to each other. This "empty shell" marriage, which is characterized by partners' disengagement and indifference, is a common antecedent of loneliness [46].

Marriage, similarly to any long-term intimate relationship, is an appropriate state for analyzing emotional loneliness separately from objective social isolation. The fact that loneliness in intimate relationships revealed itself not as a unitary concept but as being comprised of three stable and valid facets, namely, detachment, hurt, and guilt, may have important clinical implications, especially given the lack of couple-based therapy techniques designed specifically for the treatment of loneliness in close relationships [47].

As our studies revealed, detachment is a major factor of romantic loneliness, and it is thus reasonable to suggest that therapeutic interventions aimed at the improvement of attachment bonding and intimacy may potentially alleviate loneliness. More specifically, interventions that strengthen intimacy, emotional security, and mutual support are likely to encourage couples in therapy to reengage emotionally, thus reducing loneliness. Additionally, focusing on strengthening attachment bonding in romantic relationships is a preventive measure against relational loneliness. By employing preventive measures, educators and practitioners can utilize ways to help couples protect themselves from emotional detachment as a protective shield from romantic loneliness.

The authors note several limitations of these studies. First, the LIRS was not validated against behavioral measures. It is unclear how self-ratings on the LIRS manifest themselves behaviorally, thus limiting the scale's ecological validity as a predictive tool for change. Future research should test the clinical utility of the LIRS to assess the level and type of relationship loneliness. Secondly, the LIRS was not examined in comparison to existing, general loneliness scales. While it is expected that the correlation would possibly be a moderate one, future research could examine it more closely. Thirdly, the interrelations between the three main subscales of the LIRS were not thoroughly examined. Different patterns of loneliness resulting from different combinations of levels of detachment, hurt, and guilt may manifest themselves in similar or different patterns of reactions to the stressful situation, thus calling for different types of psychological interventions. Finally, the LIRS was developed and validated with Israeli participants. This may, at present, limit the generalization of the application of this scale to other cultures. Future studies are needed in order to test the generalizability of the measurement model by testing it with other native English-speaking populations.

Author Contributions: Methodology, E.B.-A.; resources, A.S.; data curation, A.R., A.S. and E.B.-A.; writing—original draft preparation, A.R. and E.B.-A.; writing—review and editing, A.R.; All authors have read and agreed to the published version of the manuscript.

Funding: This research received no external funding.

Institutional Review Board Statement: The institutional review board indicated that our research project was approved, that consent need not be signed, and that it adheres to ethical guidelines. The study was conducted in accordance with the Declaration of Helsinki, and approved by the Institutional Review of the College of Academic Studies in Israel.

Informed Consent Statement: Not applicable.

Data Availability Statement: The raw data supporting the conclusions of this article will be made available by the authors without undue reservation.

Conflicts of Interest: The authors declare no conflict of interest.

Appendix A Loneliness in Intimate Relationships—Final Version (Studies 3A and 3B)

Table A1. Please indicate the degree to which each statement describes what you may have felt or thought during a specific period or situation in which you felt lonely in an intimate relationship.

		Totally Not Describes My Situation					Totally Describes My Situation
		1	2	3	4	5	6
1	I felt a deep sense of pain						
2	I felt hurt						
3	I felt insulted						
4	I was very tense						
5	My husband/partner had no time for me						
6	I felt that I was not fulfilling my part in the relationship						

Table A1. *Cont.*

		Totally Not Describes My Situation	Totally Describes My Situation
7	I felt guilty for my misdeeds in the marriage/relationships		
8	I invested in the relationship without getting back		
9	I felt that I was not worthy of his love		
10	I felt that I was not important to him		
11	I felt that I could not continue like this		
12	I wondered whether we are suitable		
13	I contemplated divorce		
14	I thought that I was infantile		

References

1. Baumeister, R.F.; Leary, M.R. The need to belong: Desire for interpersonal attachments as a fundamental human motivation. *Psychol. Bull.* **1995**, *117*, 497–529. [CrossRef] [PubMed]
2. McCarthy, B.; Ginsberg, R.L.; Cintron, J.A. Primary prevention the first two years of marriage. *J. Fam. Psychother.* **2008**, *19*, 143–156. [CrossRef]
3. Laurenceau, J.P.; Feldman-Barrett, L.; Rovine, M.J. The interpersonal process model of intimacy in marriage: A daily-diary and multilevel modeling approach. *J. Fam. Psychol.* **2005**, *19*, 314–323. [CrossRef] [PubMed]
4. Strong, B.; De Valut, C.; Cohen, T.F. *The Marriage and Family Experience: Intimate Relationships in a Changing Society*, 11th ed.; Wadsworth: Belmont, CA, USA, 2011.
5. Cohen, S.; Gottlieb, B.H.; Underwood, L.G. Social relationships and health: Challenges for measurement and interventions. *Adv. Mind-Body Med.* **2000**, *17*, 129–141.
6. Pinquart, M. Loneliness in married, widowed, divorced, and never-married older adults. *J. Soc. Pers. Relatsh.* **2003**, *20*, 31–53. [CrossRef]
7. Hassebrauck, M.; Fehr, B. Dimensions of relationship quality. *Pers. Relatsh.* **2002**, *9*, 253–270. [CrossRef]
8. Tornstam, L. Loneliness in marriage. *J. Soc. Pers. Relatsh.* **1992**, *9*, 197–217. [CrossRef]
9. Segrin, C.; Flora, J. Perceptions of relational histories, marital quality, and loneliness when communication is limited: An examination of married prison inmates. *J. Fam. Commun.* **2001**, *1*, 151–173. [CrossRef]
10. Barbour, A. Research report: Dyadic loneliness in marriage. *J. Group Psychother. Psychodrama Sociom.* **1993**, *46*, 70–72.
11. Rokach, A.; Brock, H. Loneliness and the effects of life changes. *J. Psychol.* **1997**, *131*, 284–298. [CrossRef]
12. Rokach, A.; Sha'ked, A. *Together and Lonely: Loneliness in Intimate Relationships—Causes and Coping*; Nova: New York, NY, USA, 2013.
13. Fincham, F.; Rogge, R. Understanding relationship quality: Theoretical challenges and new tools for assessment. *J. Fam. Theory Rev.* **2010**, *2*, 227–242. [CrossRef]
14. Locke, H.J.; Wallace, K.M. Short Marital-Adjustment and Prediction Tests: Their reliability and validity. *Marriag. Fam. Living* **1959**, *21*, 251–255. [CrossRef]
15. Sarason, I.G.; Sarason, B.R.; Solky-Butzel, J.A.; Nagle, L.C. Assessing the quality of personal relationships. *J. Soc. Pers. Relatsh.* **1997**, *14*, 339–356.
16. Humbad, M.N.; Donnellan, M.B.; Klump, K.L.; Burt, S.A. Development of the Brief Romantic Relationship Interaction Coding Scheme (BRRICS). *J. Fam. Psychol.* **2011**, *25*, 759–769. [CrossRef] [PubMed]
17. Graham, J.M.; Diebels, K.J.; Barnow, Z.B. The reliability of relationship satisfaction: A reliability generalization meta-analysis. *J. Fam. Psychol.* **2011**, *25*, 39–48. [CrossRef] [PubMed]
18. Bozoglan, B. The psychometric properties of the Scale of Retired Spousal Intrusion. *Eur. J. Psychol. Assess.* **2015**, *1*, 1–7. [CrossRef]
19. Russell, D.; Cutrona, C.E.; Rose, J.; Yurko, K. Social and emotional loneliness: An examination of Weiss's typology of loneli-ness. *J. Personal. Soc. Psychol.* **1984**, *46*, 1313–1321. [CrossRef]
20. De Jong-Gierveld, J. A 6-item scale for overall, emotional, and social loneliness. *Res. Aging* **2006**, *28*, 582–598. [CrossRef]
21. Schmidt, N.; Sermat, V. Measuring loneliness in different relationships. *J. Personal. Soc. Psychol.* **1983**, *44*, 1038–1047. [CrossRef]
22. De Jong-Gierveld, J. Developing and testing a model of loneliness. *J. Personal. Soc. Psychol.* **1987**, *53*, 119–128. [CrossRef]
23. Asher, S.R.; Wheeler, V.A. Children's loneliness: A comparison of rejected and neglected peer status. *J. Consult. Clin. Psychol.* **1985**, *534*, 500–505. [CrossRef]
24. Rokach, A. Offense type and the experience of loneliness. *Int. J. Offender Ther. Comp. Criminol.* **2000**, *44*, 549–556. [CrossRef]
25. Cramer, K.M.; Ofosu, H.B.; Barry, J.E. An abbreviated form of the social and emotional loneliness scale for adults (SELSA). *Personal. Individ. Differ.* **2000**, *28*, 1125–1131. [CrossRef]
26. Russell, D. UCLA Loneliness Scale: Reliability, validity, and factor structure. *J. Personal. Assess.* **1996**, *66*, 20–40. [CrossRef] [PubMed]

27. DiTommaso, E.; Spinner, B. The development and initial validation of the social and emotional loneliness scale for adults (SELSA). *Personal. Individ. Differ.* **1993**, *14*, 127–134. [CrossRef]
28. Di Tommaso, E.; Brannen, C.; Best, L.A. Measurement and validity characteristics of the short version of the Social and Emo-tional Loneliness Scale for adults. *Educ. Psychol. Meas.* **2004**, *6*, 99–119. [CrossRef]
29. Tabachnick, B.G.; Fidell, L.S. *Using Multivariate Statistics*, 6th ed.; Allyn and Bacon: Boston, MA, USA, 2013.
30. Dinno, A. Exploring the sensitivity of Horn's parallel analysis to the distributional form of random data. *Multivar. Behav. Res.* **2009**, *44*, 362–388. [CrossRef]
31. IBM Corp. *IBM SPSS Statistics for Windows, Version 27.0*; IBM Corporation: Armonk, NY, USA, 2020.
32. Russell, D.; Peplau, L.A.; Cutrona, C.E. The revised UCLA Loneliness Scale: Concurrent and discriminant validity evidence. *J. Personal. Soc. Psychol.* **1980**, *39*, 472–480. [CrossRef]
33. Vassar, M.; Crosby, J.W. A reliability generalization study of coefficient alpha for the UCLA Loneliness Scale. *J. Personal. Assess.* **2008**, *90*, 601–607. [CrossRef]
34. Ryan, M.; Hill, R.M.; Rey, Y.; Marin, C.; Sharp, C.; Green, K.L. Evaluating the Interpersonal Needs Questionnaire: Compari-son of the reliability, factor structure, and predictive validity across five versions. *Suicide Life-Threat. Behav.* **2015**, *3*, 302–314.
35. Van Orden, K.A.; Curkowica, K.C.; Witte, T.K.; Joiner, T.E. Thwarted belongingness and perceived burdensomeness: Con-struct validity and psychometric properties of the Interpersonal Needs Questionnaire. *Psychol. Assess.* **2012**, *24*, 197–215. [CrossRef] [PubMed]
36. Beck, A.T.; Steer, R.A.; Brown, G.K. *Manual for the Beck Depression Inventory–II*; Psychological Corporation: San Antonio, TX, USA, 1996.
37. Whisman, M.A.; Judd, C.M.; Whiteford, N.T.; Gelhorn, H.L. Measurement invariance of the Beck Depression Inventory–Second Edition (BDI-II) across gender, race, and ethnicity in college students. *Personal. Assess.* **2013**, *20*, 419–428. [CrossRef] [PubMed]
38. Cozby, P.C. *Methods in Behavioral Research*; McGraw-Hill: Boston, MA, USA, 2012.
39. Vangelisti, A.L. (Ed.) *Feeling Hurt in Close Relationships*; Cambridge University Press: Boston, MA, USA, 2009.
40. DeWall, C.N.; MacDonald, G.; Webster, G.D.; Masten, C.L.; Baumeister, R.F.; Powell, C.; Eisenberger, N.I. Acetaminophen reduces social pain: Behavioral and neural evidence. *Psychol. Sci.* **2010**, *21*, 931–937. [CrossRef] [PubMed]
41. Keller, S. How do I love thee? Let me count the properties. *Am. Philos. Q.* **2000**, *37*, 163–173.
42. Holt-Lunstad, J.; Smith, T.B.; Layton, J.B. Social relationships and mortality risk: A meta-analytic review. *PLoS Med.* **2010**, *7*, e1000316. [CrossRef] [PubMed]
43. Weiss, R. *Loneliness: The Experience of Emotional and Social Isolation*; MIT Press: Cambridge, UK, 1973.
44. Gottman, J.M. *The Marriage Clinic: A Scientifically Based Marital Therapy*; W. W. Norton: New York, NY, USA, 1999.
45. Cacioppo, J.T.; Cacioppo, S. Metrics of scholarly impact. *Meas. Interdiscip. Res. Perspect.* **2012**, *10*, 154–156. [CrossRef]
46. Perlman, D.; Peplau, L.A. Loneliness. In *Encyclopedia of Mental Health*; Friedman, H., Ed.; Academic Press: San Diego, CA, USA, 1998; Volume 2, pp. 571–581.
47. Sha'ked, A. Addressing loneliness in romantic relationships. In *Treating Loneliness: Therapeutic and Psychological Interventions*; Sha'ked, A., Rokach, A., Eds.; Routledge: New York, NY, USA, 2015.

International Journal of
Environmental Research and Public Health

MDPI

Article

Association between Social Isolation and Loneliness with Estimated Atherosclerotic Cardiovascular Disease Risk in a UK Biobank Population-Based Study

Alexandre Vallée

Department of Epidemiology-Data-Biostatistics, Delegation of Clinical Research and Innovation (DRCI), Foch Hospital, 92150 Suresnes, France; al.vallee@hopital-foch.com

Abstract: Objective: The association of cardiovascular (CV) risk with social isolation and loneliness remains poorly studied. The purpose of this cross-sectional study was to investigate the associations between social isolation and loneliness with estimated 10-year atherosclerotic cardiovascular disease (ASCVD) risk. Methods: Among 302,553 volunteers of the UK Biobank population, social isolation and loneliness were assessed with a questionnaire. Associations between social isolation and loneliness with ASCVD risk were estimated using multiple gender regressions. Results: Men presented a higher estimated 10-year ASCVD risk (8.63% vs. 2.65%, $p < 0.001$) and higher proportions of social isolation (9.13% vs. 8.45%, $p < 0.001$) and loneliness (6.16% vs. 5.57%, $p < 0.001$) than women. In all covariate-adjusted models, social isolation was associated with an increased ASCVD risk in men ($B = 0.21$ (0.16; 0.26), $p < 0.001$) and women ($B = 0.12$ (0.10; 0.14), $p < 0.001$). Loneliness was associated with an increased ASCVD risk in men ($B = 0.08$ (0.03; 0.14), $p = 0.001$) but not in women ($p = 0.217$). A significant interaction was observed between social isolation and loneliness with ASCVD risk in men ($p = 0.009$) and women ($p = 0.016$). After adjustment for all covariates, both social isolation and loneliness were significantly associated with ASCVD risk in men ($B = 0.44$ (0.28; 0.61), $p < 0.001$) and women ($B = 0.20$ (0.12; 0.29), $p < 0.001$). Conclusion: Social isolation was associated with a higher estimated 10-year ASCVD risk in both genders but only loneliness among men. Social isolation and loneliness can be considered potential added risk factors for CV risk. Health policies should address these notions in prevention campaigns, in addition to traditional risk factors.

Keywords: social isolation; loneliness; gender; education; income; cardiovascular disease; cardiovascular risk; atherosclerosis; atherosclerotic cardiovascular disease

1. Introduction

Cardiovascular (CV) disease is one of the main causes of morbidity and mortality worldwide [1]. The impact of CV disease is major in terms of economic burden [2]. Understanding and identifying non-traditional risk factors could improve preventive health strategies. In 2016, a systematic review showed that participants with poor social determinants had a 30% more likely risk of cardiac and stroke events [3]. Even if no established definition exists, social isolation and loneliness are associated with the ability of individuals to form satisfying and meaningful relationships and social interactions and to be adaptative in social situations and interactions with other people, services and institutions [4]. Social isolation is a measure of the absence of social interactions or infrequent social contact with other people. Loneliness is the subjective negative notion of feeling isolated [5]. In recent years, social isolation has become a major public health issue [6]. The association between CV disease and social isolation and loneliness remains inconsistent, with studies showing no association [7], association with non-fatal CV events [8], or associations with CV events [4,7,9,10]. However, few studies have focused on large populations [11]. The link between social isolation and CV disease could be modulated by the atherosclerotic pathway [12]. To date, it remains unclear if these relationships are independent of biological factors [13]. Thus, in this cross-sectional study, I evaluated estimated 10-year atherosclerotic cardiovascular disease (ASCVD) risk [14,15] to investigate social isolation and loneliness associations among the general UK Biobank population.

2. Methods

2.1. UK Biobank Population

The UK Biobank cohort comprised 9.1 million eligible individuals, 8.6 million of which did not respond or did not provide consent. Thus, at baseline, the UK Biobank included 502,478 Britons (5.5% of the total UK Biobank cohort), aged 38–73 years, across 22 UK cities from the UK National Health Service Register between 2006 and 2010, 90 M of which were linked to national health registries. Participants responded to questionnaires and a computer-assisted interview, and they were subject to physical and functional measures and blood, urine, and saliva sampling [16]. Data included personalized information of the participants, including socio-economic, behavior and lifestyle, mental health battery, clinical diagnoses and therapies, genetics, imaging and physiological biomarkers from blood and urine samples. The cohort protocol can be found in the literature [17,18].

2.2. Ethical Considerations

All participants provided electronic informed consent, and the UK Biobank received ethical approval from the Northwest Multi-center Research Ethics Committee (MREC) covering the whole of the UK. The study was conducted according to the guidelines of the Declaration of Helsinki and approved by the Northwest Haydock Research Ethics Committee (protocol code: 21/NW/0157, date of approval: 21 June 2021). For details, see https://www.ukbiobank.ac.uk/learn-more-about-uk-biobank/about-us/ethics (Accessed on 30 November 2022).

2.3. Study Population

We included 399,067 volunteers of the UK Biobank without missing data and without previous CV events to calculate the estimated 10-year ASCVD risk. CV diseases were defined as including heart attack, angina, and stroke, as diagnosed by a doctor and reported in questionnaires. Of these, I excluded 97,517 for missing data. We therefore analyzed the data of 301,550 volunteers (Figure 1).

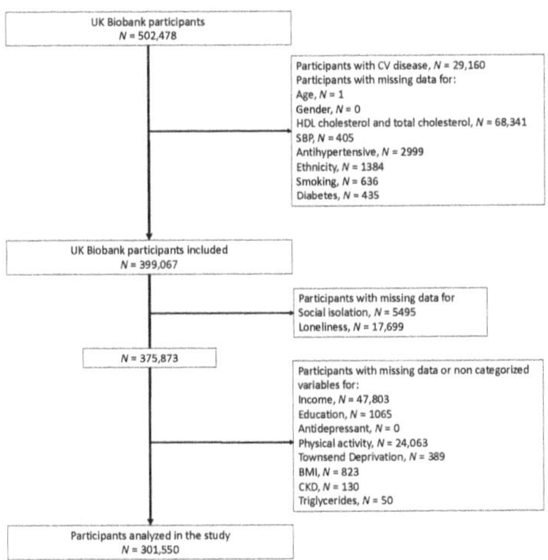

Figure 1. Flowchart.

2.4. Estimated 10-Year ASCVD Risk

Estimated 10-year ASCVD risk was evaluated using the Pooled Cohort Equations (PCE) model [14,15]. The PCE model was used to express ASCVD risk in a continuous percentage. The estimated 10-year absolute risk of ASCVD was set to be characterized by death due to coronary heart disease, nonfatal myocardial infarction or fatal or nonfatal stroke over a 10-year period in participants free of established CV diseases. The PCE allowed for the derivation of sex- and race-specific estimates of the 10-year risk for ASCVD for adults aged 40 to 79 years. Parameters included in the PCE were age, gender, Black people, tobacco smoking, total and high-density lipoprotein cholesterol, treated or untreated systolic blood pressure, and diabetes. A PCE score of 7.5% or greater indicated that a participant was at a high ASCVD risk, and participants with a PCE score of less than 7.5% were considered at low risk [19,20].

2.5. Social Isolation and Loneliness

Social isolation and loneliness were assessed with scales that were used in previous UK Biobank studies [7,9,11].

The social isolation scale contained three questions (1) "Including yourself, how many people are living together in your household?"; (2) "How often do you visit friends or family or have them visit you?"; and (3) "Which of the following (leisure/social activities) do you engage in once a week or more often? You may select more than one"), where certain answers were given one point (1 point for no participation in social activities at least weekly, 1 point for living alone, and 1 point for friend and family visits less of than once a month), and all other answers were given 0 point. This resulted in a scale ranging from 0 to 3, where a person was defined as socially isolated if she/he had two or more points.

Loneliness was measured with two questions: "Do you often feel lonely?" (no = 0; yes = 1) and "How often are you able to confide in someone close to you?" (0 = almost daily to once every few months; 1 = never or almost never). An individual was defined as lonely if she/he answered positively to both questions (score 2).

2.6. Covariates

Systolic and diastolic blood pressure (SBD, DBP) were measured twice at the assessment center with an automated BP device (Omron 705 IT electronic blood pressure monitor; OMRON Healthcare Europe B.V. Kruisweg 577 2132 NA Hoofddorp) or manually with a sphygmomanometer equipped with an inflatable cuff in association with a stethoscope if the blood pressure device failed to measure the BP or if the largest inflatable cuff of the device did not fit around the individual's arm [21].

Diabetes status was defined on either receiving anti-diabetic medication, diabetes diagnosed by a doctor, or a fasting glucose concentration of $\geq$7 mmol/L [22]. Medications were characterized by the question: "Do you regularly take any of the following medications?".

The biological parameters are detailed in the UK Biobank protocol [23].

The estimated glomerular filtration rate (eGFR) was calculated based on the Chronic Kidney Disease Epidemiology Collaboration equation (eGFR-CKD-EPI), as follows:

$$\begin{aligned} eGFR = {} & 141 \times \left(minimum\ of\ 1\ or\ standardized \frac{Scr}{\kappa} \right)^{\alpha} \\ & \times \left(maximum\ of\ 1\ or\ standardized \frac{Scr}{\kappa} \right)^{-1.209} \\ & \times [0.993]^{age} \times (1.018\ if\ female) \end{aligned}$$

where κ is 0.7 in females and 0.9 in males and α is −0.329 in females and −0.411 in males. eGFR <60 mL/min/1.73 m^2 indicated chronic kidney disease (CKD)).

The body mass index was calculated as weight (in kg) divided by $height^2$ (meters).

Education level was defined in three categories: high (college or university degree), intermediate (A/AS levels or equivalent, O levels/GCSEs or equivalent, or other professional qualifications such as nursing and teaching), and low (none of the afore mentioned categories).

Income level was defined as: high level (greater than £52,000 per year), moderate level (between £18,000 and £51,999 per year), and low level (less than £18,000 per year).

Townsend deprivation index scores were derived from national census data about car ownership, household overcrowding, owner occupation, and unemployment aggregated for postcodes of residence [24].

Current tobacco smokers were defined as participants who responded "yes, on most or all days" or "yes, only occasionally" at the question "do you smoke tobacco now".

Antidepressant medication use was included in the analyses due to the association between depression and social isolation [25]. The list of antidepressant drugs is available at [26].

Physical activity was self-reported, measured with a revised version of the International physical activity questionnaire (IPAQ) [27] completed on a tablet computer during examination. Patients were asked to state how many days they were engaged in more than 10 min of walking, moderate physical activity, and vigorous physical activity in a typical week. Individuals were then asked for how many minutes they were engaged in each of the activities on a typical day. Self-reported physical activity data were processed using the method of Bradbury et al. [28] based on the IPAQ guidelines [29]. Walking, moderate physical activity, and vigorous physical activity were scored at 2.3, 3.0 and 7.0 excess metabolic equivalents of tasks (METs), respectively [29]. Then, the time spent in each of the activities on a typical day was multiplied by the typical number of days doing the exercise and the respective MET scores to assess METs per week. A daily physical activity of less than 10 min was recorded as 0, and self-reported values of more to 1260 min per week (equivalent to an average of 3 h a day) were cut off at 1260 min according to the IPAQ guidelines [27]. Participants who answered "do not know" or "prefer not to answer" to any of the self-reported physical activity questions were excluded from the analysis. MET hours per week were categorized as low: <10.0; moderate: 10.0 to 49.9; and high: ≥50 MET hours/week) [29].

2.7. Statistical Analysis

The characteristics of the study population were described as the means with standard deviations (SDs) for continuous variables. Categorical variables were described as numbers and proportions. Comparisons between groups were performed using Student's test for continuous variables. Pearson's $\chi 2$ test was used for categorical variables. This study explored the association between social isolation and loneliness with estimated 10-year ASCVD risk levels and secondly with a high risk of CV (an estimated 10-year ASCVD risk of more than 7.5%). Associations between social isolation and loneliness with estimated 10-year ASCVD risk were examined with multiple linear regression models computing regression coefficients (*B*) and their 95% confidence intervals (95% CIs) and then with multiple logistic regression models with odds ratio (ORs) and 95% confidence intervals to estimate the 10-year ASCVD risk of more than 7.5%. First, the gender models were adjusted for age. Second, the gender models were adjusted for age, antidepressant medication, education, income level, couple, physical activity, Townsend deprivation quintiles, BMI, CKD, and triglycerides. These adjustments were justified by their relationship with ASCVD risk and CV risk: education [30], income [31], couple [32], physical activity [33], Townsend deprivation [34], BMI [35], CKD [36] and triglycerides [37].

The "no poor social isolation and no loneliness" participant group was considered as the reference group in the analyses. Statistics were calculated using SAS software (version 9.4; SAS Institute, Carry, NC, USA). A p-value < 0.05 was considered statistically significant.

3. Results

Among the 301,550 participants, social isolation affected 26,454 (8.77%) and loneliness affect 17,555 (5.82%).

Men presented a higher estimated 10-year ASCVD risk than women (8.63% vs. 2.65%, $p < 0.001$), a higher proportion of high education levels (38.44% vs. 36.23%, $p < 0.001$) and a higher proportion of high-income levels (31.37% vs. 25.29%, $p < 0.001$). Men also showed higher proportions of social isolation (9.13% vs. 8.45%, $p < 0.001$) and loneliness (6.11% vs. 5.56%, $p < 0.001$) (Table 1).

Table 1. Characteristics of the study population according to gender.

	Men N = 142,302		Women N = 159,248		p-Value
Age (years) (mean, SD)	56.08	8.16	55.49	7.97	<0.001
Estimated 10-year ASCVD risk (%) (mean, SD)	8.63	6.70	2.65	3.02	<0.001
High level of ASCVD risk (>7.5%)	65,626	46.12%	9624	6.04%	<0.001
Physical activity					<0.001
High	33,194	23.33%	30,749	19.31%	
Moderate	72,998	51.30%	85,003	53.38%	
Low	36,110	25.38%	43,496	27.31%	
BMI (kg/m^2) (mean, SD)	27.65	4.11	26.82	5.05	<0.001
BMI					<0.001
High	33,783	23.74%	34,710	21.80%	
Moderate	71,379	50.16%	58,088	36.48%	
Low	37,140	26.10%	66,450	41.73%	
Couple	111,442	78.35%	109,783	68.96%	<0.001
Education					<0.001
High	54,698	38.44%	57,688	36.23%	
Moderate	61,500	43.22%	73,934	46.43%	
Low	26,104	18.34%	27,626	17.35%	
Income					<0.001
High	44,646	31.37%	40,272	25.29%	
Moderate	73,146	51.40%	83,464	52.41%	
Low	24,510	17.22%	35,512	22.30%	
Townsend deprivation quintiles					<0.001
Q1	29,276	20.57%	31,110	19.54%	
Q2	28,828	20.26%	31,527	19.80%	
Q3	28,307	19.89%	32,004	20.10%	
Q4	27,655	19.43%	32,623	20.49%	
Q5	28,236	19.84%	31,984	20.08%	
Antidepressant medication	6209	4.36%	13,967	8.77%	<0.001
Antihypertensive medication	28,179	19.80%	23,651	14.85%	<0.001
Diabetes	9835	6.91%	7115	4.47%	<0.001
Black people	461	0.32%	750	0.47%	<0.001
Current smoking	16,685	11.74%	13,832	8.70%	<0.001
HDL cholesterol (mmol/L) (mean, SD)	1.29	0.31	1.61	0.37	<0.001
Total cholesterol (mmol/L) (mean, SD)	5.59	1.09	5.88	1.11	<0.001
Triglycerides (mmol/L) (mean, SD)	1.97	1.15	1.52	0.84	<0.001
SBP (mmHg) (mean, SD)	138.97	15.84	126.76	17.41	<0.001
eGFR (mL/min/1.73 m^2) (mean, SD)	98.15	26.65	132.67	33.65	<0.001
Chronic kidney disease	5723	4.02%	913	0.57%	<0.001
Social isolation	12,999	9.13%	13,455	8.45%	<0.001
Loneliness	8698	6.11%	8857	5.56%	<0.001
Both social isolation and loneliness	2213	1.56%	1722	1.08%	<0.001

SD: standard deviation.

In both genders, participants with social isolation showed higher levels of ASCVD risk than the reference groups (for men with social isolation, the mean ASCVD risk = 9.26% vs. 8.57%, $p < 0.001$; for women with social isolation, the mean ASCVD risk was 3.23% vs. 2.60%, $p < 0.001$) (Figure 2). No univariable difference was observed for loneliness among men (mean ASCVD risk = 8.60% vs. 8.63%, $p = 0.717$), but a significant association among women was observed (mean ASCVD risk = 2.91% vs. 2.64%, $p < 0.001$) (Figure 2).

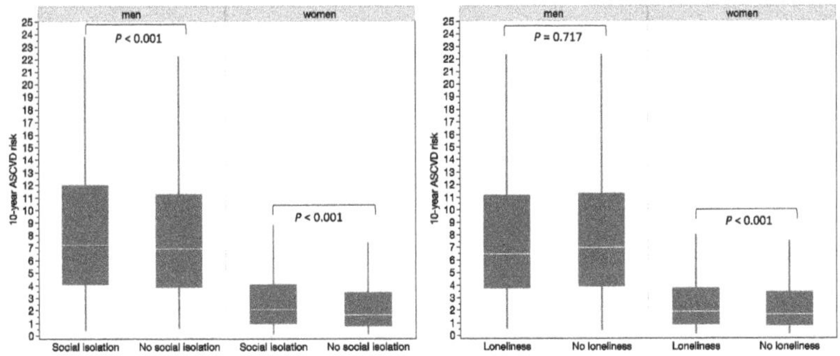

Figure 2. Estimated 10-year ASCVD risk according to gender and social isolation and loneliness status (white line: median; grey area: 25th to 75th percentile).

However, in both genders, participants with social isolation and loneliness showed lower high income and high educational level rates than the reference groups ($p < 0.001$).

When considering the overall population, both social isolation and loneliness showed significant associations with estimated 10-year ASCVD risk, as did social isolation ($B = 0.14$ (0.11; 0.17), $p < 0.001$) and not loneliness ($B = 0.02$ (−0.01; 0.05), $p = 0.198$), with a significant p-value for the interaction between social isolation and loneliness and gender ($p < 0.001$).

Compared with the reference group, men with social isolation were associated with a higher estimated 10-year ASCVD risk ($B = 0.41$ (0.37; 0.47), $p < 0.001$) in the age-adjusted model. Adjustment for all covariates did not affect this association ($B = 0.21$ (0.16; 0.26), $p < 0.001$). The same results were observed for analyses of high ASCVD risk with all covariates adjusted (OR = 1.14 [1.08–1.20], $p < 0.001$) (Table 2).

Table 2. Multiple linear and logistic regression models for estimated 10-year ASCVD risk among men (all covariates adjusted: age, education, income level, physical activity, couple, antidepressant medication, Townsend deprivation index, BMI, triglycerides, and CKD). The reference was the reference group.

	Continuous Estimated 10-Year ASCVD Risk				Estimated 10-Year ASCVD Risk Superior to 7.5%			
Men	Age-Adjusted Model		All Covariate-Adjusted Model		Age-Adjusted Model		All Covariate-Adjusted Model	
	Beta (95% CI)	p-Value	Beta (95% CI)	p-Value	OR 95% CI	p-Value	OR 95% CI	p-Value
Loneliness	0.30 (0.24; 0.36)	<0.001	0.08 (0.03; 0.14)	0.001	1.19 [1.12–1.26]	<0.001	1.01 [0.95–1.07]	0.735
Social isolation	0.41 (0.37; 0.47)	<0.001	0.21 (0.16; 0.26)	<0.001	1.30 [1.24–1.36]	<0.001	1.14 [1.08–1.20]	<0.001
Both social isolation and loneliness *	0.90 (0.73; 1.08)	<0.001	0.44 (0.28; 0.61)	<0.001	1.54 [1.38–1.72]	<0.001	1.15 [1.02–1.29]	0.028

* Analysis was performed independently of loneliness and social isolation.

Compared with the reference group, men with loneliness were associated with a higher estimated 10-year ASCVD risk ($B = 0.30$ (0.24; 0.36), $p < 0.001$) in the age-adjusted model and after adjustment for all covariates ($B = 0.08$ (0.03; 0.14), $p = 0.001$). However, after adjustment for all covariates, no association between loneliness and high ASCVD risk was observed ($p = 0.735$). Loneliness and social isolation showed a significant interaction

(p = 0.009) with ASCVD risk. When considering men with both social isolation and loneliness, the relationship with continuous ASCVD risk was higher than social isolation and loneliness alone (after adjustment for all covariates: B = 0.44 (0.28; 0.61), p < 0.001) but similar ORs with social isolation alone when considering an ASCVD risk of more than 7.5% (OR = 1.15 [1.02–1.29], p = 0.028) (Table 2).

In women, compared with the reference group, social isolation was associated with a higher estimated 10-year ASCVD risk in men (B = 0.22 (0.20; 0.24), p < 0.001) in the age-adjusted model. Adjustment for all covariates did not affect the association (B = 0.12 (0.10; 0.14), p < 0.001).

The same results were observed when I performed analyses of high ASCVD risk with all covariates adjusted (OR = 1.37 [1.27–1.49], p < 0.001) (Table 3).

Table 3. Multiple linear and logistic regression models for estimated 10-year ASCVD risk among women (all covariates adjusted: age, education, income level, physical activity, couple, antidepressant medication, Townsend deprivation index, BMI, triglycerides, and CKD). The reference was the reference group.

	Continuous Estimated 10-Year ASCVD Risk				Estimated 10-Year ASCVD Risk Superior to 7.5%			
Women	Age-Adjusted Model		All Covariate-Adjusted Model		Age-Adjusted Model		All Covariate-Adjusted Model	
	Beta (95%CI)	p-Value	Beta (95%CI)	p-Value	OR 95% CI	p-Value	OR 95% CI	p-Value
Loneliness	0.08 (0.06; 0.11)	<0.001	0.01 (−0.01; 0.03)	0.217	1.25 [1.14–1.37]	<0.001	1.09 [0.99–1.20]	0.058
Social isolation	0.22 (0.20; 0.24)	<0.001	0.12 (0.10; 0.14)	<0.001	1.62 [1.51–1.73]	<0.001	1.37 [1.27–1.49]	<0.001
Both social isolation and loneliness *	0.39 (0.30; 0.48)	<0.001	0.20 (0.12; 0.29)	<0.001	2.39 [2.02–2.83]	<0.001	1.81 [1.52–2.16]	<0.001

* Analysis was performed independently of loneliness and social isolation.

Compared with the reference group, women with loneliness were associated with a higher estimated 10-year ASCVD risk (B = 0.08 (0.06; 0.11), p < 0.001) in the age-adjusted model but not after adjustment for all covariates (p = 0.217). This relationship remained insignificant after adjustment for all covariates with high ASCVD risk (p = 0.058). Loneliness and social isolation showed a significant interaction (p = 0.016) with ASCVD risk. When considering women with both social isolation and loneliness, the relationship with continuous ASCVD risk was higher than social isolation and loneliness alone (after adjustment for all covariates: B = 0.20 (0.12; 0.29), p < 0.001) and when considering an ASCVD risk of more than 7.5% (OR = 1.82 [1.52–2.16], p < 0.001) (Table 3).

4. Discussion

The main findings of this study were that social isolation was associated with a higher estimated 10-year ASCVD risk in both genders, but only loneliness was associated with a higher estimated 10-year ASCVD risk in men. A significant trend was found between loneliness and CV risk in women (p = 0.134).

In this study, I found that men showed a higher ASCVD risk than women, which is consistent with the literature [11,38–41]. As observed in previous studies, we found a significantly higher proportion of social isolation and loneliness in men than in women [42,43]. Moreover, my findings are consistent with the literature where social isolation and loneliness have been associated with CV diseases [3,7,11,13,44]. A previous study from the National Health and Nutrition Examination Survey among 2616 Americans showed that loneliness was associated with coronary heart disease (CHD) incidence in women but not in men [44]. The results of the English Longitudinal Study of Ageing (ELSA) showed that loneliness was associated with heart disease and stroke incidence [3,45]. Moreover, previous studies from the UK Biobank study showed that social isolation was associated with CHD and stroke [9], but another study found no association between loneliness and acute myocardial infarction and a significant association between social isolation, but not loneliness, with mortality [7].

According to previous studies, the relationship between social isolation and CV disease could be stronger than the association between loneliness and CV disease [7,11]. We observed similar findings in my study, where the combination of both social isolation and loneliness showed higher combined effects on CV risk than loneliness in men and both social isolation and loneliness in women.

Social isolation and loneliness are associated with diminutions in physical activity [46], higher proportions of tobacco smoking [47], poor diets [48], and the higher consumption of alcohol [49]. Having social isolation or loneliness may have indirect action in CV disease prevention by reducing good health behavior. Nevertheless, these interactions remain too complex to highlight and clearly explain.

Several social isolation and loneliness pathways that affect health have been identified [6]. It remains crucial to identify all these pathways to develop specific and personalized health policies [6]. Social isolation and loneliness are major risk factors for mental illnesses, such as depression [50], anxiety, and suicidal behavior [51]. Moreover, social isolation and loneliness are considered poor outcomes of CV diseases [6,51].

A possible biological pathway associating social isolation and loneliness with CV risk was found to be the immune system, which activates the inflammatory process [6,52]. Cytokine production was found to be associated with loneliness through the increased production of interleukin IL-6, IL-1bB, tumor necrosis factor alpha (TNF-alpha), fibrinogen, and monocyte chemoattractant protein 1 (MCP-1) [53]. Nevertheless, no association between CRP and loneliness has been observed [54]. In parallel to inflammation, oxidative stress could be another possible biological pathway to explain the relationship between loneliness and CV risk [55].

Loneliness interferes with cardiometabolic changes by increasing blood pressure [6,53], heart rate [53], vascular resistance [53] and hypertension [56]. The psychosocial stress generated by loneliness could change gut microbiota The activation of the hypothalamic pituitary adrenal (HPA) axis leads to decreases in microbial diversity [57], thus leading to an increased risk of CV disease [58].

Few studies have investigated the interaction between social isolation and loneliness. Nevertheless, loneliness activates the HPA axis and leads to increases in the perception of social isolation [50,59]. The HPA axis sets a "flight or fight" response into motion by producing cortisol, the stress hormone, at higher levels upon awakening [59]. Chronic stress leads to chronically increased cortisol rates, which are correlated with CV disease incidence [60].

Strengths and Limitations

The major strength of the study was the large sample size of the UK Biobank cohort. The cross-sectional design limited the ability to establish a causality relationship, so reverse causation cannot be ruled out. The UK Biobank study presented a low 5.5% response rate, suggesting the possibility of participants' bias. However, given the large sample size and high internal validity, these limitations were unlikely to affect the observed associations [61–63]. Moreover, the study investigation was focused on middle-aged UK participants, so my results cannot be generalized to other age and ethnic populations. Nevertheless, the UK Biobank uses standardized protocols to collect data. This standardization ensures the replication of data collection for all participants regardless of when, where and by whom it was performed and adds external validity to my findings. Nevertheless, my study had many limitations: socio-economic, medical history, comorbidity, and social isolation and loneliness data were collected with self-reported questionnaires or by physicians during medical examination in health centers. The adjustment of both income and education may be considered potential biases due their significant interaction relationships with ASCVD risk. No clear information about thyroid disease was collected in this study, so it cannot be considered a possible cofounding factor.

5. Conclusions

Both social isolation and loneliness and their combination can be considered potential added risk factors for CV risk. Thus, health policies should address these concepts in prevention campaigns, in addition to traditional risk factors. Further studies should be performed to investigate the gender differences in social isolation and loneliness and their implications in CV prevention and management. Moreover, specific information addressed to health professionals may be targeted [64] to promote the prevention and treatment of CV diseases among individuals with social isolation and loneliness.

Funding: This research has been conducted using the UK Biobank Resource under Application Number 55917.

Institutional Review Board Statement: The study was conducted according to the guidelines of the Declaration of Helsinki and approved by the Northwest Haydock Research Ethics Committee (protocol code: 21/NW/0157, date of approval: 21 June 2021).

Informed Consent Statement: Written informed consent has been obtained from the patients.

Data Availability Statement: The data that support the findings of this study are available on request from the corresponding author. The data are not publicly available due to privacy or ethical restrictions.

Acknowledgments: The author thanks Polly Gobin for English corrections.

Conflicts of Interest: The author declares no conflict of interest for this research.

References

1. Mendis, S.; Puska, P.; Norrving, B.; World Health Organization; World Heart Federation; World Stroke Organization. *Global Atlas on Cardiovascular Disease Prevention and Control; World Health Organization*; World Health Organization: Geneva, Switzerland, 2011.
2. Bloom, D.; Cafiero, E.; Jané-Llopis, E.; Abrahams-Gessel, S.; Bloom, L.; Fathima, S.; Feigl, A.; Gaziano, T.; Hamandi, A.; Mowafi, M.; et al. *The Global Economic Burden of Noncommunicable Diseases*; "The Global Economic Burden of Noncommunicable Diseases" PGDA Working Papers 8712, Program on the Global Demography of Aging; Harvard University: Cambridge, MA, USA, 2012.
3. Valtorta, N.K.; Kanaan, M.; Gilbody, S.; Ronzi, S.; Hanratty, B. Loneliness and Social Isolation as Risk Factors for Coronary Heart Disease and Stroke: Systematic Review and Meta-Analysis of Longitudinal Observational Studies. *Heart* **2016**, *102*, 1009–1016. [CrossRef]
4. Freak-Poli, R.; Ryan, J.; Neumann, J.T.; Tonkin, A.; Reid, C.M.; Woods, R.L.; Nelson, M.; Stocks, N.; Berk, M.; McNeil, J.J.; et al. Social Isolation, Social Support and Loneliness as Predictors of Cardiovascular Disease Incidence and Mortality. *BMC Geriatr.* **2021**, *21*, 711. [CrossRef] [PubMed]
5. *Social Isolation and Loneliness in Older Adults: Opportunities for the Health Care System*; National Academies Press: Washington, DC, USA, 2020; ISBN 978-0-309-67100-2.
6. Hodgson, S.; Watts, I.; Fraser, S.; Roderick, P.; Dambha-Miller, H. Loneliness, Social Isolation, Cardiovascular Disease and Mortality: A Synthesis of the Literature and Conceptual Framework. *J. R. Soc. Med.* **2020**, *113*, 185–192. [CrossRef] [PubMed]
7. Hakulinen, C.; Pulkki-Råback, L.; Virtanen, M.; Jokela, M.; Kivimäki, M.; Elovainio, M. Social Isolation and Loneliness as Risk Factors for Myocardial Infarction, Stroke and Mortality: UK Biobank Cohort Study of 479,054 Men and Women. *Heart Br. Card. Soc.* **2018**, *104*, 1536–1542. [CrossRef] [PubMed]
8. Chang, S.-C.; Glymour, M.; Cornelis, M.; Walter, S.; Rimm, E.B.; Tchetgen Tchetgen, E.; Kawachi, I.; Kubzansky, L.D. Social Integration and Reduced Risk of Coronary Heart Disease in Women: The Role of Lifestyle Behaviors. *Circ. Res.* **2017**, *120*, 1927–1937. [CrossRef] [PubMed]
9. Smith, R.W.; Barnes, I.; Green, J.; Reeves, G.K.; Beral, V.; Floud, S. Social Isolation and Risk of Heart Disease and Stroke: Analysis of Two Large UK Prospective Studies. *Lancet Public Health* **2021**, *6*, e232–e239. [CrossRef] [PubMed]
10. Golaszewski, N.M.; LaCroix, A.Z.; Godino, J.G.; Allison, M.A.; Manson, J.E.; King, J.J.; Weitlauf, J.C.; Bea, J.W.; Garcia, L.; Kroenke, C.H.; et al. Evaluation of Social Isolation, Loneliness, and Cardiovascular Disease Among Older Women in the US. *JAMA Netw. Open* **2022**, *5*, e2146461. [CrossRef]
11. Elovainio, M.; Hakulinen, C.; Pulkki-Råback, L.; Virtanen, M.; Josefsson, K.; Jokela, M.; Vahtera, J.; Kivimäki, M. Contribution of Risk Factors to Excess Mortality in Isolated and Lonely Individuals: An Analysis of Data from the UK Biobank Cohort Study. *Lancet Public Health* **2017**, *2*, e260–e266. [CrossRef]
12. Knox, S.S.; Uvnäs-Moberg, K. Social Isolation and Cardiovascular Disease: An Atherosclerotic Pathway? *Psychoneuroendocrinology* **1998**, *23*, 877–890. [CrossRef]
13. Steptoe, A.; Shankar, A.; Demakakos, P.; Wardle, J. Social Isolation, Loneliness, and All-Cause Mortality in Older Men and Women. *Proc. Natl. Acad. Sci. USA* **2013**, *110*, 5797–5801. [CrossRef]

14. Mozaffarian, D.; Benjamin, E.J.; Go, A.S.; Arnett, D.K.; Blaha, M.J.; Cushman, M.; de Ferranti, S.; Després, J.-P.; Fullerton, H.J.; Howard, V.J.; et al. Heart Disease and Stroke Statistics–2015 Update: A Report from the American Heart Association. *Circulation* **2015**, *131*, e29–e322. [CrossRef] [PubMed]
15. Yadlowsky, S.; Hayward, R.A.; Sussman, J.B.; McClelland, R.L.; Min, Y.-I.; Basu, S. Clinical Implications of Revised Pooled Cohort Equations for Estimating Atherosclerotic Cardiovascular Disease Risk. *Ann. Intern. Med.* **2018**, *169*, 20–29. [CrossRef] [PubMed]
16. Sudlow, C.; Gallacher, J.; Allen, N.; Beral, V.; Burton, P.; Danesh, J.; Downey, P.; Elliott, P.; Green, J.; Landray, M.; et al. UK Biobank: An Open Access Resource for Identifying the Causes of a Wide Range of Complex Diseases of Middle and Old Age. *PLoS Med.* **2015**, *12*, e1001779. [CrossRef] [PubMed]
17. Bycroft, C.; Freeman, C.; Petkova, D.; Band, G.; Elliott, L.T.; Sharp, K.; Motyer, A.; Vukcevic, D.; Delaneau, O.; O'Connell, J.; et al. The UK Biobank Resource with Deep Phenotyping and Genomic Data. *Nature* **2018**, *562*, 203–209. [CrossRef] [PubMed]
18. Vallée, A. Arterial Stiffness Determinants for Primary Cardiovascular Prevention among Healthy Participants. *J. Clin. Med.* **2022**, *11*, 2512. [CrossRef]
19. Goff, D.C.; Lloyd-Jones, D.M.; Bennett, G.; Coady, S.; D'Agostino, R.B.; Gibbons, R.; Greenland, P.; Lackland, D.T.; Levy, D.; O'Donnell, C.J.; et al. 2013 ACC/AHA Guideline on the Assessment of Cardiovascular Risk: A Report of the American College of Cardiology/American Heart Association Task Force on Practice Guidelines. *J. Am. Coll. Cardiol.* **2014**, *63*, 2935–2959. [CrossRef] [PubMed]
20. Nonterah, E.A.; Boateng, D.; Crowther, N.J.; Klipstein-Grobusch, K.; Oduro, A.R.; Agongo, G.; Mohamed, S.F.; Boua, P.R.; Choma, S.S.R.; Norris, S.A.; et al. Carotid Atherosclerosis, Microalbuminuria, and Estimated 10-Year Atherosclerotic Cardiovascular Disease Risk in Sub-Saharan Africa. *JAMA Netw. Open* **2022**, *5*, e227559. [CrossRef] [PubMed]
21. UK Biobank. Arterial Pulse-Wave Velocity. Available online: https://Biobank.Ndph.Ox.Ac.Uk/Ukb/Ukb/Docs/Pulsewave.Pdf (accessed on 30 November 2022).
22. Emerging Risk Factors Collaboration. Diabetes Mellitus, Fasting Blood Glucose Concentration, and Risk of Vascular Disease: A Collaborative Meta-Analysis of 102 Prospective Studies. *Lancet Lond. Engl.* **2010**, *375*, 2215–2222. [CrossRef]
23. UK Biobank Biomarker Assay Quality Procedures: Approaches Used to Minimise Systematic and Random Errors (and the Wider Epidemiological Implications). Available online: https://Biobank.Ctsu.Ox.Ac.Uk/Crystal/Crystal/Docs/Biomarker_issues.Pdf2019 (accessed on 30 November 2022).
24. Townsend, P. Deprivation*. *J. Soc. Policy* **1987**, *16*, 125–146. [CrossRef]
25. Noguchi, T.; Saito, M.; Aida, J.; Cable, N.; Tsuji, T.; Koyama, S.; Ikeda, T.; Osaka, K.; Kondo, K. Association between Social Isolation and Depression Onset among Older Adults: A Cross-National Longitudinal Study in England and Japan. *BMJ Open* **2021**, *11*, e045834. [CrossRef]
26. Davis, K.A.S.; Cullen, B.; Adams, M.; Brailean, A.; Breen, G.; Coleman, J.R.I.; Dregan, A.; Gaspar, H.A.; Hübel, C.; Lee, W.; et al. Indicators of Mental Disorders in UK Biobank—A Comparison of Approaches. *Int. J. Methods Psychiatr. Res.* **2019**, *28*, e1796. [CrossRef] [PubMed]
27. Craig, C.L.; Marshall, A.L.; Sjöström, M.; Bauman, A.E.; Booth, M.L.; Ainsworth, B.E.; Pratt, M.; Ekelund, U.; Yngve, A.; Sallis, J.F.; et al. International Physical Activity Questionnaire: 12-Country Reliability and Validity. *Med. Sci. Sports Exerc.* **2003**, *35*, 1381–1395. [CrossRef] [PubMed]
28. Bradbury, K.E.; Guo, W.; Cairns, B.J.; Armstrong, M.E.G.; Key, T.J. Association between Physical Activity and Body Fat Percentage, with Adjustment for BMI: A Large Cross-Sectional Analysis of UK Biobank. *BMJ Open* **2017**, *7*, e011843. [CrossRef] [PubMed]
29. O'Donnell, J.; Smith-Byrne, K.; Velardo, C.; Conrad, N.; Salimi-Khorshidi, G.; Doherty, A.; Dwyer, T.; Tarassenko, L.; Rahimi, K. Self-Reported and Objectively Measured Physical Activity in People with and without Chronic Heart Failure: UK Biobank Analysis. *Open Heart* **2020**, *7*, e001099. [CrossRef]
30. Henderson, K.; Kaufman, B.; Rotter, J.S.; Stearns, S.; Sueta, C.A.A.; Foraker, R.; Ho, P.M.; Chang, P.P. Socioeconomic Status and Modification of Atherosclerotic Cardiovascular Disease Risk Prediction: Epidemiological Analysis Using Data from the Atherosclerosis Risk in Communities Study. *BMJ Open* **2022**, *12*, e058777. [CrossRef]
31. Nahodyl, L.; Vilchez, L.; Mesa, R.A.; Tremblay, J.; Elfassy, T. Abstract P232: Associations Between Income And Education With ASCVD Risk, NHANES, 1999–2018. *Circulation* **2022**, *145*, AP232. [CrossRef]
32. Dhindsa, D.S.; Khambhati, J.; Schultz, W.M.; Tahhan, A.S.; Quyyumi, A.A. Marital Status and Outcomes in Patients with Cardiovascular Disease. *Trends Cardiovasc. Med.* **2020**, *30*, 215–220. [CrossRef]
33. Rao, P.; Belanger, M.J.; Robbins, J.M. Exercise, Physical Activity, and Cardiometabolic Health: Insights into the Prevention and Treatment of Cardiometabolic Diseases. *Cardiol. Rev.* **2022**, *30*, 167–178. [CrossRef]
34. Foster, H.M.E.; Celis-Morales, C.A.; Nicholl, B.I.; Petermann-Rocha, F.; Pell, J.P.; Gill, J.M.R.; O'Donnell, C.A.; Mair, F.S. The Effect of Socioeconomic Deprivation on the Association between an Extended Measurement of Unhealthy Lifestyle Factors and Health Outcomes: A Prospective Analysis of the UK Biobank Cohort. *Lancet Public Health* **2018**, *3*, e576–e585. [CrossRef]
35. Khera, R.; Pandey, A.; Ayers, C.R.; Carnethon, M.R.; Greenland, P.; Ndumele, C.E.; Nambi, V.; Seliger, S.L.; Chaves, P.H.M.; Safford, M.M.; et al. Performance of the Pooled Cohort Equations to Estimate Atherosclerotic Cardiovascular Disease Risk by Body Mass Index. *JAMA Netw. Open* **2020**, *3*, e2023242. [CrossRef]

36. Chronic Kidney Disease Prognosis Consortium; Matsushita, K.; van der Velde, M.; Astor, B.C.; Woodward, M.; Levey, A.S.; de Jong, P.E.; Coresh, J.; Gansevoort, R.T. Association of Estimated Glomerular Filtration Rate and Albuminuria with All-Cause and Cardiovascular Mortality in General Population Cohorts: A Collaborative Meta-Analysis. *Lancet Lond. Engl.* **2010**, *375*, 2073–2081. [CrossRef] [PubMed]
37. Nordestgaard, B.G. Triglyceride-Rich Lipoproteins and Atherosclerotic Cardiovascular Disease: New Insights From Epidemiology, Genetics, and Biology. *Circ. Res.* **2016**, *118*, 547–563. [CrossRef] [PubMed]
38. Zibaeenejad, F.; Mohammadi, S.S.; Sayadi, M.; Safari, F.; Zibaeenezhad, M.J. Ten-Year Atherosclerosis Cardiovascular Disease (ASCVD) Risk Score and Its Components among an Iranian Population: A Cohort-Based Cross-Sectional Study. *BMC Cardiovasc. Disord.* **2022**, *22*, 162. [CrossRef]
39. Okunrintemi, V.; Valero-Elizondo, J.; Patrick, B.; Salami, J.; Tibuakuu, M.; Ahmad, S.; Ogunmoroti, O.; Mahajan, S.; Khan, S.U.; Gulati, M.; et al. Gender Differences in Patient-Reported Outcomes Among Adults With Atherosclerotic Cardiovascular Disease. *J. Am. Heart Assoc.* **2018**, *7*, e010498. [CrossRef] [PubMed]
40. Jędrychowska, M.; Januszek, R.; Plens, K.; Surdacki, A.; Bartuś, S.; Dudek, D. Impact of Sex on the Follow-up Course and Predictors of Clinical Outcomes in Patients Hospitalised Due to Myocardial Infarction with Non-Obstructive Coronary Arteries: A Single-Centre Experience. *Kardiol. Pol.* **2019**, *77*, 198–206. [CrossRef] [PubMed]
41. Sielski, J.; Kaziród-Wolski, K.; Jurys, K.; Wałek, P.; Siudak, Z. The Effect of Periprocedural Clinical Factors Related to the Course of STEMI in Men and Women Based on the National Registry of Invasive Cardiology Procedures (ORPKI) between 2014 and 2019. *J. Clin. Med.* **2021**, *10*, 5716. [CrossRef] [PubMed]
42. Umberson, D.; Lin, Z.; Cha, H. Gender and Social Isolation across the Life Course. *J. Health Soc. Behav.* **2022**, *63*, 319–335. [CrossRef]
43. Elovainio, M.; Komulainen, K.; Sipilä, P.N.; Pulkki-Råback, L.; Alonso, L.C.; Pentti, J.; Nyberg, S.T.; Suominen, S.; Vahtera, J.; Lipsanen, J.; et al. Association of Social Isolation and Loneliness with Risk of Incident Hospital-Treated Infections: An Analysis of Data from the UK Biobank and Finnish Health and Social Support Studies. *Lancet Public Health* **2023**, *8*, e109–e118. [CrossRef]
44. Thurston, R.C.; Kubzansky, L.D. Women, Loneliness, and Incident Coronary Heart Disease. *Psychosom. Med.* **2009**, *71*, 836–842. [CrossRef]
45. Bu, F.; Zaninotto, P.; Fancourt, D. Longitudinal Associations between Loneliness, Social Isolation and Cardiovascular Events. *Heart* **2020**, *106*, 1394–1399. [CrossRef]
46. Schrempft, S.; Jackowska, M.; Hamer, M.; Steptoe, A. Associations between Social Isolation, Loneliness, and Objective Physical Activity in Older Men and Women. *BMC Public Health* **2019**, *19*, 74. [CrossRef]
47. Wootton, R.E.; Greenstone, H.S.R.; Abdellaoui, A.; Denys, D.; Verweij, K.J.H.; Munafò, M.R.; Treur, J.L. Bidirectional Effects between Loneliness, Smoking and Alcohol Use: Evidence from a Mendelian Randomization Study. *Addict. Abingdon Engl.* **2021**, *116*, 400–406. [CrossRef] [PubMed]
48. Leigh-Hunt, N.; Bagguley, D.; Bash, K.; Turner, V.; Turnbull, S.; Valtorta, N.; Caan, W. An Overview of Systematic Reviews on the Public Health Consequences of Social Isolation and Loneliness. *Public Health* **2017**, *152*, 157–171. [CrossRef] [PubMed]
49. Canham, S.L.; Mauro, P.M.; Kaufmann, C.N.; Sixsmith, A. Association of Alcohol Use and Loneliness Frequency Among Middle-Aged and Older Adult Drinkers. *J. Aging Health* **2016**, *28*, 267–284. [CrossRef] [PubMed]
50. Lee, S.L.; Pearce, E.; Ajnakina, O.; Johnson, S.; Lewis, G.; Mann, F.; Pitman, A.; Solmi, F.; Sommerlad, A.; Steptoe, A.; et al. The Association between Loneliness and Depressive Symptoms among Adults Aged 50 Years and Older: A 12-Year Population-Based Cohort Study. *Lancet Psychiatry* **2021**, *8*, 48–57. [CrossRef]
51. Park, C.; Majeed, A.; Gill, H.; Tamura, J.; Ho, R.C.; Mansur, R.B.; Nasri, F.; Lee, Y.; Rosenblat, J.D.; Wong, E.; et al. The Effect of Loneliness on Distinct Health Outcomes: A Comprehensive Review and Meta-Analysis. *Psychiatry Res.* **2020**, *294*, 113514. [CrossRef]
52. Eisenberger, N.I.; Moieni, M.; Inagaki, T.K.; Muscatell, K.A.; Irwin, M.R. In Sickness and in Health: The Co-Regulation of Inflammation and Social Behavior. *Neuropsychopharmacology* **2017**, *42*, 242–253. [CrossRef]
53. Brown, E.G.; Gallagher, S.; Creaven, A.-M. Loneliness and Acute Stress Reactivity: A Systematic Review of Psychophysiological Studies. *Psychophysiology* **2018**, *55*, e13031. [CrossRef]
54. Smith, K.J.; Gavey, S.; RIddell, N.E.; Kontari, P.; Victor, C. The Association between Loneliness, Social Isolation and Inflammation: A Systematic Review and Meta-Analysis. *Neurosci. Biobehav. Rev.* **2020**, *112*, 519–541. [CrossRef]
55. Cole, S.W.; Capitanio, J.P.; Chun, K.; Arevalo, J.M.G.; Ma, J.; Cacioppo, J.T. Myeloid Differentiation Architecture of Leukocyte Transcriptome Dynamics in Perceived Social Isolation. *Proc. Natl. Acad. Sci. USA* **2015**, *112*, 15142–15147. [CrossRef]
56. Li, H.; Xia, N. The Role of Oxidative Stress in Cardiovascular Disease Caused by Social Isolation and Loneliness. *Redox Biol.* **2020**, *37*, 101585. [CrossRef] [PubMed]
57. Makris, A.P.; Karianaki, M.; Tsamis, K.I.; Paschou, S.A. The Role of the Gut-Brain Axis in Depression: Endocrine, Neural, and Immune Pathways. *Horm. Athens Greece* **2021**, *20*, 1–12. [CrossRef] [PubMed]
58. Kazemian, N.; Mahmoudi, M.; Halperin, F.; Wu, J.C.; Pakpour, S. Gut Microbiota and Cardiovascular Disease: Opportunities and Challenges. *Microbiome* **2020**, *8*, 36. [CrossRef] [PubMed]
59. Quadt, L.; Esposito, G.; Critchley, H.D.; Garfinkel, S.N. Brain-Body Interactions Underlying the Association of Loneliness with Mental and Physical Health. *Neurosci. Biobehav. Rev.* **2020**, *116*, 283–300. [CrossRef]

60. Iob, E.; Steptoe, A. Cardiovascular Disease and Hair Cortisol: A Novel Biomarker of Chronic Stress. *Curr. Cardiol. Rep.* **2019**, *21*, 116. [CrossRef]
61. Richiardi, L.; Pizzi, C.; Pearce, N. Commentary: Representativeness Is Usually Not Necessary and Often Should Be Avoided. *Int. J. Epidemiol.* **2013**, *42*, 1018–1022. [CrossRef]
62. Rothman, K.J.; Gallacher, J.E.J.; Hatch, E.E. Why Representativeness Should Be Avoided. *Int. J. Epidemiol.* **2013**, *42*, 1012–1014. [CrossRef]
63. Vallée, A. Association Between Lipids and Arterial Stiffness for Primary Cardiovascular Prevention in a General Middle-Aged European Population. *Front. Cardiovasc. Med.* **2022**, *9*, 899841. [CrossRef]
64. Holt-Lunstad, J.; Smith, T.B. Loneliness and Social Isolation as Risk Factors for CVD: Implications for Evidence-Based Patient Care and Scientific Inquiry. *Heart Br. Card. Soc.* **2016**, *102*, 987–989. [CrossRef]

International Journal of
Environmental Research and Public Health

MDPI

Article

Loneliness before and after COVID-19: Sense of Coherence and Hope as Coping Mechanisms

Michal Einav [1,2] and Malka Margalit [1,3,*]

1 Behavioral Sciences Department, Peres Academic Center, Rechovot 7610202, Israel; einav.michal@gmail.com
2 Behavioral Sciences Department, The Academic College of Tel-Aviv-Yaffa, Tel-Aviv 6818218, Israel
3 School of Education, Tel Aviv University, Tel-Aviv 6997505, Israel
* Correspondence: malka@tauex.tau.ac.il

Abstract: The COVID-19 pandemic posed a major threat to public health, with long-lasting consequences for the daily habits and practices of people around the world. The combination of hazardous health conditions and extensive changes to people's daily routines due to lockdowns, social restrictions, and employment uncertainty have led to mental health challenges, reduced levels of subjective wellbeing, and increased maladaptive behaviors and emotional distress. Nevertheless, some studies have reported increased adaptive functioning and resilience after the pandemic, suggesting a more complex pattern of effects. The goals of the current study were to explore the role of two coping variables, sense of coherence and hope, in people's emotional wellbeing and adaptation in dealing with loneliness before and after such a stressful period. In a cross-sectional study, 974 Israeli participants (sample 1: 540 participants before the pandemic; sample 2: 434 participants after the pandemic restrictions) answered online questionnaires about their loneliness, hope and sense of coherence levels before and after the pandemic. While the two groups did not differ in their levels of hope, the participants in the group before COVID-19 reported lower levels of loneliness and sense of coherence. However, the results also indicated that although the COVID-19 pandemic was related to increased levels of loneliness, the participants' sense of coherence mediated this increase and their levels of hope moderated it. The theoretical contribution of these findings is discussed, as well as interventional implications and future directions.

Keywords: loneliness; hope; sense of coherence; COVID-19; coping resources

1. Introduction

Coping mechanisms are essential tools for individuals to deal with the stresses and challenges of life, specifically during times of hardship such as a global pandemic [1,2]. The COVID-19 pandemic has brought about unprecedented levels of uncertainty, fear, and anxiety throughout the world [3–6], emphasizing the critical role of effective coping strategies for promoting wellbeing and mental health. Past research has highlighted the critical role of various coping mechanisms in reducing stress and anxiety, providing a sense of control and stability during a time of uncertainty, helping manage anxious thoughts and negative emotions, promoting positive thinking and behavior, and encouraging social connections [7–9]. Focusing on coping mechanisms and promoting resilience has become particularly important, considering the emotional consequences of day-to-day changes and life threats during the COVID-19 pandemic.

The current study seeks to shed light on the coping mechanisms people used to mitigate the negative consequences of the COVID-19 pandemic. The results help us identify the factors that may predict resilience during times of major life-threatening distress.

2. Loneliness

Loneliness has been defined as the aversive emotional outcome experienced when a discrepancy exists between the interpersonal relationships people want to have, and those they currently experience [10]. Numerous studies have focused on the harmful consequences of prolonged loneliness, such as emotional distress, depression, and anxiety [11]. Left untended, loneliness may have serious consequences for people's cognitive processes, emotions, behavior, and health.

The COVID-19 epidemic affected interpersonal and community interactions. Personal social contacts were dramatically reduced, to prevent the spread of the virus. The alternative remote forms of communication that were developed in place of face-to-face communication are regarded as more superficial and less intimate than personal social interactions [12].

Meta-analyses of the research surrounding the pandemic have examined the links between loneliness and the pandemic. However, surprisingly, they have yielded inconclusive results. Whereas some studies reported overall elevated levels of loneliness, as one might expect [12–14], others indicated that people's levels of loneliness remained relatively stable [15,16].

In an attempt to identify the factors that account for the disparities in these findings, studies have generally focused on the risk factors that might account for these inconsistent reports. For example, researchers have established a positive association between low socioeconomic status and poor health and increased loneliness [17,18]. Similarly, mental health challenges such as depression, stress, anxiety, sleep disorders, and substance abuse were also associated with increased loneliness during the pandemic [18,19]. These studies concluded that individuals with various health and socioeconomic difficulties were at an increased risk of higher levels of loneliness during the pandemic. However, there is limited research on the role of the factors related to resilience, such as coping resources, in the links between the epidemic and loneliness.

The current study examines the significance of coping mechanisms using Antonovsky's salutogenic model. This health promotion paradigm emphasizes the factors that help people maintain their health and wellbeing rather than the factors that cause illness or distress [20]. Developed by Antonovsky, it is based on the belief that people have an innate drive to maintain their health and wellbeing, even in the face of adversity [21]. The term "salutogenic" comes from the Latin word "salus", which means "health", and "genesis", which means "creation". This dynamic construct proposes that people are not fully healthy or completely sick, but constantly move along a continuum between illness and health [20]. During periods of stress and uncertainty such as the pandemic, many people focused on the disease, its diagnosis, and impacts. Therefore, this emphasis on health promotion has a unique value. These attempts to identify how people can stay healthy and thrive, even during stressful times, can be empowering [21,22]. Therefore, rather than focusing solely on detecting or preventing adversity, the salutogenic model has been used extensively in a variety of settings, including healthcare [23], education [24], and workplace [25] health promotion programs, to help individuals and communities maintain and enhance their health and wellbeing. In line with this model's tenets, the current study explores the role of two key resources: sense of coherence and hope.

2.1. Sense of Coherence (SOC)

Sense of coherence is considered a key factor in Antonovsky's salutogenic approach that emphasizes the importance of promoting health [20,21]. SOC is defined as a person's general orientation towards the world as comprehensible, manageable, and meaningful [20]. Thus, sense of coherence has three components. The first is people's ability to understand their environment as ordered, consistent, and structured. Second, people expect their resources to enable them to meet their needs. Some of these resources may be under their own control, whereas others, such as professional support or the support of friends, may be available from other people. The third aspect refers to meaningfulness: the consideration of many aspects of their life as important and worthy of emotional commitment, engagement, and investment. Therefore, sense of coherence does not refer to a particular style of coping. Rather, it involves a broad repertoire of coping strategies from which people can choose the appropriate one in any given situation [21].

We posited that sense of coherence might be an important resource for coping with the pandemic because of COVID-19's perception as a significant, unrelenting crisis. Earlier research has examined sense of coherence as a major factor in protecting people's mental health. For example, studies established a relationship between lower levels of sense of coherence and higher levels of psychological distress [26]. In contrast, higher levels of sense of coherence were strongly associated with fewer symptoms of anxiety and depression [27]. In addition, sense of coherence buffered work-related burnout [28], a finding of particular significance, considering the increased vulnerability that medical teams faced due to exposure to the disease, their physical and emotional burdens, lack of resources, and exposure to death. This pattern of results, establishing the mediating role of sense of coherence in the relationship between pandemic experiences and psychological wellbeing, was also found in the general population, predicting mental health difficulties as well as future related anxiety [22,29]. In effect, major life changes during the pandemic disrupted people's ability to consider future opportunities, a significant factor in wellbeing [30]. Therefore, we also examined the role of hopeful thinking about the future, assessed in people's ability to identify their goals and plan for the future.

2.2. Hope

Hopeful thinking enables individuals to set goals, plan paths to achieving these goals, and gather the motivation and personal energy to follow them [31]. Hope theory emphasizes that it is a constant, structured, goal-oriented cognitive set. According to this premise, hopeful thinking incorporates two interrelated patterns of thinking: agentic thinking and pathways thinking. The first addresses the driving force in defining and achieving one's goals, whereas the latter is focused on planning the paths to success and considering alternatives to possible barriers to achieving it [32]. Hence, researchers have proposed hope as a resilience factor, promoting people's wellbeing and supporting their ability to cope effectively with stress [33,34].

Given the ongoing stress that the COVID-19 pandemic created, studies have investigated the role of hope as a protective factor during it. Recent studies have reported that hope is related to fundamental indicators of mental health such as satisfaction with life and a sense of meaningfulness [35], transcendent values and spiritual moorings [36], as well as resilience and behaviors to prevent stress [37]. One study of particular interest in this regard indicated that hope moderates the relationship between psychological distress and depression as well as between distress and insomnia. Thus, research has established the ability of hope to activate mechanisms that moderate psychological distress, especially in times of elevated fear and uncertainty [37–40].

2.3. The Current Study

The purpose of this study is to clarify the relationship between people's reactions to the pandemic and their feelings of loneliness, and the role of hope and SOC in these relationships. Research has already demonstrated the role of SOC as a mediator in the relationship between various types of distress and outcomes [27–30] as well as the role of hope in moderating this relationship [41,42]. These studies presented SOC as a mediator with a direct path to the outcome. People who have higher levels of SOC are expected to be less lonely. Nevertheless, the early research on hope presented it as a mediator in several studies. Given that the anxiety and distress following COVID-19 caused many people to have difficulty thinking about and planning for their future, we hypothesize that experiencing medium and high levels of hope will activate SOC, leading people to feel less lonely. Thus, we expect people with medium and high levels of hope to have higher levels of SOC, which, in turn, will predict lower levels of loneliness [38]. Therefore, in line with the salutogenic approach [20], the current study has two main purposes: (1) to compare people's levels of loneliness, SOC and hope before and after the pandemic and (2) to examine the mediating role of SOC and the moderating role of hope, as two key personal resources, in the relationship between the two periods and loneliness. We hypothesize that the availability of personal resources, specifically, sense of coherence and hope, will predict people's levels of loneliness.

3. Method

3.1. Procedure

We utilized a cross-sectional repeated design consisting of two independent samples, one before and one after the pandemic's restrictions and lockdown policies. The sample before the pandemic was collected between December 2017 and March 2018 as part of a larger study. The sample after the pandemic was collected during the end of January 2021, after the end of several periods of lockdowns, when life in Israel returned to normal. The college's ethics committee approved these studies, and informed consent was obtained from all participants. Participation was voluntary and without compensation.

3.2. Participants

To test our hypothesis, we combined a sample of 974 Israeli participants from two samples: 540 participants before the pandemic and 434 participants after it. We used convenience sampling and sent the questionnaires to the participants via an electronic link on Qualtrics. Of those who participated before the pandemic, 59.4% (N = 321) were males, and after the pandemic, 54.4% (N = 236) were males. On average, the participants were 37.25 years old (SD = 11.86), and a large percentage (75.2%) had a university degree. The remaining participants (24.8%) had a high school diploma or technical education. Comparisons between the periods did not reveal significant differences in the proportions of the respondents by age, gender, or education.

3.3. Measures

We used several established measures to assess the respondents with regard to our variables.

Loneliness. We used the Hebrew adaptation [43] of the loneliness scale [44] consisting of 11 statements that describe social and emotional loneliness (e.g., "I miss having a really close friend"). The respondents were asked to indicate the degree to which they agreed with each statement on a 5-point Likert scale ranging from 1 (not at all) to 5 (exactly like it). Cronbach's α reliability for the scale was 0.83.

Sense of Coherence. To assess sense of coherence [20,21] we used the short version of the self-report scale that taps three components: comprehensibility, manageability, and meaningfulness. The 10 statements were assessed on 7-point Likert-type scales. For example, the statement, "Until now your life has had: ... " was rated on descriptors ranging from 1 ("no clear goals or purpose at all") to 7 ("very clear goals and purpose"). Cronbach's α reliability for the scale was 0.70.

Hope. We used the Hebrew adaptation [45] of the State Hope Scale [31] consisting of six statements assessing hopeful thinking (e.g., "Even when others want to give up, I know I can find ways to solve the problem"). The respondents were asked to indicate the degree to which they agreed with each statement on a 6-point Likert scale ranging from 1 (never) to 6 (always). Cronbach's α reliability for the scale was 0.87.

3.4. Data Analysis

As a preliminary analysis, we performed a MANOVA and calculated Pearson's correlations. The hypothesized moderated mediation model (see Figure 1) was tested in a single model using a bootstrapping approach to assess the significance of the indirect effects at differing levels of the moderator [46]. The periods (before/after COVID-19) were the predictor variable, with sense of coherence as the mediator, and age and gender as covariates. The outcome variable was loneliness and hope was the moderator. Moderated mediation analyses tested the conditional indirect effect of the moderating variable (i.e., hope) on the relationship between the predictor (i.e., periods before/after the pandemic) and the outcome variable (i.e., loneliness) via a potential mediator (i.e., sense of coherence). The

PROCESS macro, model 8, v 4.0 [47] in SPSS ver. 28 with bias-corrected 95% confidence intervals was used to test the significance of the indirect (i.e., mediated) effects moderated by hope, meaning the conditional indirect effects. This model tested the moderating effect on the predictor to mediator path (i.e., path a) and on the outcomes path. An index of moderated mediation was used to test the significance of the moderated mediation, meaning the difference in the indirect effects on three levels of hope [48]. Significant effects were supported by the absence of zero within the confidence intervals.

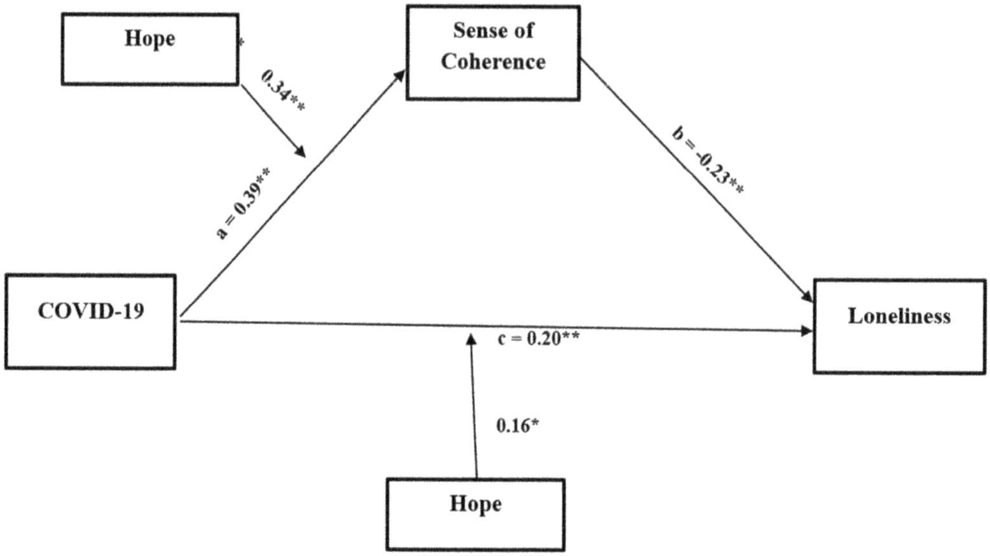

Figure 1. Direct and indirect effect of pandemic periods on loneliness through sense of coherence with three levels of hope moderating the path between periods and sense of coherence, and between periods and loneliness. a′= Low: 0.13*; Medium: 0.39**; High: 0.65**; c′ = Low: −0.08; Medium: 0.20**; High: 0.33**. Note: * $p < 0.05$; ** $p < 0.01$.

4. Results

4.1. Preliminary Analyses

In order to explore differences in the research variables during the two periods, we performed a one-way MANOVA with the periods (before/after the pandemic) as the independent variables, and loneliness, hope, and sense of coherence as the dependent variables. Age and gender were controlled. A main effect for the periods emerged F (3, 967) = 30.49, $p = 0.001$, partial $\eta^2 = 0.086$. A univariate analysis yielded a main effect for loneliness (before COVID-19: M = 2.37, SD = 0.81, after COVID-19, M = 2.48 SD = 0.73, F (1, 973) = 5.57, $p = 0.002$, partial $\eta^2 = 0.006$) and sense of coherence (before COVID-19: M = 4.41, SD = 0.76, after COVID-19, M = 4.80, SD = 0.82, F (1, 973) = 60.54, $p = 0.001$, partial $\eta^2 = 0.059$), but not for hope.

Pearson's correlations between the research measures were also calculated, revealing negative correlations between sense of coherence and loneliness (r = −0.27, $p < 0.01$), negative correlations between loneliness and hope (r = −0.32, $p < 0.01$), and positive correlations between hope and sense of coherence (r = 0.39, $p < 0.01$).

4.2. Moderated Mediation Analyses

Using the PROCESS macro model, the hypothesized moderated mediation model (model 8) was tested. In accordance with our model in Figure 1, there were significant relationships between the pandemic periods and loneliness (path c: B = 0.20, se = 0.05, t = 4.26, p = 0.00, CI = 0.1100; 0.2981). In addition, sense of coherence mediated these relationships in path A (the path of the periods to sense of coherence: B = 0.39, se = 0.05, t = 8.69, p = 0.00, CI = 0.2993; 4738) and path B (the path of sense of coherence to loneliness: B = −0.22, se = 0.03, t = −6.71, p = 0.00, CI = −2894; −1584). Hope moderated the effect of COVID-19 with sense of coherence (Interaction B = 0.34, se = 0.06, t = 5.61, p = 0.00, CI = 0.2197; 0.4560) and COVID-19 with loneliness (Interaction B = 0.16, se = 0.06, t = 2.52, p = 0.01, CI = 0.0352; 0.2844). The overall moderated mediation model was supported by the index of moderated mediation = −0.0756 (95% CI = −0.1146; 0.0415).

As Figure 2 indicates, overall, there was a greater sense of coherence after the pandemic. However, individuals with higher levels of hope reported a stronger sense of coherence than those with lower levels of hope (Low hope: B = 0.13*, Medium hope: B = 0.39**, High hope: B = 0.65**). Figure 3 demonstrates that after COVID-19, people felt lonelier than before it. However, in both periods, individuals with medium to high levels of hope reported less loneliness than those who felt less hopeful (Low hope: B = −0.08, Medium hope: B = 0.20**, High hope: B = 0.33**). Thus, after the pandemic period, people tended to feel lonelier than before it. However, that feeling was mediated by their sense of coherence and moderated by their levels of hope. Therefore, while COVID-19 predicted higher levels of sense of coherence, those with more hope were less lonely than those who felt less hopeful.

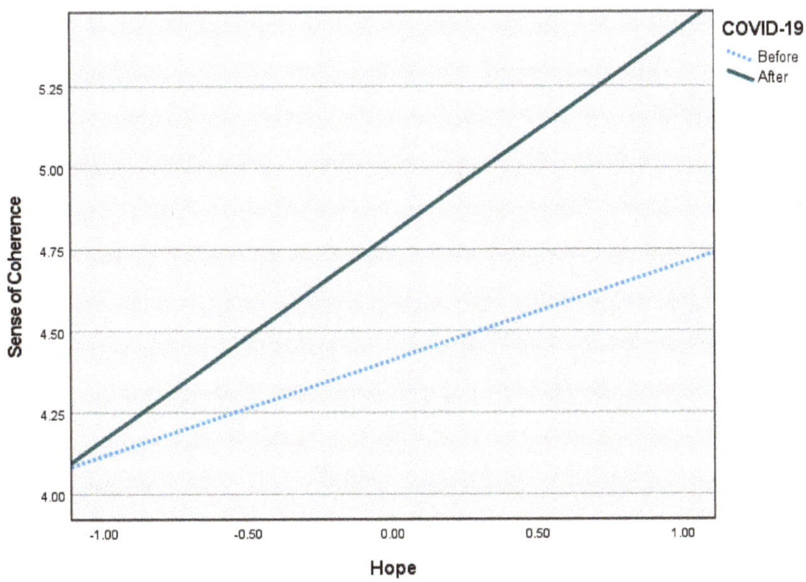

Figure 2. Hope as a moderator that differentiated sense of coherence levels during the periods.

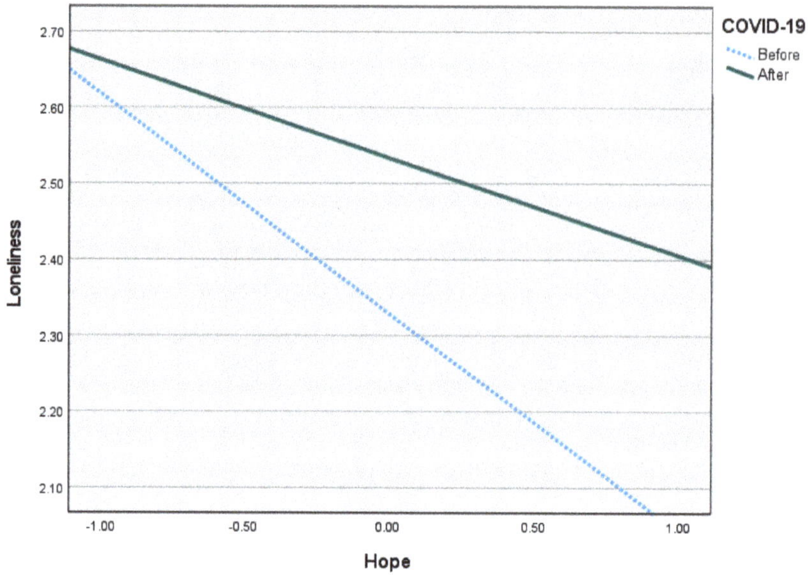

Figure 3. Hope as a moderator that differentiated loneliness levels during the periods.

5. Discussion

The COVID-19 pandemic brought about significant changes in the way individuals live their lives, including social distancing, lockdowns, and isolation. These changes have had a profound impact on people's mental health, with many experiencing increased feelings of loneliness [12].

Consistent with past research [13,14], the results of the current study indicated that the COVID-19 pandemic was related to increased levels of loneliness. In other words, many participants reported feeling lonelier after the pandemic than before it. This finding supports previous studies and emphasizes the harmful social consequences of the pandemic, which forced individuals to endure prolonged periods of social distancing and isolation.

However, some studies also indicated that the link between the pandemic and loneliness varied among people [15,16]. In an attempt to explore these interpersonal variations, our findings revealed that SOC and hope mediated and moderated this link, respectively. Rather than focusing on issues related to the disease of COVID-19 and the distress it created, we utilized the salutogenic approach and explored the factors that empowered people to deal with the situation and promoted their health.

Within this construct, as a personal strength, SOC may enable people to understand and make sense of the world around them. Thus, when faced with a crisis, those who could rely on their sense of coherence were less paralyzed by stress. They were better able to deal with the adversity and be more resistant to loneliness. They were also able to continue the move towards maintaining and improving their mental health.

The results also indicated that hope moderated the links between the pandemic periods and sense of coherence and those between the pandemic periods and loneliness. Therefore, those individuals whose SOC reflected the impact of the distress were able to benefit from medium and high levels of hopeful thinking. They were able to activate their SOC and thus minimize their feelings of loneliness in the face of adversity. This finding further establishes the importance of hope as a fundamental personal activating strength that enables people to have a vision of the future even in the face of a challenging, immobilizing present. It is the basis of the ability to cope with, adjust to, and endure difficult times.

Together, these results emphasize the contribution of the salutogenic approach to promoting wellbeing. Both sense of coherence and hope can help people develop a sense of purpose and meaning in life, which can reduce feelings of loneliness. Studies have documented these links, emphasizing the valuable relationship between sense of coherence and the ability to find life meaningful [49,50] as well as the facilitating effect of the latter on loneliness [51,52]. Given these findings, individuals with a strong sense of coherence may be better able to make sense of the changes brought on by COVID-19 and adapt to new ways of connecting with others. Similarly, those who have hope for the future may be more likely to seek out social connections and find ways to maintain those connections during times of social distancing. Overall, having a strong sense of coherence and hope can be beneficial for coping with loneliness after COVID-19. Thus, from an empirical standpoint, interventions that strengthen these qualities, such as workshops on developing hopeful thinking, cognitive behavioral therapy, or mindfulness-based stress reduction techniques are positive steps for improving people's wellbeing. For instance, studies have documented how intervention programs designed to improve people's levels of hope [53,54] can help them deal with the stress and challenges of the COVID-19 pandemic. These interventions may target hope-based cognitive strategies for positive thinking, problem solving, and goal setting, providing people with the tools to manage the stress and uncertainty of the pandemic. Additionally, such interventions can help reduce negative emotions such as helplessness and apprehension, which may be exacerbated by the pandemic, by promoting positive emotions and outlooks during challenging times. Lastly, with regard to loneliness specifically, interventions to increase people's levels of hope can help them build social support networks by strengthening their participatory communication and active listening skills, encouraging the inclusion of the feelings of others, and motivating participants to reach out to friends, family or colleagues.

Taking a broader point of view, the COVID-19 pandemic is an extreme example of an adverse situation affecting individuals and communities alike. Allocating resources to develop and strengthen people's resilience will help them avoid the detrimental effects of crises and grow even stronger in the future. As our results suggested, the availability and accessibility of coping mechanisms are significant in dealing with adversity. They can help reduce the negative effects of stress, build resilience, develop problem-solving skills, foster social support, and minimize loneliness. By utilizing effective coping mechanisms, individuals can better manage the challenges they face and maintain their mental health and wellbeing.

6. Limitations and Future Directions

This study has several limitations. First, it was based on self-reported, correlational research, potentially raising concerns regarding causality and social desirability bias. In addition, our cross-sectional study used two convenience samples based on online questionnaires. The two samples were collected in an identical manner. We ensured the anonymity of the participants by using online questionnaires, but doing so limited the personal information available to us. Thus, future studies should validate the results by using observational methods, in-depth interviews, or a combination of research methods. In addition, we collected the second sample soon after people returned to their normal life. Future studies should investigate the long-term impacts of the pandemic and the role of the resilience factors we explored. Additional resilience factors, both intrapersonal ones (e.g., attachment style) and interpersonal ones (e.g., family and social support), may extend our understanding of people's resilience and adjustment to adverse situations.

Author Contributions: Conceptualization, M.E. and M.M.; methodology, M.E. and M.M.; software, M.E. and M.M.; validation, M.E. and M.M.; formal analysis, M.E. and M.M.; investigation, M.E. and M.M.; resources, M.E. and M.M.; data curation, M.E. and M.M.; writing—original draft preparation, M.E. and M.M.; writing—review and editing, M.E. and M.M.; visualization, M.E. and M.M.; supervision, M.E. and M.M.; project administration, M.E. and M.M.; funding acquisition, M.E. and M.M. All authors have read and agreed to the published version of the manuscript.

Funding: This research received no external funding.

Institutional Review Board Statement: The study was conducted in accordance with the Declaration of Helsinki, and approved by the Institutional Review Board (or Ethics Committee) of Peres Academic Center (protocol code 230 and 373, date of approval 13 November 2017 and 18 December 2020.).

Informed Consent Statement: Informed consent was obtained from all subjects involved in the study.

Data Availability Statement: The data presented in this study are available on request from the corresponding author. The data are not publicly available due to participants' privacy concerns.

Conflicts of Interest: The authors declare no conflict of interest.

References

1. Rana, I.A.; Bhatti, S.S.; Aslam, A.B.; Jamshed, A.; Ahmad, J.; Shah, A.A. COVID-19 risk perception and coping mechanisms: Does gender make a difference? *Int. J. Disaster Risk Reduct.* **2021**, *55*, 102096. [CrossRef]
2. Kim, S.C.; Sloan, C.; Montejano, A.; Quiban, C. Impacts of coping mechanisms on nursing students' mental health during COVID-19 lockdown: A cross-sectional survey. *Nurs. Rep.* **2021**, *11*, 36–44. [CrossRef]
3. Vindegaard, N.; Benros, M.E. COVID-19 pandemic and mental health consequences: Systematic review of the current evidence. *Brain Behav. Immun.* **2020**, *89*, 531–542. [CrossRef]
4. Usher, K.; Durkin, J.; Bhullar, N. The COVID-19 pandemic and mental health impacts. *Int. J. Ment. Health Nurs.* **2020**, *29*, 315–318. [CrossRef]
5. Mancini, A.D. Heterogeneous mental health consequences of COVID-19: Costs and benefits. *Psychol. Trauma* **2020**, *12*, S15–S16. [CrossRef]
6. Banks, J.; Fancourt, D.; Xu, X. Mental health and the COVID-19 pandemic. In *World Happiness Report; New York: Sustainable Development Solutions Network;* 2021; pp. 107–130, ISBN 978-1-7348080-1-8.
7. Maresca, G.; Corallo, F.; Catanese, G.; Formica, C.; Lo Buono, V. Coping strategies of healthcare professionals with burnout syndrome: A systematic review. *Medicina* **2022**, *58*, 327. [CrossRef] [PubMed]
8. Freire, C.; Ferradás, M.D.M.; Regueiro, B.; Rodríguez, S.; Valle, A.; Núñez, J.C. Coping strategies and self-efficacy in university students: A person-centered approach. *Front. Psychol.* **2020**, *11*, 841. [CrossRef] [PubMed]
9. Martínez, J.P.; Méndez, I.; Ruiz-Esteban, C.; Fernández-Sogorb, A.; García-Fernández, J.M. Profiles of burnout, coping strategies and depressive symptomatology. *Front. Psychol.* **2020**, *11*, 591. [CrossRef]
10. Peplau, L.A.; Perlman, D. *Loneliness: A Sourcebook of Current Theory, Research and Therapy;* Wiley: New York, NY, USA, 1982.
11. Park, M.; Cook, A.R.; Lim, J.T.; Sun, Y.; Dickens, B.L. A systematic review of COVID-19 epidemiology based on current evidence. *J. Clin. Med.* **2020**, *9*, 967. [CrossRef] [PubMed]
12. Banerjee, D.; Rai, M. Social isolation in COVID-19: The impact of loneliness. *Int. J. Soc. Psychiatry.* **2020**, *66*, 525–527. [CrossRef] [PubMed]
13. Buecker, S.; Horstmann, K.T. Loneliness and social isolation during the COVID-19 pandemic. *Eur. Psychol.* **2022**, *26*, 251–397. [CrossRef]
14. Li, L.Z.; Wang, S. Prevalence and predictors of general psychiatric disorders and loneliness during COVID-19 in the United Kingdom. *Psychiatry Res.* **2020**, *291*, 113267. [CrossRef]
15. Luchetti, M.; Lee, J.H.; Aschwanden, D.; Sesker, A.; Strickhouser, J.E.; Terracciano, A.; Sutin, A.R. The trajectory of loneliness in response to COVID-19. *Am. Psychol.* **2020**, *75*, 897–908. [CrossRef] [PubMed]
16. Stefana, A.; Youngstrom, E.A.; Hopwood, C.J.; Dakanalis, A. The COVID-19 pandemic brings a second wave of social isolation and disrupted services. *Eur. Arch. Psychiatry Clin. Neurosci.* **2020**, *270*, 785–786. [CrossRef] [PubMed]
17. Bu, F.; Steptoe, A.; Fancourt, D. Loneliness during a strict lockdown: Trajectories and predictors during the COVID-19 pandemic in 38,217 United Kingdom adults. *Soc. Sci. Med.* **2020**, *265*, 113521. [CrossRef]
18. Pan, Y.; Yang, Z.; Han, X.; Qi, S. Family functioning and mental health among secondary vocational students during the COVID-19 epidemic: A moderated mediation model. *Pers Individ Dif.* **2021**, *171*, 110490. [CrossRef]
19. De Lange, A.M.G.; Kaufmann, T.; Quintana, D.S.; Winterton, A.; Westlye, L.T.; Ebmeier, K.P. Risk factors associated with loneliness, social isolation, and neuroticism in the UK Biobank cohort. *PsyArXiv* **2020**.
20. Antonovsky, A. *Unraveling the Mystery of Health: How People Manage Stress and Stay Well;* Jossey-Bass Publishers: San Francisco, CA, USA, 1987; Volume 175.
21. Mittelmark, M.B.; Bauer, G.F.; Vaandrager, L.; Pelikan, J.M.; Sagy, S.; Eriksson, M.; Lindstrrom, B.; Magistretti, C.M. *The Handbook of Salutogenesis*, 2nd ed.; Springer Nature: Berlin/Heidelberg, Germany, 2022.
22. Mana, A.; Bauer, G.F.; Meier Magistretti, C.; Sardu, C.; Juvinyà-Canal, D.; Hardy, L.J.; Catz, O.; Tušl, M.; Sagy, S. Order out of chaos: Sense of coherence and the mediating role of coping resources in explaining mental health during COVID-19 in 7 countries. *SSM Mental Health* **2021**, *1*, 100001. [CrossRef]
23. Langeland, E.; Vinje, F. Applying Salutogenesis in mental healthcare settings. In *The Handbook of Salutogenesis*, 2nd ed.; Springer Nature: Berlin/Heidelberg, Germany, 2022; pp. 433–439.
24. Dooris, M.; Doherty, S.; Orme, J. Applying Salutogenesis in higher education. In *The Handbook of Salutogenesis*, 2nd ed.; Springer Nature: Berlin/Heidelberg, Germany, 2022; pp. 307–319.

25. Jenny, G.J.; Bauer, G.F.; Vinje, H.F.; Brauchli, R.; Vogt, K.; Torp, S. Applying Salutogenesis in the workplace. In *The Handbook of Salutogenesis*, 2nd ed.; Springer Nature: Berlin/Heidelberg, Germany, 2022; pp. 321–336.
26. Gómez-Salgado, J.; Domínguez-Salas, S.; Romero-Martín, M.; Ortega-Moreno, M.; García-Iglesias, J.J.; Ruiz-Frutos, C. Sense of coherence and psychological distress among healthcare workers during the COVID-19 pandemic in Spain. *Sustainability* **2020**, *12*, 6855. [CrossRef]
27. Schmuck, J.; Hiebel, N.; Rabe, M.; Schneider, J.; Erim, Y.; Morawa, E.; Jerg-Bretzke, L.; Beschoner, P.; Albus, C.; Hannemann, J.; et al. Sense of coherence, social support and religiosity as resources for medical personnel during the COVID-19 pandemic: A web-based survey among 4324 health care workers within the German Network University Medicine. *PLoS ONE* **2021**, *16*, e0255211. [CrossRef]
28. Navarro Prados, A.B.; Jiménez García-Tizón, S.; Meléndez, J.C. Sense of coherence and burnout in nursing home workers during the COVID-19 pandemic in Spain. *Health Soc. Care Community* **2022**, *30*, 244–252. [CrossRef]
29. Barni, D.; Danioni, F.; Canzi, E.; Ferrari, L.; Ranieri, S.; Lanz, M.; Iafrate, R.; Regalia, C.; Rosnati, R. Facing the COVID-19 pandemic: The role of sense of coherence. *Front. Psychol.* **2020**, *11*, 578440. [CrossRef] [PubMed]
30. Dadaczynski, K.; Okan, O.; Messer, M.; Rathmann, K. University students' sense of coherence, future worries and mental health: Findings from the German COVID-HL-survey. *Health Promot. Int.* **2022**, *37*, daab070. [CrossRef] [PubMed]
31. Snyder, C.R. Hope theory: Rainbows in the mind. *Psychol. Inq.* **2002**, *13*, 249–275. [CrossRef]
32. Margalit, M.; Schmidt-Barad, T.; Einav, M. Individual and interpersonal aspects of hope and people with developmental disabilities. In *The Positive Psychology of Personal Factors: Implications for Understanding Disability*; Lexington Books: New York, NY, USA, 2022; Volume 107.
33. Gallagher, M.W.; Lopez, S.J. *The Oxford Handbook of Hope*; Oxford University Press: Oxford, UK, 2018.
34. Einav, M.; Margalit, M. The hope theory and specific learning disorders and/or attention deficit disorders (SLD/ADHD): Developmental perspectives. *Curr. Opin. Psychol.* **2022**, *48*, 101471. [CrossRef] [PubMed]
35. Trzebiński, J.; Cabański, M.; Czarnecka, J.Z. Reaction to the COVID-19 pandemic: The influence of meaning in life, life satisfaction, and assumptions on world orderliness and positivity. *J. Loss Trauma* **2020**, *25*, 544–557. [CrossRef]
36. Walsh, F. Loss and resilience in the time of COVID-19: Meaning making, hope, and transcendence. *Fam. Process* **2020**, *59*, 898–911. [CrossRef]
37. Yao, Y.; Lin, M.; Ni, J.; Ni, J. Hope Buffers the Effect of Fear of COVID-19 on Depression among College Students: Insomnia as a Mediator. *Int. J. Environ. Res. Public Health* **2023**, *20*, 3245. [CrossRef]
38. Geiger, K.A.; Kwon, P. Rumination and depressive symptoms: Evidence for the moderating role of hope. *Personal. Individ. Differ.* **2010**, *49*, 391–395. [CrossRef]
39. Karababa, A. The Moderating Role of Hope in the Relationship Between Maladaptive Perfectionism and Anxiety Among Early Adolescents. *J. Genet. Psychol.* **2020**, *181*, 159–170. [CrossRef] [PubMed]
40. Zhang, R.; Zhao, L.; Han, X.; Wu, S.; Liu, X. Moderating role of hope in the relationship between perceived discrimination and life satisfaction among left-behind children in China. *Soc. Behav. Personal.* **2020**, *48*, 1–8. [CrossRef]
41. Yıldırım, M.; Arslan, G. Exploring the associations between resilience, dispositional hope, preventive behaviors, subjective well-being, and psychological health among adults during early stage of COVID-19. *Curr. Psychol.* **2022**, *41*, 5712–5722. [CrossRef] [PubMed]
42. Laslo-Roth, R.; George-Levi, S.; Margalit, M. Hope during the COVID-19 outbreak: Coping with the psychological impact of quarantine. *Couns. Psychol. Q.* **2021**, *34*, 771–785. [CrossRef]
43. Iecovich, E. Psychometric properties of the Hebrew version of the de Jong Gierveld loneliness scale. *Educ. Gerontol.* **2013**, *39*, 12–27. [CrossRef]
44. De Jong Gierveld, J.; van Tilburg, T. A 6-item scale for overall, emotional and social loneliness confirmatory tests on survey data. *Res. Aging* **2006**, *28*, 582–598. Available online: http://roa.sagepub.com/cgi/reprint/28/5/582 (accessed on 27 March 2023). [CrossRef]
45. Lackaye, T.; Margalit, M. Comparisons of achievement, effort and self-perceptions among students with learning disabilities and their peers from different achievement groups. *J. Learn. Disabil.* **2006**, *39*, 432–446. [CrossRef]
46. Hayes, J.R. *The Complete Problem Solver*; Routledge: London, UK, 2013.
47. Hayes, A.F. Partial, conditional, and moderated mediation: Quantification, inference, and interpretation. *Commun. Monogr.* **2018**, *85*, 4–40. [CrossRef]
48. Hayes, A.F. An index and test of linear moderated mediation. *Multivariate Behav. Res.* **2015**, *50*, 1–22. [CrossRef]
49. Winger, J.G.; Adams, R.N.; Mosher, C.E. Relations of meaning in life and sense of coherence to distress in cancer patients: A meta-analysis. *Psycho-Oncology* **2016**, *25*, 2–10. [CrossRef] [PubMed]
50. Sales, A.; Pinazo-Hernandis, S.; Martinez, D. Effects of a reminiscence program on meaning of life, sense of coherence and coping in older women living in nursing homes during COVID-19. *Healthcare* **2022**, *10*, 188. [CrossRef]
51. Wang, X.; Sun, Y.; Kramer, T. Ritualistic consumption decreases loneliness by increasing meaning. *J. Mark Res.* **2021**, *58*, 282–298. [CrossRef]
52. Tomšik, R. Relationship of loneliness and meaning of life among adolescents. In Proceedings of the Current Trends in Educational Science and Practice VIII: International Proceedings of Scientific Studies, Nitra, Slovakia, June 2015; pp. 66–79.

53. Burles, M.; Bally, J.M.; Holtslander, L.; Zimmer, M.; Hodgson-Viden, H. Supporting parental caregivers of seriously ill children: Findings from a feasibility and acceptability study of a hope intervention. *Child Health Care* **2022**, *51*, 1–19. [CrossRef]
54. Chan, K.; Wong, F.K.; Lee, P.H. A brief hope intervention to increase hope level and improve well-being in rehabilitating cancer patients: A feasibility test. *SAGE Open Nurs.* **2019**, *5*, 2377960819844381. [CrossRef] [PubMed]

International Journal of
Environmental Research and Public Health

MDPI

Article

Impact of COVID-19-Related Social Isolation on Behavioral Outcomes in Young Adults Residing in Northern Italy

Alessandra Patrono [1,2,*], Azzurra Invernizzi [2], Donatella Placidi [3], Giuseppa Cagna [3], Stefano Calza [1], Manuela Oppini [3], Elza Rechtman [2], Demetrios M. Papazaharias [2], Abraham Reichenberg [4], Roberto G. Lucchini [3,5], Maurizio Memo [1], Elisa Ongaro [3], Matteo Rota [1], Robert O. Wright [2], Stefano Renzetti [3] and Megan K. Horton [2]

1 Department of Molecular and Translational Medicine, University of Brescia, 25121 Brescia, Italy
2 Department of Environmental Medicine and Public Health, Icahn School of Medicine at Mount Sinai, New York, NY 10029, USA
3 Department of Medical and Surgical Specialties, Radiological Sciences and Public Health, University of Brescia, 25121 Brescia, Italy
4 Department of Psychiatry, Icahn School of Medicine at Mount Sinai, New York, NY 10029, USA
5 Department of Environmental Health Sciences, Robert Stempel College of Public Health and Social Work, Florida International University, Miami, FL 33199, USA
* Correspondence: alessandra.patrono@unibs.it

Abstract: Social isolation affects our emotions, behavior and interactions. Worldwide, individuals experienced prolonged periods of isolation during the first wave of the COVID-19 pandemic when authorities-imposed restrictions to reduce the spread of the virus. In this study, we investigated the effects of social isolation on emotional and behavioral outcomes in young adults from Lombardy, Italy, a global hotspot of COVID-19. We leveraged baseline (pre-social isolation) and follow-up (mid- or post-isolation) data collected from young adults enrolled in the ongoing, longitudinal Public Health Impact of Metals Exposure (PHIME) study. At baseline, 167 participants completed the ASEBA questionnaires (ASR/YSR) by web link or in person; 65 completed the ASR 12–18 weeks after the onset of restrictions. Using the sign test and multiple linear regression models, we examined differences in ASR scores between baseline and follow-up adjusting for sex, age, pre-pandemic IQ and time with social restrictions (weeks). Further, we examined interactions between sex and time in social isolation. Participants completed the ASR after spending an average of 14 weeks in social isolation (range 12–18 weeks). Thought problems increased between baseline and follow-up (median difference 1.0; 1st, 3rd quartile: −1.0, 4.0; $p = 0.049$). Among males, a longer time in social isolation (≥14 weeks) was associated with increased rule-breaking behaviors of 2.8 points. These results suggest the social isolation related to COVID-19 adversely impacted mental health. In particular, males seem to externalize their condition. These findings might help future interventions and treatment to minimize the consequences of social isolation experience in young adults.

Keywords: social isolation; mental health; COVID-19; young adults

1. Introduction

The COVID-19 pandemic has led to unprecedented social distancing behavior to limit the spread of the virus [1,2]. These measures impacted the general population, not only those found to be infected or exposed to the disease. Social distancing measures can effectively counter the spread of the disease [3], but can have an unprecedented impact on mental health and psychological well-being.

In Italy, the Lombardy area was the epicenter of the infection and one of the first places in the Western world confronted with COVID-19. No medications or vaccinations were available during the first wave of COVID-19. Therefore, the Italian government implemented a non-pharmacological measure referred to as lockdown, a forced and prolonged period of social restrictions, distancing and isolation [4,5] to stem the spread of infection. Lockdown social isolation refers to the "inadequate quality and quantity of social relationships with other people at the individual, group, community level and the wider social environment in which human interaction occurs" [6]. Italy was the first country to enter a COVID-19-related lockdown [7]. The lockdown and social isolation began in northern Italy on 23 February 2020 [8]. Increasingly restrictive decrees followed gradually up to 9 March 2020, and the restraining measures were extended throughout Italy from 11 March 2020 [9]. In Italy, during this period, only essential activities and shops were accessible (i.e., medical services, grocery stores), individuals were allowed to leave their homes only for demonstrated needs, such as for health reasons, shopping for basic needs and for work (if it was not possible to work from home) [7]. Social gatherings were minimized or prohibited [10]. The restriction measures in Italy have gradually decreased starting with a more extensive opening of shops, the permission to leave one's home to reach relatives and the possibility of being able to attend social events and equipped with a mask. On 11 June, the containment measures were eased again but conditions of distancing, the use of masks and the discouragement of social situations were maintained. Our investigation took place when participants were subjected to socially restrictive conditions and had recently been subjected to social isolation.

Although these restrictive measures successfully prevented more serious consequences of the COVID-19 pandemic, the social isolation may have resulted in mental health conditions [4]. Extended social isolation conditions related to COVID-19 have been associated with short- and long-term psychosocial and mental health consequences among all ages of the population [11]. The magnitude of the impact is influenced by many risk factors such as gender [12], age [13], economic disadvantage [14] and pre-existing health conditions [15]. In general, sex (female), age (individuals 18–30 years and over 60 years of age) and education (higher education) were associated with the highest levels of mental health problems following COVID-19-related social isolation [16,17] such as anxiety, sleep disorders and depression [16].

Although several studies have focused on mental health assessment in different subgroups of the population and especially investigated the effect of social restrictions in the elderly [10], there are few studies that have longitudinal data (baseline and follow-up) of the impact of COVID-19-related social isolation on the mental health of healthy young adults. In this study, we examine the impact of COVID-19-related social isolation on emotional and behavioral outcomes among healthy young adults living in northern Italy (Province of Brescia), one of the first global hotspots of COVID-19. Using information on behavioral outcomes collected prior to and following participants' experience of social isolation, we aim to quantify the impact of social isolation on young adult mental health to inform future interventions to minimize or eliminate the consequences of social isolation experience in healthy young adults.

2. Materials and Methods

2.1. Participants

Participants were part of the Public Health Impact of Metals Exposure (PHIME) study, an ongoing longitudinal cohort study of adolescents in the Province of Brescia, northern Italy. PHIME was designed to assess cognitive and behavioral function in adolescents and young adults with environmental exposure to neurotoxic metals. Participants were never to have received a psychological or neuropsychological diagnosis. Other enrollment, inclusion and exclusion criteria for the PHIME study are described in detail elsewhere [18–21]. Upon enrollment, PHIME participants participated in a baseline in-person visit consisting of self- and interviewer-assisted questionnaires capturing sociodemographic characteristics (i.e., sex, date of birth, residential address, parental education and occupation) and neurodevelopmental outcomes including the Kaufman Brief Intelligence Test, second edition (K-BIT 2) [22] for IQ and the Achenbach System of Empirically Based Assessment (ASEBA) Youth Self Report (YSR) [23] or (ASEBA) Adult Self Report (ASR) [24] for behavioral and emotional regulation (Section 2.3). As part of the PHIME study, 167 participants (ages 19.3 years $\pm$ 2.3) completed the YSR or the ASR in person with a trained psychologist prior to the beginning of COVID-19-related social isolation (on average, the first visit was performed 81.8 $\pm$ 43.2 weeks prior to the first day of social isolation). To assess the impact of social isolation on emotional and behavioral outcomes, we re-administered the ASR via an online platform (REDCap®, Research Electronic Data Capture, Vanderbilt University, Nashville, TN, USA) 12–18 weeks following the onset of social isolation measures (on average, the subjects answered the questionnaire after 13.4 $\pm$ 1.4 weeks). We distributed the web link to all 167 PHIME participants who completed the baseline assessment; 40% (65/167) of participants completed the online ASR. During the second time point, no information relating to the SES and the IQ was collected again, as these variables were considered stable over a short time after the first administration.

Eligible participants received a detailed description of the study procedures before consenting to participate. The parents of the minors during the baseline phase received an informed consent form to be signed. The Institutional Review Boards of the Ethical Committee of Brescia, the Icahn School of Medicine at Mount Sinai and the University of California, Santa Cruz approved all PHIME study protocols.

2.2. ASEBA Young and Adult Self Report (YSR and ASR) Questionnaires

The Achenbach System of Empirically Based Assessment (ASEBA) offers a comprehensive approach to assessing adaptive and maladaptive functioning. During the baseline PHIME visit, adolescent participants (ages 15–17 years; n = 45) completed the Youth Self Report (YSR) questionnaire [23,25] and adult participants (ages 18–25 years; n = 122) completed the Adult Self Report (ASR) questionnaire [26]. The YSR questionnaire is designed for self-reporting in the 11–17 years age range; the ASR is appropriate for adults ages 18–59 years. ASR questionnaires evaluate the following clinical areas: (I) Anxious/ Depressed; (II) Withdrawn; (III) Somatic Complaints; (IV) Thought Problems; (V) Attention Problems; (VI) Aggressive Behavior; (VII) Rule-Breaking Behavior; (VIII) Intrusive. An Internalization Problem Composite Scale is aggregated from the individual symptoms scales: Anxiety (18 items), Withdrawn (9 items) and Somatic Complaints (12 items). An Externalizing Problem Composite Scale is composed of: Aggressive Behavior (15 items), Rule-Breaking Behavior (14 items) and Intrusive Behavior (6 items). The other scales concern Attention Problems (15 items) and Thought Problems (10 items). The scale Other Problems (21 elements) includes elements that do not frame any syndrome. The remaining 11 items measure adaptive functioning. For the following study, we used the version validated on the Italian population.

The clinical scales investigated by the ASR are comparable to those of the YRS with some changes related to the adaptation of the items by age. In the YSR version, the component of Depression is investigated both by scale I and II; the ASR scale VIII Intrusive corresponds to the YSR scale V, Thought Problems.

Since the seven ASR syndromes have YSR-rated counterparts, questionnaire scores can be directly compared [27]. A score from 0 (behavior/problem absent) to 2 (behavior/problem present) is applied to each item that makes up the individual scales considered in the YSR/ASR questionnaires. Each scale will then assume a numerical value which is transformed into a T score in a range from 50 to 100. Scores between 50 and 64 are considered normal; scores between 65 and 70 are considered borderline; scores above 70 are considered clinically significant.

Both the YSR and ASR yield a Total Problems score indicating the overall psychopathological assessment of the individual (a higher score indicates greater psychopathology). Symptomatic scales correlate with the DSM-oriented diagnosis (i.e., ASR depressive symptoms correlate with DSM-diagnosed depression).

2.3. Covariate Data

Sociodemographic data (i.e., participant sex and age, and parental occupation and education) were collected at the baseline assessment through questionnaires. Intelligence quotient (IQ) was measured using the Kaufman Brief Intelligence Test, 2nd edition (KBIT-2) [28], a short measure of verbal and non-verbal intelligence for children, adolescents and adults, aged 4 to 90 years. The verbal and non-verbal scores yield a composite IQ score that can be considered as a measure of general intelligence with good correlations with other tests of intellectual functioning [28]. An index of family socioeconomic status (SES; low, medium or high) was calculated from parental age, occupation and education [29].

2.4. Statistical Analysis

Descriptive statistics were used to assess the distribution of variables; continuous variables are analyzed using the median and the first and third quartiles because of the skewed distribution and, for categorical variables, we used absolute frequencies and percentages. Student's *t*-tests with Welch's correction for continuous variables and chi-squared (χ^2) tests for categorical variables were used to examine differences in demographic characteristics across the participants. The time spent in social isolation was calculated in weeks starting from the start of social isolation (9 March 2020) and the date the participants completed the follow-up ASR online. Time spent in isolation was calculated based on the median (14 weeks); low = less than 14 weeks between the initiation of the first restrictions and the follow-up questionnaire response, high = greater than or equal to 14 weeks between onset of social isolation and follow-up questionnaire response. Figure 1 describes the distribution of time spent in social isolation starting from the first day of social isolation to the last day when a response to the questionnaire was collected. Most of the data were collected around 12 weeks from the start of the social isolation (n = 24, 36.9%) while the last responses were received after around 18 weeks (n = 2, 3.1%).

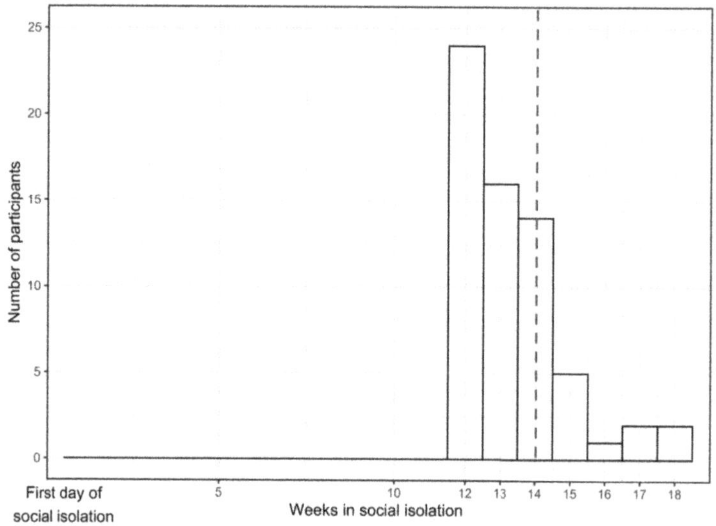

Figure 1. Time elapsed in social isolation. In total, 65 participants answered the questionnaire (axis y). The amount of time spent in isolation (axis x) was calculated as the number of weeks elapsed between the start of social isolation (3 September 2020) and the administration of the follow-up ASR. The red dashed line indicates the median (14 weeks). We categorized this variable as low (<14 weeks in social isolation) and high ($\geq$14 weeks in social isolation) based on the median weeks spent in social isolation prior to assessment.

We used the sign test, a non-parametric test to assess differences between paired observations, to assess the difference between YSR/ASR symptoms before and after social isolation. The choice of the sign test was also driven by the non-symmetric distribution of differences. We then examined how the amount of time in social isolation, defined as the time elapsed between the first day of social restrictions and the follow-up visit, impacted differences in YSR/ASR scores. We applied a linear regression model to examine how time elapsed in isolation (independent variable) predicted the change in YSR/ASR scores, adjusting for age, sex, baseline SES and IQ. We then determined whether the associations between time in social isolation and the change in ASR scores differed by sex through a multiplicative interaction term. Statistical significance level was set at 5% for all tests. All the statistical analyses were performed with R (version 4.1.0).

3. Results

3.1. Sociodemographic Characteristics

Sociodemographic characteristics of PHIME participants included in this study are presented in Table 1. In total, 65 participants (26 male, 19.8 +/− 2.4 years) repeated the ASR during or following the social isolation (i.e., follow-up). Participants experienced an average of 14.6 +/− 9.5 weeks with social restrictions before completing the follow-up ASR questionnaire (Figure 1). The average IQ was 106.1 (SD 9.7). No YSR/ASR scores indicated problematic behaviors at baseline or follow-up (Supplementary Table S1). Sociodemographic characteristics and baseline ASR scores of those participants who completed the online follow-up assessment did not differ from those who did not complete the assessment. The amount of time (weeks) spent in social isolation ranged from 12–18 weeks, the average time spent in isolation was 14 weeks (Figure 1).

Table 1. Sociodemographic characteristics of PHIME participants included in this study at baseline and follow-up (n = 65).

Characteristics	Baseline (n = 65)
Age (years)	
mean ± sd	19.8 (2.4)
Sex (n, %)	
Male	26 (40%)
Female	39 (60%)
Socioeconomic status (n, %)	
Low	
Medium	17 (26.2%)
High	32 (49.2%)
IQ	16 (24.6%)
Mean ± sd	106.1 (9.7)

Note: Mean, standard deviation (sd), range (minimum and maximum values) and percentage (%) are reported.

3.2. Social Isolation and Behavioral Outcomes

We observed no differences in Total Problems reported at baseline and follow-up (Figure 2A). Participants reported significantly more Thought Problems at follow-up (sign test; 51.5 (50.0, 55.8) vs. 53.5 (51.0, 58.0), $p = 0.049$; Figure 2B). None of the other ASR scales differed significantly between baseline and follow-up (Table S1).

3.3. Length of Social Isolation and Behavioral Outcomes

Though not significant, we observed a trend between spending a longer amount of time in social isolation (<14 compared to ≥14 weeks) and an increase of 1.73 points in Rule-Breaking Behaviors was found (linear regression, $\beta = 1.73$; 95% confidence interval (CI): −0.03, −3.48, $p = 0.053$).

We did not observe significant differences between baseline and follow-up in the other YSR/ASR symptom scales or internalizing/externalizing composite scales (Figure S1).

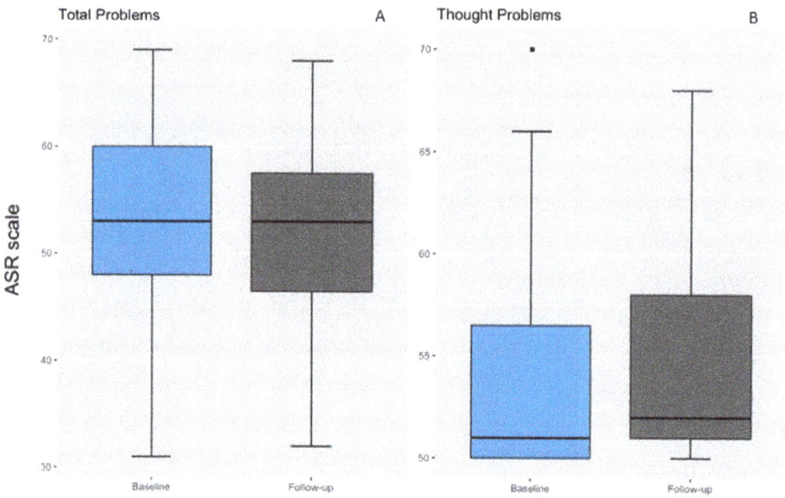

Figure 2. Differences in ASR score between baseline and follow-up. The boxplot shows YSR/ASR scores for Total Problems (**A**) and Thought Problems (**B**) at baseline (blue box) and follow-up (gray box). The error bars are the 95% confidence interval, the bottom and top of the box are the 25th and 75th percentiles, the line inside the box is the 50th percentile (median), and any outliers are shown as open circles. No differences are shown in Total Problems score scales between baseline and follow-up. Thought Problems are significantly higher in the follow-up assessment, with an overall clinical worsening in the post-social isolation period. The sign test was applied to test the difference between baseline and follow-up.

3.4. *Sex-Specific Effects of Social Isolation on Behavioral Outcomes*

In the interaction between time and sex analysis (Table S3), the amount of time spent in social isolation was significantly associated with increased Rule-Breaking Behavior in males only (i.e., average change in Rule-Breaking Behavior among males with a higher social isolation time = 2.8, 95%CI 0.06, 5.5, $p = 0.046$; Figure 3). Male participants who spent more time in social isolation (≥14 weeks) reported a 3-point increase in Rule-Breaking Behavior compared to males who spent less time (<14 weeks) in social isolation. No differences in the association between the time elapsed in social isolation and ASR scores were found for female participants.

3.5. *Results of the Other Clinical Scales*

As shown in Figure S1, the other clinical scales investigated did not show significant differences between baseline and follow-up. The total scale on externalized problems and internalizing problems is also stable, demonstrating how the impact of social isolation has been specific and circumscribed.

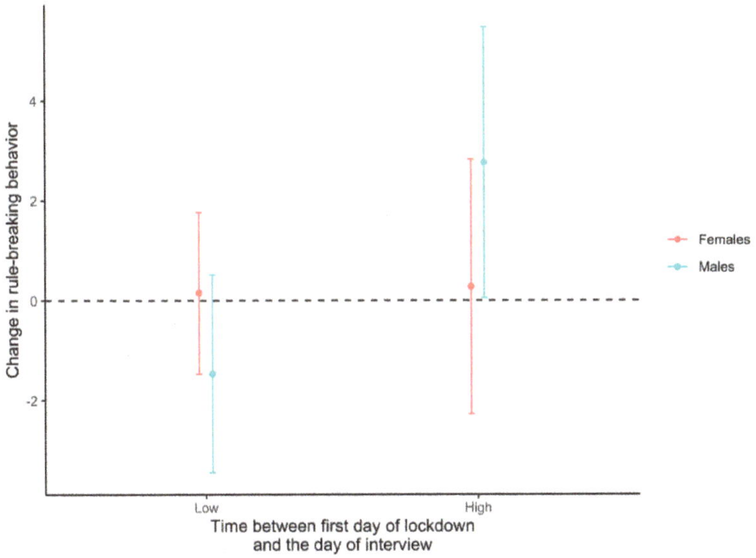

Figure 3. Sex-specific effects of social isolation and Rule-Breaking Behavior. Results from the linear regression model including an interaction term between time in social isolation and sex. Here are displayed the marginal effects of the time spent in social isolation (<14 weeks vs. ≥14 weeks vs. low) on the difference in the ASR Rule-Breaking Behavior score by sex. The model was adjusted by age (years), SES and IQ. The statistical significance for males with a longer time spent in social isolation is $p = 0.046$.

4. Discussion

In this study, we assess the impact of COVID-19-related social isolation on baseline (pre-isolation) and follow-up (mid- or post-isolation) behavioral outcomes in young adults enrolled in an ongoing longitudinal PHIME cohort study in northern Italy. Our findings suggest that social isolation is associated with increased Thought Problems. Further, the length of time spent in social isolation more adversely impacts males compared to females; males who spend more time in social isolation reported more Rule-Breaking Behavior.

In our study, males reported higher Rule-Breaking Behavior scores after social isolation than females. Further, spending a longer amount of time in social isolation increased the severity of Rule-Breaking Behavior scores (i.e., more time, more rule breaking). The construct of Rule-Breaking Behavior is defined as "non-compliance with the applicable regulatory expectations of the group" [30] and is related to disinhibition [31]. The general construct of rule breaking is considered a transitory factor within the behavior and mediated by the environmental situation [32,33]. Our findings in males contribute to the literature on social isolation and behavioral outcomes as most of the previous studies focus on female mood disorders related to the pandemic and social isolation [34]. Our data are fairly consistent with studies that broadly analyze gender differences in typical traits in mental disorders, with a higher frequency of behavioral outcomes in males [35] although these series may have been influenced by bias [36,37].

The worsening of these clinical scales, with regard to the social isolation period, is theoretically and clinically significant and reflects the need to implement intervention dynamics aimed at containing or preventing long-term effects. Creating free and easily accessible support networks for young adults is a solution that should be promoted. These networks, which can also be created online, could be facilitated by general practitioners and psychologists at the local level in the places most frequented by young adults, including university institutions. In particular, in view of the delivery of online therapies, the approaches of cognitive behavioral therapy, dialectical behavioral therapy and mind–

body practice techniques have emerged as valid strategies to counteract the emerging symptomatology [38]. Thinking problems and anxiety levels may have been supported by the growing phenomenon of cyberchondria: a behavior characteristic of an excessive online search for medical information associated with rising levels of health anxiety [39]. Furthermore, previous research has found that receiving health information from the internet was associated with poorer psychological well-being [40]. This may become particularly true in a pandemic era, leading the World Health Organization to speak of two major threats to public health: the pandemic and the infodemic [31].

Our unique study design and population, located in one of the first global hotspots of the first wave of the COVID-19 pandemic, provided the opportunity to examine the impact of the pandemic-related social isolation on healthy young adults. Our findings suggesting that males may be more vulnerable to the impacts of social isolation on Rule-Breaking Behavior could help direct targeted interventions. In general, males are less likely to seek therapeutic interventions to treat mental health or mood-related disorders [41]. Based on the externalizing symptomatology that drives male behavior, initiatives that focus more on attention to functioning than on emotionality should be considered. General practitioners must be instructed to differentiate gender-specific alarm bells for subsequent referral to specialist treatment.

5. Limitations

The sample is relatively small and the participation rate was modest (40%) but we have a unique sample: healthy young adults living in one of the main COVID-19 disease hotspots in Europe at the beginning of the pandemic. We were able to collect the information during two time points in a period of time sufficient to evaluate behavioral changes due to social isolation. The low compliance could have driven a selection bias, with a possible tendency toward responses to the questionnaire only by the most emotionally affected subjects with a tendency of the most affected subjects to be interested in participating in the survey. However, although the sample is not very large, it assumes importance due to the possibility of being able to compare the scores with the previous administration of the questionnaire. Another limitation is the lack of information on COVID-19 infection and its possible impact of emotional and behavioral outcomes. At the time of our follow-up, accessibility of antigen and antibody verification of the presence of the disease was limited and took place only in the presence of symptoms. Rapid testing was not widespread. The socioeconomic data were not collected in the two time points, only in the first time point. Future investigations could investigate this aspect further.

6. Conclusions

To conclude, this study demonstrates how COVID-19 social restriction policies negatively impacted on mental and behavioral health in healthy young adults. The worsening of clinical scales of ASR, with regard to the pandemic period, is theoretically and clinically significant and reflects the need to implement intervention dynamics aimed at containing or preventing long-term effects of social isolation. Future studies are needed to understand how targeted interventions, based on the results of this and other similar research, can address changes in public health well-being.

Supplementary Materials: The following supporting information can be downloaded at: https://www.mdpi.com/article/10.3390/ijerph192416496/s1, Figure S1: Differences in all ASR score between baseline and follow up; Table S1: Complete ASR scores at the baseline and follow-up visit; Table S2: Interaction between sociodemographic variables and ASR scales; Table S3. Association between time in social isolation and the ASR scales by sex. Relationship between the time spent in social isolation and the psychopathological outcomes at the follow-up visit by sex. Models were adjusted by age, SES and IQ.

Author Contributions: Conceptualization, A.P. and D.P.; Data curation, D.M.P. and S.R.; Investigation, G.C., M.O. and E.O.; Supervision, M.K.H.; Visualization, A.I.; Writing—original draft, A.P. and S.R.; Writing—review and editing, A.I., D.P., S.C., E.R., A.R., R.G.L., M.R., R.O.W., S.R., M.M. and M.K.H. All authors have read and agreed to the published version of the manuscript.

Funding: This research received no external funding.

Institutional Review Board Statement: The Institutional Review Boards of the Ethical Committee of Brescia, the Icahn School of Medicine at Mount Sinai and the University of California, Santa Cruz approved all PHIME study protocols.

Informed Consent Statement: Informed consent was obtained from all subjects involved in the study.

Data Availability Statement: Not applicable.

Acknowledgments: National Institutes of Environmental Health Sciences (NIEHS) grant numbers R01 ES019222, R01 ES013744, P30ES023515, and the European Union through its Sixth Framework Programme for RTD (contract number FOOD-CT-2006-016253). Thanks to "Honors Center of Italian University—Centro interuniversitario per la formazione internazionale—H2CU" for supporting the exchange period at Mount Sinai in New York by contributing to the implementation of the research work.

Conflicts of Interest: The authors declare no conflict of interest.

References

1. Schulze, A.; Biermann, M.; Atanasova, K.; Unterseher, F.; Winkler, L.; Bohus, M.; Lis, S. Social Touch, Social Isolation, and Loneliness in Borderline Personality Disorder during the COVID-19 Pandemic. *Front. Psychiatry* **2022**, *13*, 876413. [CrossRef] [PubMed]
2. Anderson, R.M.; Heesterbeek, H.; Klinkenberg, D.; Hollingsworth, T.D. How Will Country-Based Mitigation Measures Influence the Course of the COVID-19 Epidemic? *Lancet* **2020**, *395*, 931–934. [CrossRef] [PubMed]
3. Glass, R.; Glass, L.; Beyeler, W.; Min, H. Targeted Social Distancing Designs for Pandemic Influenza. *Emerg. Infect. Dis.* **2006**, *12*, 1671–1681. [CrossRef] [PubMed]
4. Pasca, L.; Zanaboni, M.P.; Grumi, S.; Totaro, M.; Ballante, E.; Varesio, C.; De Giorgis, V. Impact of COVID-19 Pandemic in Pediatric Patients with Epilepsy with Neuropsychiatric Comorbidities: A Telemedicine Evaluation. *Epilepsy Behav.* **2021**, *115*, 107519. [CrossRef]
5. Shen, K.; Yang, Y.; Wang, T.; Zhao, D.; Jiang, Y.; Jin, R.; Zheng, Y.; Xu, B.; Xie, Z.; Lin, L.; et al. Diagnosis, Treatment, and Prevention of 2019 Novel Coronavirus Infection in Children: Experts' Consensus Statement. *World J. Pediatr.* **2020**, *16*, 223–231. [CrossRef]
6. Zavaleta, D.; Samuel, K.; Mills, C. *Social Isolation: A Conceptual and Measurement Proposal*; Oxford Poverty and Human Development Initiative: Oxford, UK, 2014.
7. Gazzetta Ufficiale. Available online: https://www.gazzettaufficiale.it/eli/id/2020/03/09/20A01558/sg (accessed on 4 August 2022).
8. Gazzetta Ufficiale. Available online: https://www.gazzettaufficiale.it/eli/id/2020/02/23/20G00020/sg (accessed on 4 August 2022).
9. Gazzetta Ufficiale. Available online: https://www.gazzettaufficiale.it/eli/id/2020/03/11/20A01605/sg (accessed on 4 August 2022).
10. Gorenko, J.A.; Moran, C.; Flynn, M.; Dobson, K.; Konnert, C. Social Isolation and Psychological Distress among Older Adults Related to COVID-19: A Narrative Review of Remotely-Delivered Interventions and Recommendations. *J. Appl. Gerontol.* **2021**, *40*, 3–13. [CrossRef] [PubMed]
11. Singh, S.; Roy, D.; Sinha, K.; Parveen, S.; Sharma, G.; Joshi, G. Impact of COVID-19 and Lockdown on Mental Health of Children and Adolescents: A Narrative Review with Recommendations. *Psychiatry Res.* **2020**, *293*, 113429. [CrossRef]
12. Özdin, Ş.B. Levels and Predictors of Anxiety, Depression and Health Anxiety during COVID-19 Pandemic in Turkish Society: The Importance of Gender. *Int. J. Soc. Psychiatry* **2020**, *66*, 504–511. [CrossRef]
13. Wilson, R.S.; Krueger, K.R.; Arnold, S.E.; Schneider, J.A.; Kelly, J.F.; Barnes, L.L.; Tang, Y.; Bennett, D.A. Loneliness and Risk of Alzheimer Disease. *Arch. Gen. Psychiatry* **2007**, *64*, 234–240. [CrossRef]
14. Aragona, M.; Barbato, A.; Cavani, A.; Costanzo, G.; Mirisola, C. Negative Impacts of COVID-19 Lockdown on Mental Health Service Access and Follow-up Adherence for Immigrants and Individuals in Socio-Economic Difficulties. *Public Health* **2020**, *186*, 52–56. [CrossRef]
15. Conti, E.; Sgandurra, G.; De Nicola, G.; Biagioni, T.; Boldrini, S.; Bonaventura, E.; Buchignani, B.; Della Vecchia, S.; Falcone, F.; Fedi, C.; et al. Behavioural and Emotional Changes during COVID-19 Lockdown in an Italian Paediatric Population with Neurologic and Psychiatric Disorders. *Brain Sci.* **2020**, *10*, 918. [CrossRef] [PubMed]

16. Volken, T.; Zysset, A.; Amendola, S.; Klein, S.A.; Huber, M.; von Wyl, A.; Dratva, J. Depressive Symptoms in Swiss University Students during the COVID-19 Pandemic and Its Correlates. *Int. J. Environ. Res. Public Health* **2021**, *18*, 1458. [CrossRef] [PubMed]
17. Xiong, J.; Lipsitz, O.; Nasri, F.; Lui, L.M.W.; Gill, H.; Phan, L.; Chen-Li, D.; Iacobucci, M.; Ho, R.; Majeed, A.; et al. Impact of COVID-19 Pandemic on Mental Health in the General Population: A Systematic Review. *J. Affect. Disord.* **2020**, *277*, 55–64. [CrossRef] [PubMed]
18. Lucchini, R.G.; Guazzetti, S.; Zoni, S.; Donna, F.; Peter, S.; Zacco, A.; Salmistraro, M.; Bontempi, E.; Zimmerman, N.J.; Smith, D.R. Tremor, Olfactory and Motor Changes in Italian Adolescents Exposed to Historical Ferro-Manganese Emission. *Neurotoxicology* **2012**, *33*, 687–696. [CrossRef] [PubMed]
19. Chiu, Y.M.; Claus, H.B.; Hsu, H.L.; Pendo, M.P.; Coull, B.A.; Austin, C.; Cagna, G.; Fedrighi, C.; Placidi, D.; Smith, D.R.; et al. Sex Differences in Sensitivity to Prenatal and Early Childhood Manganese Exposure on Neuromotor Function in Adolescents. *Environ. Res.* **2017**, *159*, 458–465. [CrossRef]
20. Lucas, E.L.; Bertrand, P.; Guazzetti, S.; Donna, F.; Peli, M.; Jursa, T.P.; Lucchini, R.; Smith, D.R. Impact of Ferromanganese Alloy Plants on Household Dust Manganese Levels: Implications for Childhood Exposure. *Environ. Res.* **2015**, *138*, 279–290. [CrossRef]
21. Bauer, J.A.; Claus, H.B.; Austin, C.; Zoni, S.; Fedrighi, C.; Cagna, G.; Placidi, D.; White, R.F.; Yang, Q.; Coull, B.A.; et al. Manganese in Teeth and Neurobehavior: Sex-Specific Windows of Susceptibility. *Environ. Int.* **2017**, *108*, 299–308. [CrossRef]
22. Kaufman, A.S.; Kaufman, N.L. *K-BIT 2: Kaufman Brief Intelligence Test*, 2nd ed.; Pearson: London, UK, 2004.
23. Achenbach, T.M.; Rescorla, L. *Multicultural Supplement to the Manual for the ASEBA School-Age Forms & Profiles: Child Behavior Checklist for Ages 6–18, Teacher's Report Form, Youth Self-Report: An Integrated System Fo Multi-Informant Assessment*; Aseba: Burlington, VT, USA, 2007; ISBN 9781932975093.
24. Achenbach, T.M.; Rescorla, L. *Manual for the ASEBA Adult Forms & Profiles: For Ages 18–59: Adult Self-Report and Adult Behavior Checklist*; Aseba: Burlington, VT, USA, 2003; ISBN 9780938565864.
25. Achenbach, T.M.; Rescorla, L.A. *Manual for the ASEBA School-Age Forms & Profiles: An Integrated System of Multi-Informant Assessment*; Aseba: Burlington, VT, USA, 2001; ISBN 9780938565734.
26. de Vries, L.P.; van de Weijer, M.P.; Ligthart, L.; Willemsen, G.; Dolan, C.V.; Boomsma, D.I.; Baselmans, B.M.L.; Bartels, M. A Comparison of the ASEBA Adult Self Report (ASR) and the Brief Problem Monitor (BPM/18-59). *Behav. Genet.* **2020**, *50*, 363–373. [CrossRef]
27. Achenbach, T.M. International Findings with the Achenbach System of Empirically Based Assessment (ASEBA): Applications to Clinical Services, Research, and Training. *Child Adolesc. Psychiatry Ment. Health* **2019**, *13*, 30. [CrossRef]
28. Cesana, G.C.; Ferrario, M.; De Vito, G.; Sega, R.; Grieco, A. Evaluation of the socioeconomic status in epidemiological surveys: Hypotheses of research in the Brianza area MONICA project. *Med. Lav.* **1995**, *86*, 16–26.
29. Abdellaoui, A.; de Moor, M.H.M.; Geels, L.M.; van Beek, J.H.D.A.; Willemsen, G.; Boomsma, D.I. Thought Problems from Adolescence to Adulthood: Measurement Invariance and Longitudinal Heritability. *Behav. Genet.* **2011**, *42*, 19–29. [CrossRef] [PubMed]
30. Burt, S.A.; Alexandra Burt, S.; Brent Donnellan, M. Personality Correlates of Aggressive and Non-Aggressive Antisocial Behavior. *Personal. Individ. Differ.* **2008**, *44*, 53–63. [CrossRef]
31. Eurosurveillance Editorial Team. Note from the editors: World Health Organization declares novel coronavirus (2019-nCoV) sixth public health emergency of international concern. *Eurosurveillance* **2020**, *25*, 200131e. [CrossRef]
32. Eley, T.C.; Lichtenstein, P.; Moffitt, T.E. A Longitudinal Behavioral Genetic Analysis of the Etiology of Aggressive and Nonaggressive Antisocial Behavior. *Dev. Psychopathol.* **2003**, *15*, 383–402. [CrossRef]
33. Tackett, J.L.; Krueger, R.F.; Iacono, W.G.; McGue, M. Symptom-Based Subfactors of DSM-Defined Conduct Disorder: Evidence for Etiologic Distinctions. *J. Abnorm. Psychol.* **2005**, *114*, 483–487. [CrossRef]
34. Almeida, M.; Shrestha, A.D.; Stojanac, D.; Miller, L.J. The Impact of the COVID-19 Pandemic on Women's Mental Health. *Arch. Womens. Ment. Health* **2020**, *23*, 741–748. [CrossRef] [PubMed]
35. Paris, J. An Overview on Gender, Personality and Mental Health. *Personal. Ment. Health* **2007**, *1*, 14–20. [CrossRef]
36. Braamhorst, W.; Lobbestael, J.; Emons, W.H.M.; Arntz, A.; Witteman, C.L.M.; Bekker, M.H.J. Sex Bias in Classifying Borderline and Narcissistic Personality Disorder. *J. Nerv. Ment. Dis.* **2015**, *203*, 804. [CrossRef]
37. Crosby, J.P.; Sprock, J. Effect of Patient Sex, Clinician Sex, and Sex Role on the Diagnosis of Antisocial Personality Disorder: Models of Underpathologizing and Overpathologizing Biases. *J. Clin. Psychol.* **2004**, *60*, 583–604. [CrossRef]
38. Riboldi, I.; Cavaleri, D.; Calabrese, A.; Capogrosso, C.A.; Piacenti, S.; Bartoli, F.; Crocamo, C.; Carrà, G. Digital mental health interventions for anxiety and depressive symptoms in university students during the COVID-19 pandemic: A systematic review of randomized controlled trials. *Rev. Psiquiatr. Salud Ment.* **2022**. In press. [CrossRef]
39. Vismara, M.; Caricasole, V.; Starcevic, V.; Cinosi, E.; Dell'Osso, B.; Martinotti, G.; Fineberg, N.A. Is cyberchondria a new transdiagnostic digital compulsive syndrome? A systematic review of the evidence. *Compr. Psychiatry* **2020**, *99*, 152167. [CrossRef] [PubMed]
40. Muse, K.; McManus, F.; Leung, C.; Meghreblian, B.; Williams, J.M.G. Cyberchondriasis: Fact or fiction? A preliminary examination of the relationship between health anxiety and searching for health information on the Internet. *J. Anxiety Disord.* **2012**, *26*, 189–196. [CrossRef] [PubMed]
41. Liddon, L.; Kingerlee, R.; Barry, J.A. Gender Differences in Preferences for Psychological Treatment, Coping Strategies, an Triggers to Help-Seeking. *Br. J. Clin. Psychol.* **2018**, *57*, 42–58. [CrossRef] [PubMed]

International Journal of
Environmental Research and Public Health

MDPI

Article

Too Close for Comfort: Stigma by Association in Family Members Who Live with Relatives with Mental Illness

Joel O. Goldberg *, Suzanne A. McKeag, Alison L. Rose, Heather Lumsden-Ruegg and Gordon L. Flett

Department of Psychology, York University, Toronto, ON M3J 1P3, Canada
* Correspondence: jgoldber@yorku.ca

Abstract: Stigma by association is described in qualitative research of family members who have relatives diagnosed with mental illness, depicting their sense of public shame for having these relationship ties. However, there have been relatively few empirical studies thus far, in part due to the isolation of family members affecting research recruitment. In order to address this gap, an online survey was administered to 124 family members, comparing those who live in the same home with their ill relative (n = 81) and those who do not (n = 43). A remarkable incidence of one in three family members reported experiencing stigma by association. Those living with an ill relative reported comparatively higher levels of stigma by association using an adapted questionnaire measure. Both groups experienced loneliness (moderate levels), but importantly, the cohabiting relatives perceived themselves as lacking support from friends and other family members. Correlational analyses revealed that those with heightened stigma by association reported heightened anti-mattering: that is, feeling that other people treat them as if they are insignificant and invisible. Anti-mattering was also associated with more loneliness and reduced social support. Our discussion focuses on the theme that family members who actually live with mentally ill relatives experience heightened social isolation that is under-recognized due to public stigma concerns, compounded by feeling their own lives do not matter to others. Public health implications are considered for the stigmatized family members who appear to be particularly marginalized.

Keywords: mental health stigma; social isolation; mattering; loneliness; stigma by association

1. Introduction

The COVID-19 pandemic with societally prescribed social restrictions [1] has served to sharpen the focus on the public health consequences of social isolation and loneliness. Previous meta-analytic work [2] has highlighted the impact of both perceived and actual social isolation on early mortality. However, within our broad society, it is individuals with serious mental illness (SMI) and their families who are often most isolated and who report a profound sense of social exclusion related to perceived stigmatization [3]. Family members who have a relative with SMI often assume demanding caregiving responsibilities that can become quite distressing [4] and place them at risk for burnout [5]. A recent mixed-methods study of family caregivers of individuals with SMI [6] poignantly depicted the extreme social isolation of these family members who were found to have exceedingly small social networks, an isolation which the authors ascribed to stigmatization. Specifically, family members reported the need to be "secretive about the (relative's) mental illness … so they reduce their social interactions". This is consistent with earlier work describing how family members feel avoided by friends, relatives, and other people in their communities. They hide their relationship with their mentally ill relative to evade stigma [7], and they believe that most people hold negative views of relatives of people with mental illnesses [8].

Corrigan and Miller [9] described how family members can experience a sense of shame, blame and contamination in their perceived stigma of being associated with their relative with SMI. This kind of stigma has been previously referred to as 'courtesy' stigma or 'family' stigma [9] but is now typically termed stigma by association [10]. Research studies of stigma by association using qualitative methods were conducted by van der Sanden et al. [11,12] in the Netherlands with Dutch family members of people with mental illness. Through interviews with family members, the authors found that 74% had experienced stigma by association [11]. Dominant themes reported included family members being blamed for the mental illness of their relative and experiencing social exclusion, which resulted both from friends, relatives, and other community members pulling away from participants and from participants withdrawing from people to avoid stigma. Additional qualitative research attests to the existence and importance of stigma by association among family members (see [13,14]).

What is unclear at present is whether family members who are actually living with versus living apart from their relative with SMI experience more stigma, more loneliness, and more isolation. Research findings thus far are mixed and are mainly restricted to qualitative reports. This is likely due, in part, to the difficulties in participant recruitment. Some research has suggested that there is a similar level of caregiver burden independent of joint household status [15,16]. Others [10] suggest more clearly that family members who actually live with their ill relatives experience a heightened caregiver burden. However, there remains a gap in the literature regarding the impact and consequences of loneliness and social isolation and stigma by association in this vulnerable group. There is a paucity of empirical studies that have been conducted in the area, which thus far has mainly been restricted to qualitative research.

The current study had two primary goals. First, we compared family members who are either living with or not cohabiting with their relative with serious mental illness to determine their relative levels of experienced stigma by association, loneliness, social support, and feelings of not mattering. Second, in the sample of family members as a whole, we examined the correlates of feelings of not mattering. We hypothesized that feelings of not mattering would be associated with elevated levels of loneliness and lower levels of social support, in accordance with past findings with young adults and other groups (see [17–20]). In addition, however, we wished to explore how feelings of not mattering might be linked with the experience of stigma by association. A link between feeling insignificant and stigma by association would be in keeping with the notion that being made to feel insignificant and invisible contributes to a more general sense of being devalued, judged, and stigmatized by others. This is thought to be felt most acutely among family members with a relative with a mental illness.

2. Methods

2.1. Participants

Participants were recruited through organizations that support family members who have relatives with mental illnesses. The Canadian Mental Health Association, the Institute for Advancements in Mental Health (formerly the Schizophrenia Society of Ontario), and Reconnect Community Health Services sent recruitment email advertisements communicating the opportunity to take part in the study. Clients who were engaged in their programs and services and had consented to receive follow-up correspondence were contacted. Additional participants were recruited through the Schizophrenia Society of York University (SSY), which promotes schizophrenia awareness and stigma reduction. The SSY posted the advertisement communicating the opportunity to take part in the study on their social media platforms (e.g., Instagram). Participants received a $5.00 (CND) coffee shop gift card as compensation for completing the study. The participants accessed the survey through the Qualtrics XM platform via an online link.

Data were collected from 254 individuals who provided informed consent and self-identified as relatives of people with serious mental illnesses, including but not limited to psychotic disorders (e.g., schizophrenia) and affective disorders (e.g., bipolar), and excluding neurocognitive disorders (e.g., dementia). Cases were removed from the data set for participants who had invalid profiles ($n = 8$) and missing data ($n = 122$). The final sample consisted of 124 relatives of people with mental illness, who spent an average of 45.3 (SD = 36.4) minutes online responding to the survey.

Participants' demographics are noted in Table 1. The family members were divided into two groups. One group was comprised of people who cohabited with their relative with mental illness (n = 81), henceforth referred to as the cohabiting group, while the other group was comprised of people who did not live with their relative with mental illness (n = 43), henceforth referred to as the non-cohabiting group. Individuals in the cohabiting group ranged from 18 to 80 years old, with a mean of 44.0 years old (SD = 17.1). Participants in the non-cohabiting group ranged from 20 to 80 years old, with a mean of 53.8 years old (SD = 17.7). The cohabiting group was significantly younger overall than the non-cohabiting group ($t(df = 78.40) = -2.91, p < 0.01$). Inspection of additional demographics showed generally comparable patterns of distributions between the groups, with the most notable differences being that those in the non-cohabiting group self-identified more as "mother/father" (44%; n = 36 versus 58%; n = 25), less as spouse/partner (11%; n = 14 versus 0%; n = 0), and more as "other" (2%; n = 2 versus 19%; n = 8).

Table 1. Participant Demographics.

Demographic	Cohabiting Family Member Group		Non-Cohabiting Family Member Group	
Participant	n = 81		n = 43	
Age in Years	M = 44.0 (SD = 17.1)		M = 53.8 (SD = 17.7)	
Female	n = 53	(65%)	n = 37	(86%)
Male	n = 27	(33%)	n = 6	(14%)
Non-binary	n = 1	(1%)	n = 0	(0%)
White/European	n = 54	(67%)	n = 32	(74%)
BIPOC	n = 27	(33%)	n = 11	(26%)
Mother/father	n = 36	(44%)	n = 25	(58%)
Sister/brother	n = 21	(26%)	n = 7	(16%)
Daughter/son	n = 11	(14%)	n = 3	(7%)
Spouse/partner	n = 11	(14%)	n = 0	(0%)
Other (e.g., aunt, cousin)	n = 2	(2%)	n = 8	(19%)

Note: BIPOC: Black, indigenous, and people of color.

The demographics for the participants' relatives with SMI are noted in Table 2. The age of the relatives with SMI was not significantly different between the groups. Consistent with participant demographics, an inspection of additional demographics of the relatives with mental illness generally showed comparable distributions between the groups. Importantly, clinical diagnoses of relatives with mental illness were relatively evenly distributed between the groups. Each participant could report more than one mental health condition. This corresponds to concurrent disorders often experienced by relatives with SMI and aligns with previous research which describes the characteristics of relatives with SMI [11].

Table 2. Demographics of Relatives with Mental Illness.

Demographic	Cohabiting Family Member Group		Non-Cohabiting Family Member Group	
Relative with Mental Illness	n = 81		n = 43	
Age in Years	M = 35.8 (SD = 13.66)		M = 40.6 (SD = 15.44)	
Female	n = 30	(37%)	n = 18	(42%)
Male	n = 48	(59%)	n = 24	(56%)
Non-binary	n = 3	(4%)	n = 1	(2%)
White/European	n = 56	(69%)	n = 30	(70%)
BIPOC	n = 25	(31%)	n = 13	(30%)

Table 2. *Cont.*

Demographic	Cohabiting Family Member Group		Non-Cohabiting Family Member Group	
Schizophrenia	$n = 32$	(40%)	$n = 17$	(40%)
Other Psychotic Disorder	$n = 34$	(42%)	$n = 13$	(30%)
Bipolar Disorder	$n = 22$	(27%)	$n = 16$	(37%)
Major Depression	$n = 14$	(17%)	$n = 10$	(23%)
Other Mental Disorder	$n = 14$	(17%)	$n = 11$	(26%)

Note: The sum of the number and percentage of mental illnesses listed exceeds 124 and 100%, respectively, as each participant could report more than one condition. BIPOC: Black, indigenous, and people of color.

2.2. Measures

Demographics were collected through a questionnaire that asked participants to report the age, gender, and race of themselves and their relative with SMI, their relationship to the relative with SMI, and their understanding of the mental illness(es) that their relative is experiencing.

- Stigma by Association Scale (SAS; adapted from Tessler & Gamach [21])

Stigma by association was measured using a 9-item SAS questionnaire originally published by Tessler and Gamach [21] as a subscale of their toolkit. We adapted the measure to specify its relevance for any family member of a person with an SMI (see Supplementary Materials). Therefore, items in the current measure substituted the term "relative" in lieu of the more general term "(NAME)" [21]. Further, minor edits were made to make items more concise and to keep the terminology about their "relative's mental illness" consistent throughout the measure. An example item from the SAS is: "I have felt the need to hide my relative's mental illness", with participants selecting one of five options on a Likert scale ranging from "Never" to "Always", scoring 1–5. The range of possible scores on the SAS is 9–45, with higher scores indicative of more stigma. A cutoff score of 27 (or higher) was established to identify those who report experiencing stigma by association. Cronbach's alpha was very good for the SAS at 0.88.

- Multidimensional Scale of Perceived Social Support (MSPSS; [22])

Perceived social support was measured using the three subscales of the 12-item MSPSS (MSPSS; [22]), which assesses support from a significant other, support from family, and support from friends. Participants were asked to indicate how they felt about a series of statements by selecting one of seven options on a Likert scale ranging from "very strongly disagree" to "very strongly agree". Sample items include the statement: "There is a special person who is around when I am in need" from the support from significant others subscale, "My family really tries to help me" from the support from family subscale, and "I can count on my friends when things go wrong" from the support from friends subscale. The range of possible scores on the MSPSS is 1–7; higher scores are associated with more social support. Cronbach's alpha was found to be very good for the MSPSS subscales, at 0.87 for the significant others scale, 0.91 for the support from family scale, and 0.91 for the support from friends scale.

- General Mattering Scale (GMS; [23])

The GMS [23] was administered to measure how much participants felt that they generally mattered to other people. Participants were asked to select one of four options, from "1 = Not at all" to "4 = A lot", in response to five statements, such as "How important do you feel you are to other people?" Scores on the GMS [23] can range from 5 to 20, with higher scores representing a greater sense of generally mattering to other people. Cronbach's alpha was found to be lower than usual (see [24]) but acceptable for the GMS at 0.66.

- Anti-Mattering Scale (AMS; [18])

Anti-mattering pertains to the feeling that others are treating the individual as unimportant and insignificant [18]. Participants were asked to select one of four options, from "1 = Not at all" to "4 = A lot", in response to five statements, such as "How often have you been made to feel by someone that they don't care about what you think or what you have to say?". AMS scores can range from 5 to 20, with higher scores representing a greater sense of being made to feel unimportant and invisible to other people. Cronbach's alpha was found to be very good for the AMS at 0.87.

- UCLA Loneliness Scale (UCLA LS; [25])

The UCLA Loneliness Scale [25] was used to evaluate how frequently participants felt lonely. Participants were presented with 20 statements, such as "I have nobody to talk to", and instructed to choose one of four responses, from "1 = I never feel this way" to "4 = I often feel this way". Scores on the UCLA Loneliness Scale [25] can range from 20 to 80, and higher scores are associated with feeling lonely more often. Cronbach's alpha was excellent for the UCLA Loneliness Scale [25] at 0.95.

Finally, participants were asked to provide a short answer to the question, "Please describe any experiences you have had with stigma as the family member of a person with mental illness."

2.3. Procedure

Participants gave their informed consent and responded to the survey online. They were administered the demographics questionnaire, the five questionnaire measures, and the short answer question noted above. In addition, participants answered other questionnaire measures and short answer questions as part of a larger ongoing program of research.

2.4. Statistical Analyses

Quantitative data were analyzed in R Studio [26]. Welch's independent *t*-tests were computed to assess differences between the cohabiting group versus the group of people who did not cohabit with their relative with mental illness on the SAS (adapted from Tessler & Gamach [21]), GMS [23], AMS [18], MSPSS subscales [22] and UCLA Loneliness Scale [25]. Correlations were computed between the dependent measures and the AMS [18].

For the qualitative analyses, keyword themes were identified in the responses in accordance with the qualitative analysis stage-by-stage process [27], with the exception that we did not have an opportunity to include the 'member checking' stage since we were unable to return to reach out to the participants.

3. Results

Means and standard deviations for the cohabiting group and non-cohabiting group on the variables examined are noted in Table 3.

Table 3. Descriptive Statistics.

Measures	Total Sample		Cohabiting Family Member Group		Non-Cohabiting Family Member Group	
	M	*SD*	*M*	*SD*	*M*	*SD*
SAS	24.49	7.77	26.11	6.60	21.44	8.91
MSPSS SO	5.13	1.35	4.85	1.29	5.63	1.31
MSPSS FM	4.40	1.48	4.15	1.47	4.85	1.41
MSPSS FR	4.79	1.41	4.52	1.40	5.28	1.30
GMS	15.01	2.77	14.68	2.60	15.63	3.01
AMS	11.89	3.95	12.20	3.63	11.29	4.48
UCLA LS	46.16	14.02	47.22	14.09	44.19	13.83

Note: SAS: Stigma by Association Scale; MSPSS SO: Multidimensional Scales of Perceived Social Support from a Significant Other; MSPSS FM: Multidimensional Scales of Perceived Social Support from Family Members; MSPSS FR: Multidimensional Scales of Perceived Social Support from Friends; GMS: General Mattering Scale; AMS: Anti-mattering Scale; UCLA LS: UCLA Loneliness Scale.

The prevalence of self-reported stigma by association in the community sample was determined to be quite high (n = 43) at a remarkable one in every three family members, based on the SAS cutoff score. It may even be higher in the general population since our sample was recruited through community organization connections. A key finding, based on the SAS (adapted from Tessler & Gamach [21]) questionnaire, was that participants who live with a relative with SMI report significantly higher levels of stigma by association (t(67.06) = 3.02, $p < 0.003$; d = 0.62). The experience of stigma by association was poignantly described in the qualitative response of a 58-year-old mother who resides with her 24-year-old son with SMI: "Raising a child has been very difficult due to stigma. Being blamed as a 'bad parent' was a frequent occurrence for years; from immediate family to strangers, to teachers, to health professionals. It was excruciatingly difficult, and contributed to chronic feelings of self-blame, feeling like a failure, feelings of helplessness, hopelessness, confusion, chaos, isolation … ". Her vivid depiction of many painful emotions tied to stigma was a theme described by other participants and clearly compounded by social isolation and rejection ("my sister has cut me off since discovering my family member's illness").

Analyses of the subscales of the Multidimensional Scale of Perceived Social Support (MSPSS; [22]) confirmed a remarkably consistent pattern in which the cohabiting family member group perceived themselves as having significantly less support from friends (t(92.17) = −3.03, $p < 0.003$; d = 0.56), family (t(89.37) = −2.56, $p < 0.011$; d = 0.48), and significant others (t(84.89) = −3.16, p = 0.002; d = 0.60). A 62-year-old mother who resides with her 32-year-old son, diagnosed with schizophrenia, shared a powerful demonstration of her lived experience of social isolation and its relationship to stigma: "A conversation happened with my son telling family that he had just gotten out of hospital and was diagnosed with schizophrenia. The long and short of it being my family has nothing to do with us now, we are avoided … I told family and they shut us out, I am so hurt and angry at their hypocrisy!"

Analysis of the General Mattering Scale (GMS; [23]) revealed a trend in which people who live with their relative with SMI experience a lower sense that their lives truly matter compared with family members who do not live with their relative (t(75.72) = −1.75, p = 0.08; d = 0.35). This sentiment was reflected by a 24-year-old daughter who resides with her father with SMI, who indicated that her experience of stigma involved "Not being able to talk about my own experiences because it is not as important as the individual with the mental illness." There were no group differences in anti-mattering (t(69.62) = 1.14, p = 0.26; d = 0.22).

Family members who reported experiencing stigma by association (based on the SAS cutoff score) were found to be experiencing moderate levels of loneliness (M = 50.5; SD = 12.7). However, mean scores did not differ significantly between the groups on the UCLA Loneliness Scale [25] (t(87.11) = 1.16, p = 0.25).

Correlations among the measures for the entire sample (n = 124 except for a very few instances of missing data) can be found in Table 4.

Table 4. Pearson Correlation Coefficients (r) for all Participants and all Measures.

Measures	SAS	MSPSS SO	MSPSS FM	MSPSS FR	GMS	AMS
MSPSS SO	−0.09					
MSPSS FM	−0.24 **	0.54 ***				
MSPSS FR	−0.23 *	0.55 ***	0.52 ***			
GMS	−0.18 *	0.39 ***	0.30 ***	0.45 ***		
AMS	0.41 ***	−0.35 ***	−0.51 ***	−0.38 ***	−0.53 ***	
UCLA LS	0.34 ***	−0.53 ***	−0.45 ***	−0.48 ***	−0.44 ***	0.59 ***

* $p < 0.05$; ** $p < 0.01$; *** $p < 0.001$. Note: SAS: Stigma by Association Scale; MSPSS SO: Multidimensional Scales of Perceived Social Support from a Significant Other; MSPSS FM: Multidimensional Scales of Perceived Social Support from Family Members; MSPSS FR: Multidimensional Scales of Perceived Social Support from Friends; GMS: General Mattering Scale; AMS: Anti-mattering Scale; UCLA LS: UCLA Loneliness Scale.

What was clear among all participants were findings that heightened stigma by association was linked to the strong sense that others treat them like they are insignificant or not truly valued, based on the AMS correlation ($r = 0.41$, $p < 0.001$). Further, there was a significant pattern of correlations between anti-mattering (AMS) and the variables of significant other (SO), family member (FM) and friend (FR) social supports (MSPSS), as well as between anti-mattering (AMS) and loneliness (UCLA Loneliness), such that those with reduced social supports and those with heightened loneliness report a significantly reduced sense that their lives matter to others. Further, heightened loneliness (UCLA Loneliness) was strongly associated with all aspects of lack of social support: that is, feeling unsupported by family members, significant others, and friends.

4. Discussion

The study found a startling one in three family members with relatives with SMI reported experiencing stigma by association. These family members were found to be experiencing, on average, at least moderate levels of loneliness in what is, to our knowledge, among the very first empirical studies of loneliness, social isolation, and stigma by association in a North American family member sample. The findings are consistent with recent research that found so-called 'loneliness in the presence of others' in family members who care for a relative with severe mental illness in Iran [6] and are also consistent with past research in Scandinavian family members [28,29]. Our findings also echo prior qualitative research that found family members of people with SMI experienced stigma by association and perceived themselves as lacking social support [7,30], particularly those who cohabited with their relatives [31].

Specifically, family members who live with a relative with SMI were found to feel significantly more social isolation compared with those family members who do not cohabit with their relative with SMI, according to family, friends, and significant other social support measures. The extent of their isolation is considerable, reflected in the striking findings that their MSPSS subscale levels were considerably lower than the original MSPSS psychometric validation studies [32] and much lower than those obtained recently from a community maternal caregiver sample [33]. The public health implications of this finding are clear, according to a study conducted in Turkey on social support in family caregivers [5]: that is, family caregivers with reduced social support are at heightened risk for burnout. Individuals who experience psychosis are themselves among the loneliest and socially isolated of adults, according to national surveys conducted in Australia [34]. The current research suggests that family members who live with relatives with SMI may also be quite marginalized in society, related to their experiences of stigma by association.

However, the findings of the current study point to the importance of 'mattering' as a key factor in the experience of lack of social support experienced by family members. Specifically, family members who are experiencing the most loneliness and who feel the most socially isolated are missing the sense that their lives truly matter to others; they are experiencing what has been termed a *double jeopardy* of feeling both lonely and unimportant [19]. This sense of mattering has been seen as a critical support for people during the COVID-19 pandemic [35], that there are true benefits from feeling that someone sees you as being important and valued.

In this regard, we extended past research that linked the new AMS measure with loneliness by showing that this association is not only present in university students (see [19]). It is also detectable among adults who have family members with serious mental illnesses. The findings align with the conclusion [18] that the anti-mattering construct has a particular focus on, and perhaps sensitivity to, feelings of being marginalized.

Examination of the qualitative responses gathered in the current study appears to mirror the social exclusion themes found in previous qualitative research [11,12], which are highlighted by the disturbing salience of the anti-mattering construct among the most stigmatized of our participants. Anti-mattering empirical findings are underscored by emotionally intense self-disclosures in participant responses about being shut out and cut off from other family members because of their relative with SMI. Feeling not listened to, feeling that what is being said is not important, and feeling like there is no opportunity to talk about their own experiences are troubling findings among these family members whose stigma reports seem poignantly linked to being ostracized even by those closest to them. This experience, for them, is too close for comfort.

There appears to be a dearth of interventions aimed at reducing stigma by association, according to a recent scoping review [36]. Future research should consider the implications of the current findings, particularly those that link societal stigma and marginalization with feelings of not mattering. Some suggested interventions have included transformative education, sharing, disclosure, social networking, and support, as well as public education, to correct misconceptions surrounding mental illness. The current findings highlight the importance of these interventions to address the specific need for heightened public mental health awareness surrounding stigma by association and the need to reach out with support to those marginalized individuals who are particularly affected by it.

One limitation of the current study relates to recruitment issues. Our sample was obtained by contacting local and nationally connected support organizations. The population of relatives of those with SMI has been particularly challenging to recruit for research participation, which is not surprising given the findings of social isolation. It is possible, and in fact quite likely, given the links of our participants to support organizations, that the prevalence of stigma by association is even higher, and the extent of loneliness and social isolation is underestimated in the broader population of family members. A further limitation is that the diagnoses of the relatives with mental illness were not independently verified; like other research in this area, we relied on family member self-reports.

5. Conclusions

The current study begins to address the gap in the existing family stigma literature by providing evidence of mental illness stigma by association, loneliness and social isolation in a North American sample. Through quantitative analyses, findings showed that the cohabiting family member group experienced higher levels of stigma by association and social isolation compared to the non-cohabiting group, though all participants experienced loneliness. The public health implications are that this is a marginalized group that is at serious risk for caregiver burnout, which would likely be exacerbated among caregivers who feel they are unappreciated and insignificant. The findings extend previous research, mainly restricted to qualitative studies, conducted in Scandinavia, Turkey, and Iran. In future studies, there is a need to examine societal interventions for reducing stigma by association as well as increasing the sense of mattering among family members, particularly those who live with a relative with SMI, because of the extent of their loneliness combined with heightened social isolation.

Supplementary Materials: The following supporting information can be downloaded at: https://www.mdpi.com/article/10.3390/ijerph20065209/s1. The Stigma by Association Scale (SAS) adapted from Reference [21] is provided in the supplementary materials.

Author Contributions: J.O.G. lab direction and supervision, writing; S.A.M. recruitment, analysis, writing; A.L.R. analysis, writing; H.L.-R. writing; G.L.F. conceptualization, writing and review. All authors have read and agreed to the published version of the manuscript.

Funding: This research received no external funding.

Institutional Review Board Statement: The study was conducted according to the guidelines of the Declaration of Helsinki and approved by the York University Human Participants Research Committee (REB Certificate #: e2021-316; 23 September 2021).

Informed Consent Statement: Informed consent was obtained from all participants involved in the study.

Data Availability Statement: The datasets presented in this article are not readily available because the requesting source must be affiliated with an academic institution. Requests to access the datasets should be directed to the corresponding author: jgoldber@yorku.ca.

Acknowledgments: We acknowledge and are grateful to the following organizations for their much valued time and efforts in the recruitment of participants: the Canadian Mental Health Association, the Institute for Advancements in Mental Health (formerly the Schizophrenia Society of Ontario), Reconnect Community Health Services, and the Schizophrenia Society of York University.

Conflicts of Interest: The authors declare no conflict of interest.

References

1. Rumas, R.; Shamblaw, A.L.; Jagtap, S.; Best, M.W. Predictors and consequences of loneliness during the COVID-19 pandemic. *Psychiatry Res.* **2021**, *300*, 113934. [CrossRef] [PubMed]
2. Holt-Lunstad, J.; Smith, T.B.; Baker, M.; Harris, T.; Stephenson, D. Loneliness and social isolation as risk factors for mortality: A meta-analytic review. *Perspect. Psychol. Sci.* **2015**, *10*, 227–237. [CrossRef] [PubMed]
3. Best, M.W.; Bowie, C.R. Social exclusion in psychotic disorders: An interactional processing model. *Schizophr. Res.* **2022**, *244*, 91–100. [CrossRef]
4. Wirsén, E.; Åkerlund, S.; Ingvarsdotter, K.; Hjärthag, F.; Östman, M.; Persson, K. Burdens experienced and perceived needs of relatives of persons with SMI—A systematic meta-synthesis. *J. Ment. Health* **2020**, *29*, 712–721. [CrossRef]
5. Kokurcan, A.; Özpolat, A.G.Y.; Gogus, A.K. Burnout in caregivers of patients with schizophrenia. *Turk. J. Med. Sci.* **2015**, *45*, 678–685. [CrossRef] [PubMed]
6. Tabatabaee, M.; Yousefi Nooraie, R.; Mohammad Aghaei, A.; Rostam-Abadi, Y.; Ansari, M.; Sharifi, S.; Sharifi, V. Loneliness in the presence of others: A mixed-method study of social networks of caregivers of patients with severe mental disorders. *Int. J. Soc. Psychiatry* **2023**, *69*, 190–199. [CrossRef]
7. Phelan, J.C.; Bromet, E.J.; Link, B.G. Psychiatric illness and family stigma. *Schizophr. Bull.* **1998**, *24*, 115–126. [CrossRef]
8. Struening, E.L.; Perlick, D.A.; Link, B.G.; Hellman, F.; Herman, D.; Sirey, J.A. Stigma as a barrier to recovery: The extent to which caregivers believe most people devalue consumers and their families. *Psychiatr. Serv.* **2001**, *52*, 1633–1638. [CrossRef]
9. Corrigan, P.W.; Miller, F.E. Shame, blame, and contamination: A review of the impact of mental illness stigma on family members. *J. Ment. Health* **2004**, *13*, 537–548. [CrossRef]
10. Östman, M. The burden experienced by relatives of those with a severe mental illness—Differences between those living with and those living apart from the patient. *J. Psychiatr. Intensive Care* **2007**, *3*, 35–43. [CrossRef]
11. Van der Sanden, R.L.M.; Stutterheim, S.E.; Pryor, J.B.; Kok, G.; Bos, A.E.R. Coping with stigma by association and family burden among family members of people with mental illness. *J. Nerv. Ment. Dis.* **2014**, *202*, 710–717. [CrossRef] [PubMed]
12. Van der Sanden, R.L.M.; Bos, A.E.R.; Stutterheim, S.E.; Pryor, J.B.; Kok, G. Stigma by association among family members of people with a mental illness: A qualitative analysis. *J. Community Appl. Soc. Psychol.* **2015**, *25*, 400–417. [CrossRef]
13. Richard-Lepouriel, H.; Aubry, J.M.; Favre, S. Is coping with sigma by association role-specific for different family members? A qualitative study with bipolar disorder patients' relatives. *Community Ment. Health J.* **2022**, *58*, 179–192. [CrossRef] [PubMed]
14. Yin, M.; Li, Z.; Zhou, C. Experience of stigma among family members of people with severe mental illness: A qualitative systematic review. *Int. J. Ment. Health Nurs.* **2020**, *29*, 141–160. [CrossRef] [PubMed]
15. Martens, L.; Addington, J. The psychological wellbeing of family members of individuals with schizophrenia. *Soc. Psychiatry Psychiatr. Epidemiol.* **2001**, *36*, 128–133. [CrossRef]
16. Laidlaw, T.M.; Coverdale, J.H.; Fallon, I.R.; Fydd, R.R. Caregiver's stresses when living together or apart from patients with chronic schizophrenia. *Community Ment. Health J.* **2002**, *38*, 303–310. [CrossRef]
17. Elliott, G.; Kao, S.; Grant, A.-M. Mattering: Empirical validation of a social-psychological concept. *Self Identity* **2004**, *3*, 339–354. [CrossRef]
18. Flett, G.L.; Nepon, T.; Goldberg, J.O.; Rose, A.L.; Atkey, S.K.; Zaki-Azat, J. The Anti-Mattering Scale: Development, psychometric properties, and associations with well-being and distress measures in adolescents and emerging adults. *J. Psychoeduc. Assess.* **2022**, *40*, 37–59. [CrossRef]
19. McComb, S.E.; Goldberg, J.O.; Flett, G.L.; Rose, A.L. The double jeopardy of feeling lonely and unimportant: State and trait loneliness and feelings and fears of not mattering. *Front. Psychol.* **2020**, *11*, 563420. [CrossRef]
20. Taylor, J.; Turner, R.J. A longitudinal study of the role and significance of mattering to others for depressive symptoms. *J. Health Soc. Behav.* **2001**, *42*, 310–325. [CrossRef]
21. Tessler, R.; Gamache, G. *Evaluating Family Experiences with Severe Mental Illness*; Human Services Research Institute: Cambridge, MA, USA, 1993; p. 87.
22. Zimet, G.D.; Dahlem, N.W.; Zimet, S.G.; Farley, G.K. The multidimensional scale of perceived social support. *J. Personal. Assess.* **1988**, *52*, 30–41. [CrossRef]
23. Marcus, F.M.; Rosenberg, M. Mattering: Its measurement and significance in everyday life. In Proceedings of the 57th Annual Eastern Sociological Society Meeting, Boston, MA, USA, March 1987.

24. Flett, G.L. *The Psychology of Mattering: Understanding the Human Need to Be Significant*; Elsevier Academic Press: Cambridge, MA, USA, 2018.
25. Russell, D.; Peplau, L.A.; Ferguson, M.L. Developing a measure of loneliness. *J. Personal. Assess.* **1978**, *42*, 290–294. [CrossRef] [PubMed]
26. R Core Team. *R: A Language and Environment for Statistical Computing*; R Foundation for Statistical Computing: Vienna, Austria, 2022; Available online: https://www.r-project.org/ (accessed on 2 January 2023).
27. Burnard, P. A method of analysing interview transcripts in qualitative research. *Nurse Educ. Today* **1991**, *11*, 461–466. [CrossRef] [PubMed]
28. Van der Sanden, R.L.M.; Bos, A.E.R.; Stutterheim, S.E.; Pryor, J.B.; Kok, G. Experiences of stigma by association among family members of people with mental illness. *Rehabil. Psychol.* **2013**, *58*, 73–80. [CrossRef] [PubMed]
29. Van der Sanden, R.L.M.; Pryor, J.B.; Stutterheim, S.E.; Kok, G.; Bos, A.E.R. Stigma by association and family burden among family members of people with mental illness: The mediating role of coping. *Soc. Psychiatry Psychiatr. Epidemiol.* **2016**, *51*, 1233–1245. [CrossRef]
30. Wahl, O.F.; Harman, C.R. Family views of stigma. *Schizophr. Bull.* **1989**, *15*, 131–139. [CrossRef]
31. Ostman, M.; Kjellin, L. Stigma by association: Psychological factors in relatives of people with mental illness. *Br. J. Psychiatry* **2002**, *181*, 494–498. [CrossRef]
32. Zimet, G.D.; Powell, S.S.; Farley, G.K.; Werkman, S.; Berkoff, K.A. Psychometric characteristics of the Multidimensional Scale of Perceived Social Support. *J. Personal. Assess.* **1990**, *55*, 610–617.
33. Li, H. Maternal-Infant Attachment and its Relationships with Postpartum Depression, Anxiety, Affective Instability, Stress, and Social Support in a Canadian Community Sample. *Psychiatr. Q.* **2023**, *94*, 9–22. [CrossRef]
34. Stain, H.J.; Galletly, C.A.; Clark, S.; Wilson, J.; Killen, E.A.; Anthes, L.; Harvey, C. Understanding the social costs of psychosis: The experience of adults affected by psychosis identified within the second Australian National Survey of Psychosis. *Aust. N. Z. J. Psychiatry* **2012**, *46*, 879–889. [CrossRef]
35. Flett, G.L.; Zangeneh, M. Mattering as a vital support for people during the COVID-19 pandemic: The benefits of feeling and knowing that someone cares during times of crisis. *J. Concurr. Disord.* **2020**, *2*, 106. [CrossRef]
36. Adu, J.; Oudshoorn, A.; Anderson, K.; Marshall, C.A.; Stuart, H.; Stanley, M. Policies and interventions to reduce familial mental illness stigma: A scoping review of empirical literature. *Issues Ment. Health Nurs.* **2021**, *2*, 1123–1137. [CrossRef] [PubMed]

International Journal of
Environmental Research and Public Health

MDPI

Article

Loneliness in Young Adult Workers

Sarah L. Wright [1,*] and Anthony G. Silard [2]

[1] Department of Management, Marketing & Entrepreneurship, University of Canterbury, Christchurch 8041, New Zealand
[2] Center for Sustainable Leadership, Luiss Business School, 00162 Rome, Italy
* Correspondence: sarah.wright@canterbury.ac.nz; Tel.: +64-3-369-3762

Abstract: Loneliness is commonly associated with older people with the majority of research and interventions focusing on loneliness in aged and aging populations. However, loneliness seems to be on the rise for young adults more so than the elderly. Our research focusses on the experiences of young workers who report feeling lonely at work. We explore individual and organisational factors that may be contributing to loneliness, and comment on the consequences of feeling lonely at work. Qualitative data from 37 young adults from Western Europe suggest that these workers feel invisible at work, have a thwarted sense of belonging to their employing organisation, and often experience relational deficiencies due to automation and individualisation of work practices.

Keywords: loneliness; social relationships at work; belongingness; young adult workers; social disconnection; work practices

1. Introduction

"I'm seen as this figure, in this role, but not as me ... it's really isolating being treated as a nothing, like you as a person don't exist" Retail worker, 23 years

"I think it's a time in life that often gets overlooked. I think school children tend to get a lot of interventions and things but once you leave school and go out into the big wide world you kind of get thrown out, and it's a time of a lot of change when you're moving away or starting a new job or going to uni, and it's just so many changes and it can be very overwhelming and very lonely." Marketing assistant, 24 years

Loneliness has historically been known to predominately afflict older people, with the majority of research and interventions focussing on loneliness in aged and aging populations. Indeed, there is a vast research literature examining the prevalence and negative outcomes of loneliness in older age [1]. However, loneliness seems to be on the rise for young adults more so than the elderly. Recent research indicates that people over 65 are now more likely than any other age group to say they *never* feel lonely, with young adults (18–25 years) across Europe [2], New Zealand [3], Australia [4], the UK [5] and USA indicating higher incidences of loneliness than their older counterparts [6]. According to a recent Cigna survey of more than 6000 workers, loneliness at work is also on the rise, but it appears to be most prevalent among younger workers (<38 years), of whom nearly half report feeling lonely when they are at work [7]. In the workplace, lonely workers tend to have lower performance ratings, are less committed and less approachable than their non-lonely co-workers [8], and take twice as much sick leave [9]. The silence of loneliness and the stigma associated with it adds to the complexity of addressing these adverse outcomes.

In view of the emerging evidence of the growing prevalence of loneliness among young adults, it is helpful to gain insight into the experience of loneliness among young workers. The current study offers a preliminary understanding of loneliness among young adult workers in Western Europe by exploring the interaction between life stage as an individual characteristic and the organisational context as a socio-environmental characteristic. Such insight will ultimately lead us to develop further research studies and design age-appropriate interventions.

Loneliness is the psychological pain of perceived relationship deficiencies [10]. Perception is critical to this definition: people can live relatively solitary lives and not feel lonely, or can have many social relationships and nevertheless feel lonely. Consequently, loneliness is more closely related to the perceived quality than the quantity of social relationships and can be devastating for one's psychological and physical health [11], even more so than obesity [12]. Loneliness is also a potent risk factor for suicide [13]; a link that is particularly evident for teenagers and young adults [14]. Feeling lonely can be particularly acute during young adulthood because this stage in life also presents the greatest risk period for the emergence of depression and magnifies the stigma of loneliness given the strong pressure to appear socially connected [15].

In addition, while the pernicious effects of rejection are felt by all age groups [16] and can cause an individual to feel like life is less meaningful [17]—even if the rejection is by a group the individual does not wish to belong to [18]—these effects can be particularly severe for young adults [19]. As such, young adults are often at greater risk for experiencing loneliness because rapid social changes are often occurring, existing support networks can be unstable, and new stressors are introduced, such as starting work and carving out an occupational or professional identity. Given this context, it seems that young adulthood is a vulnerable time for loneliness.

Importantly for the current research, young adulthood represents an era where the individual strives to form and maintain social bonds and meaningful relationships with non-family members, and explores independence and multiple facets of their potential occupational identity. We know from prior research that having social support and a sense of belonging during emerging adulthood is an important foundation for positive physical and mental health [20]. As such, studying the transition and exploration during emerging adulthood are not new avenues to explore in loneliness research. However, what is novel is the contemporary labour market young adults enter and the individual variation of their experiences. The psychology of working framework [21] is a theoretical model that can help frame the sociocultural aspects of contemporary work experiences and shape how organisational contexts can be a major influence on an individual's psychological wellbeing. The core assumptions of the psychology of working model are that work (i) has a major influence on well-being, (ii) is intertwined with other life spheres, (iii) is shaped by socioeconomic, political, and historical factors, (iv) encompasses both paid and unpaid activities, (v) is important for workers and nonworkers who want to work, and (vi) can potentially satisfy fundamental human needs. The current study adopts these assumptions, with special emphasis on the role of work as a vehicle that shapes relational experiences.

Young adult workers are entering the workforce amidst new ways of working—in part driven by the pandemic [22]—which may be contributing to loneliness in this age group. Contemporary ways of working are also likely to see the continuing rise of digitalization, automation and individuation in young adult working lives that can increase social isolation (e.g., remote work, virtual work, piece-rate and gig-economy jobs, platform work). These changes in the way work is conducted is accompanied by changes in employment contracts to accommodate more flexible working arrangements (e.g., causal work, temporary/fixed-term/variable contracts, or self-employment). Such work often comprises a lot of time spent alone socially distant from coworkers or in temporary employment rather than in socially connected workplaces, and may increase feelings of disconnection and loneliness. Additionally, the fragmentation of the traditional '9-to-5' workday shared with coworkers in-person and the rise of virtual and precarious work in the 'gig' economy [23] often mean a lot of time spent alone with less meaningful face-to-face interactions that might thwart the environment emerging adults need to build fulfilling social bonds. Researching the psychosocial consequences of this evolution of work is important, including studying feelings of loneliness that emerges while working. We know much about the personal factors that predispose people to loneliness (especially in childhood and older adulthood) but the interpersonal and contextual factors are much less understood, making targeted evidence-driven interventions and evaluation problematic.

Technology and social media are often touted as both the blame and remedy for youth loneliness. However, there is growing recognition that the underpinnings of loneliness are more complex and interact with environmental factors in multifaceted ways. Available evidence suggests that different age groups experience loneliness differentially in various contexts [24], and can arise from psychosocial tasks and relationships unique to that period. This evidence suggests that it is important to study life stage *and* context when understanding loneliness in the workplace. However, context is not often considered a property of loneliness, and the workplace context is given even less consideration when understanding the nature of the experience. Although data from online and media surveys [25] indicate the majority of workers feel lonely and 53% would give up some compensation for more meaningful relationships with colleagues [26], very little academic research explores how the nature of contemporary labour is contributing to loneliness. Because of the stigma and feelings of personal failure associated with loneliness, not all young adults will seek help. The stigma and associated inhibition of disclosing feelings of loneliness may be highlighted in a social context such as the workplace where interactions are often coupled with power and status differentials, which are often not in the young adult's control or influence. In view of the increasing prevalence of loneliness among young adults in general, it is important to gain a better understanding of work and its intersection with loneliness that is unique to this developmental period [27]. Our primary research objective is to understand the experiences and consequences of loneliness at work for young adults. Our more speculative goal is to generate an awareness that loneliness is a political, economic, and social reality, rather than simply an individual problem.

2. Method

2.1. Research Design

Existing research on loneliness often associates the experience with a mental illness such as depression or social anxiety and is therefore perceived as an individual deficit. Loneliness is rarely studied from the perspective of those whom are often in the company of others, e.g., in a collective workplace (physical or virtual). Therefore, this preliminary study seeks to explore the meaning of this particular aspect of loneliness in organisational contexts. Because human existence in organisations is fundamentally interpersonal and exists in a push and pull of intersubjectivity, we used qualitative methods to explore the meaning of young worker loneliness and to begin to understand the role organisations (systems, processes, and the people that engage in them), play in its development and maintenance.

Some time ago, Rook [28] argued that researchers should take a differentiated view of loneliness and incorporate these distinctions into research methodologies. However, it is evident that most research on workplace loneliness is quantitative (e.g., [8,29–34]). We chose a qualitative inductive research design given the exploratory nature of the study and our interest in the participants' experiences of loneliness. This approach helped us respond to our research objective of understanding the experience of participants rather than using standardised measures of loneliness to determine hypothesized predictions. We felt this approach would allow us to more fully understand the reasons why young workers identify as lonely, as the feelings of loneliness may differ widely depending on the experiences of the young worker and have various consequences.

2.2. Procedure

We used the data collection service provider, Prolific, to recruit participants aged 18–25 years who were employed at least part-time in a work environment interacting with other people. Prolific was used for several reasons: (i) because we wanted to pre-screen participants for their age, employment status, and degree of loneliness before they participated in the qualitative study (i.e., workers were screened for and excluded from participating if they were older than 25 years, were unemployed, and responded 'never' or 'hardly ever' to the question how often they felt lonely at work); (ii) participants could remain completely anonymous using only their Prolific ID as an identifier, (iii) the questions required responses of a private and sensitive nature and thus we wanted separation from any particular sponsoring or employing organisation, and (iv) the Prolific pool of participants has shown to be of a good quality [35]. The survey was open for seven days in November 2021. Participants could choose where and on what device to complete the survey so their responses were private without fear of organizational monitoring. From a possible 40 respondents, we analysed 37 useable responses. Participants were from Portugal, Spain, Italy, England, and Poland; 14 were female, 22 were male, 1 was non-binary, with an average age of 22 years. Each participant was offered £10 to participate in the study. Informed consent was obtained prior to participation, and no information on participant identity was collected at any time. The study was reviewed and approved by the University of Canterbury Human Ethics Committee (HEC 2020/113).

We used Qualtrics to create an online anonymous survey and to collect data on participant's experiences of loneliness in their work. Anonymous online surveys are a suitable medium to collect data on sensitive topics such as loneliness [36], and allow for the disclosure of potentially negative depictions of the respondent's workplace, supervisor, or coworkers because of the assured anonymity. We also felt interviews with a stranger on a highly sensitive and stigmatised subject matter such as loneliness may result in socially desirable responses.

In the online survey, we provided information on the nature of the study and sought informed consent before proceeding. Participants could opt-out at any time during the survey. We asked several warm-up questions about the nature of the participant's role, and then the following study-specific open-ended questions to elicit as much detail as possible. Example questions include: *I want you to think about a time when you have felt especially lonely at work. Tell me about that time [where were you working at the time, what tasks were you doing, who else (if anyone) were you working with, why do you think it was an especially lonely time?]. What do you do when you feel lonely at work? How does loneliness affect you? What do you think are the reasons for your loneliness?*

2.3. Data Analysis

All of the analysis was carried out using the verbatim text from the survey data. The length of the entries varied depending on the stories and scenarios described by the participants. Word count averaged 588 words for each participant and each took on average 46 min to complete the survey. Thematic analysis was carried out based on the procedure described by Braun and Clarke [37]. To summarise, we (i) read the text several times to build familiarity with the data, both across the entries and within each participant's responses; (ii) created a set of broad themes, (iii) reviewed the themes for meaning and succinctness, and (iv) described the final three themes with exemplar anonymised quotes to support them. The initial coding and identification of themes was repeated by a doctoral student (not involved in the data collection) who was blind to the initial analysis. This process helped strengthen the reliability of the analysis. The labels and description of the final themes were discussed between the researchers and agreed upon after multiple rounds of discussion and analysis. Quotes reported in this paper are verbatim without grammatical correction.

3. Results and Discussion

Thematic analysis of the data from lonely workers suggested three main themes, which we labelled 'feeling unheard and unseen at work', 'thwarted belongingness', and 'individuation of work'.

3.1. Theme 1: Feeling Unheard and Unseen at Work

> *"I'd like to be of use at work, and be comfortable enough that someone higher up would want to speak with me and, like, see you, and you're sort of actually having those conversations go in different directions and then realise that others at work don't really listen to you"*—Oil data analyst, 23 years

Visibility at work can be thought of as the degree to which an employee is "fully regarded and recognised by others" [38] (p. 63). Several participants wrote about work environments where they did not feel they mattered, that they experienced little care or positive attention, or felt directly undermined. Their invisibility was noticeable and distressing. The experiences typically reflected two phenomena; one relating to perceived deficiencies in the participant's character resulting in them feeling invisible or unnoticed (i.e., something is wrong with me), and another of other organizational members in the environment excluding them (i.e., no one notices me).

> *"When I feel really lonely at work ... you kind of think there's something wrong with you and you think you're lonely because no one likes you and because you don't matter and no one cares"* Cook, 20 years

> *"There are certain times when, for instance, a certain thing must be done that can be "more difficult", so [my supervisor] decides to ask my [coworker] about it instead of me, or for him to do my work instead of me, while choosing to ignore me and the things I pitch in, only because "I'm the new one". That feels odd, like I go unnoticed, and besides, it also feels like she [the supervisor] never trusts me"* Accounting assistant, 22 years

Dispersed through the participant's entries were elements of a lack of care in not being seen or heard, feeling misunderstood or that the person does not matter to anyone at work.

> *"no one really talks or interacts with me and I felt really lonely and unwanted"* Warehouse worker, 22 years

> *"If I call in sick, no one would bother wondering what's wrong ... and then I'm blasted when I go back to work for taking sick ... no one cares"* Check-in assistant, 23 years

> *" ... I lost a family member and was upset [at work], but I knew not to tell any of my coworkers. I felt lonely because nobody knew and nobody cared and I really wanted someone with who I could share my problems"* Salesperson, 25 years

A useful framework to help explain these observations is Buber's [39] 'I and Thou' theory, which describes how people treat each other and how they learn to interact with others. Buber distinguishes between seeing people as I–It where people are used as a goal or tool toward an outcome, or I–Thou where the other is acknowledged and treated as a meaningful human being. It appears from our data that many lonely workers are in environments where people are treated as a means to an end.

When prompted to think about their loneliest experience, one participant commented that the worst aspect of that experience was

> *"not being able to express myself, my feelings, or raise issues ... I felt completely ignored"* [in relation to a team decision that affected their work] Graphics creator, 24 years

Another commented of the inability to talk with others about her feelings:

> *" ... nobody even notices you need help with [tasks], so it kind of hit me really hard that nobody even listens or even notices. I felt really lonely because it felt like there is some kind of magical barrier between us and we couldn't really even talk about it"* Recruitment coordinator, 23 years

Jung [40] argued long ago that being lonely is not merely social isolation, but rather it includes not being heard or understood: "Loneliness does not come from having no people about one, but from being unable to communicate the things that seem important to oneself, or from holding views which others find inadmissible" (p. 356). This insight seems to resonate for many young adults in the contemporary workforce, in that they feel 'overlooked', 'ignored', or 'silenced'. Furthermore, it was evident in the data that employees were not strategically managing their level of visibility by hiding parts of who they are, which may be a strategy exercised in more senior roles to establish and maintain professional distance [38].

In reporting the experiences of being unseen or unheard in the experience of loneliness, we are cognisant that lonely people tend to have a cognitive bias and heightened awareness of social threat [41]. Therefore, our sample of lonely workers is likely to experience and report some social interactions as more threatening or abrasive than non-lonely workers. Respondents wrote about a lack of felt care from others in the organisation, or feeling undervalued or unappreciated. It is unclear from our data whether this lack of felt care stems from a lack of reciprocity (i.e., lonely individuals are less able to capitalise on the benefits of interpersonal interaction due to heightened levels of social rejection) or the withdrawal from others that isolates them further and results in their failing to pick up on caring cues. The sad irony, though, of not having a voice or feeling invisible at work is that young lonely workers may not gain the experience of interpersonal and group interactions that might foster social skill development as they mature in their working lives. As a result, they may develop less skill in appropriately disclosing their experiences of relational deficiency, further reinforcing their distress and heightened sense of social threat. A consequence of this vicious cycle [42] is that young workers may ultimately miss the opportunity to build trusting and fulfilling relationships at work.

3.2. Theme 2: Thwarted Belongingness

This theme describes participants feeling disconnected from the social fabric of the organisation, which is both elemental to their loneliness and a consequence from it. Frequently, this was simply a result of age or other individual differences leading to participants feeling alienated from the in-group and not 'fitting-in'.

> *" . . . here's what I believe: Most of the times, it is as though I feel like an odd one out, like I can hardly relate to others in terms of what I'm currently experiencing: I'm the youngest at work, and my coworkers can be a bit hard to confide in, at times, so it feels like I don't have that many people to talk to"* Accounting assistant, 22 years

> *Since I was the latest "addition" to the office sometimes I feel left out with my coworkers since they have been working together for many many years and I just arrived like a few months ago, they have their own inside jokes and besides since they are men and I'm the only woman in the office it's kinda hard for me to catch up whilst talking whenever we get to be together. At those times when they are talking/sharing experiences or memories is when i feel alone"* Administrative worker, 24 years

Not surprisingly for a sample of lonely workers, most of the participants reported various degrees of feeling only superficially connected to others at work, or being directly ostracised from the social fabric of the organisation.

> *"At that moment everyone stopped talking and laughing and stared at me like if I had to say something wrong. I immediately shut up and one of the girls said "what are you laughing about? This is a personal joke, you don't even know him". And I just answered "Oh, I do know him from X" and then I left. I felt like the biggest idiot on earth and went to the bathroom to cry a little. I was so humiliated and ashamed that it took me a couple of minutes to recompose myself. No one ever mentioned anything about that moment again"* Hospitality frontline worker, 23 years

> *"we had a hard morning and by 3 p.m we was working yet without eat. We had a break in work and we had to choose how to eat without leave the service alone. all my co-workers choose eat together and leave me alone in service. I felt that no one likes my company and that's why they choose me to be alone"* Nurse intern, 25 years

> *"I feel lonely whenever I hear them [coworkers] laugh outside my office, it makes me wish I could have someone to relate"* Polygraph processer, 24 years

> *"I can get a bit desperate for connection with others"* Postal worker, 22 years

Social isolation is in itself a neutral experience. It is the affective component, the *'desperation'* and *'wish'* for connection that is part of the experience of loneliness, coupled with the distress of social disconnection. For this reason, loneliness can be considered a subjective rather than objective sense of social isolation. Thwarted belongingness is a "psychologically painful mental state that results when the fundamental need for connectedness is unmet" [43] (p. 2). This state is evident with many of our lonely workers. The cognitive and affective effort to process, interpret and understand the implications of being social excluded [44] (p. 841) can inhibit self-regulation of socially accepted behaviours [45] and can manifest as being ostracised from the group. As mentioned earlier, these effects of ostracism can be especially painful for young adults. This is seen in the above quote where the nurse intern realises that there must be something about their behaviour which is creating social exclusion.

For some participants, there are tentative links between workplace incivility, ostracism and thwarted belongingness.

> *"There was one time when I accidently dropped a customer's item and we couldn't find it (it was a microSD card) and it was really stressful for me, especially because the customer was starting to get angry and stress out and my coworkers were pressuring me a lot. I eventually found it but I felt really bad about it and my coworkers didn't communicate with me for the rest of the day"* Retail worker, 20 years

Without a sense of belonging to the group or workplace, there is no protective buffer for the young worker between the experience of incivility or the 'silent treatment' and feelings of ostracism. In fact, a quarter of participants used the words "anger" or "angry" in expressing narratives about their interactions with other coworkers or superiors, and corresponding with the first theme many participants conflated this hostile or ostracising behaviour with something being "wrong" with them. Such treatment or negative affective experiences can result in feelings of exclusion from the social milieu of the organisation.

According to Hagerty et al. [46] there are three main individual antecedents in developing a sense of belonging: the potential and desire for meaningful involvement, the potential for shared characteristics, and energy for involvement. Our data shows some evidence of the first two factors being thwarted in young workers' experiences (i.e., the desperation and wish for social connection, and the feelings of not fitting in due to age or some other perceived personal deficiencies). Energy for involvement is a code that emerged in the data both from the participant's perspective and from those they work with. That is, there is a bidirectional element—a lack of effort by others at work to connect with the referent when they are lonely coupled with a lack of effort on the referent's behalf to connect with others.

> *"When I feel really alone at work, I try to put on some wireless headphones at work and listen to some music at a low level, I usually go to the bathroom a little more often to clear up my feelings of loneliness"* Administrative worker, 24 years

> *"I'm the new one, so I do feel lonely most of the time, because noone talks to me and when that happens I feel bad and decide to distract myself with my cellphone"* Check-in assistant, 23 years

> *"Often I want to talk to someone and then I just go "Nooo they don't really care, I shouldn't bother them" and I just don't"*. Recruitment coordinator, 23 years

As per the last two comments, there seems to be a reward and punishment mechanism built into social interaction that derails a sense of belonging. That is, social interaction is not rewarding for the individual, therefore they gravitate toward solitary engagement or acknowledge mechanisms in place whereby people are inhibited from interacting:

> *"I felt more loneliness when I have my break lunch, it's really annoying that our business has different rest times for each one. I eat total alone, sometimes is okay but the rest of*

the time I felt it's not fair. They are breaking our labor relation, in my opinion" Dental assistant, 24 years

"Having social relationship at work is really important, but my job is a bit restrictant about interacting with others (excepting phone calls)" Telemarketer, 24 years

The regular, continuous social interaction that can often provide a rich source of reward and social learning in organisations, in these instances, is obstructed. Through their examples, several participants mentioned work practices that inhibited social connection, such as solitary break times to keep operations moving, unpredictable work schedules, and limited collaborative activities. Focussing solely on work tasks can implicitly remove the permission to interact, and therefore stymie the opportunity for social connection.

Thwarted belongingness was also encapsulated by a lack of social support felt during times of work challenges, resulting in the worker feeling alone and vulnerable.

"At work I feel like there is so much to figure out, and who I can ask because I don't know everything yet. I just turned up and was kind of left alone. I wasn't sure what do to do and that felt quite lonely" Call centre workers, 23 years

"I would say that the most lonely I feel when there is a very stressful day or situation at work and there is nobody around I could talk to to let the steam out" Recruitment coordinator, 23 years

"I like to have the support of the workers when I have doubts about something I haven't learned how to do, so if no one is available to help me, I feel lonely" Product promoter, 22 years

Social support is a central feature in the experience of belonging, particularly in endeavours of shared activities [47]. Furthermore, our sense of support can be adversely affected by interpersonal moments that undermine belonging needs [48]. It is important to note that while a lack of social support is a strong antecedent to loneliness, it is not the experience of loneliness itself. Rather, social support represents a set of interpersonal behaviours (or perceptions of behaviours) that are distinguishable from loneliness. Our data suggest that the affective experiences derived from a lack of social support, particularly those situations that arise from needing help, contribute to a sense of thwarted belongingness, which in turn contributes to lonely feelings.

3.3. Theme 3: Automation and Individuation of Work

Although much of what participants discussed as their experience of loneliness was related to real and perceived social disconnection and thwarted belonging needs, once we delved deeper it became apparent that the underpinnings of work-related loneliness are more complex than simply social disconnection. This final theme was the most diverse in terms of participant experiences of their working conditions, and took some discussion to agree upon as a defined theme. The range of work experiences were varied among participants and ranged from feeling powerless or disempowered at work (in itself not unusual for young or low-level employees) through to a lack of self-determination over *how* one works, and the repetitive, menial nature of many tasks performed by participants. We focussed on the narrative around the disconnecting nature of the work itself, and how the characteristics of their tasks resulted in loneliness.

"I have to work and concentrate on what I am doing. so I really couldn't communicate with anyone" IT worker, 20 years

"My loneliness in my job depends whether or not I sort mail by hand or by machine. When sorting by hand I feel like I have more time to interact with my colleagues. The problem is that I generally sort mail by machine a lot more. When sorting by machine I don't really have the opportunity to interact much with others because the job is too intensive in order for any socializing to happen. I therefore often feel a bit tired and lonely during my hours at work" Postal worker, 22 years

Our analysis shows that high demands at work were not considered problematic per se, unless accompanied by a lack of control and relational disconnection. For some workers a lack of ability to form relational connections due to the intensification of individualised work was problematic and led to feelings of loneliness.

> *" ... we are constantly immersed in whatever we're doing on our computers; most of what I do is digital, so there isn't much interaction with people, which can make it especially difficult to feel as though I am part of something"* Accounting assistant, 22 years

> *"I often feel lonely during work because I start working at maximum speed and in full concentration, so I do not have time to talk to other people"* Sim racer, 20 years

Our data suggest that the frequency of informal contact between coworkers can be a significant factor in the organic formation of relationships. In other words, workers often create bonds through the simple act of day-to-day chit-chat [49]. Even though many workers felt that their work did not allow for socialising due to time or task restrictions, there was also a sentiment expressed that their loneliness arose because of the lack of informal relational connections (such as chit-chat).

> *"The loneliness that I have isn't just about human contact. It's how that contact looks. Most of workers in my job, even in my team don't really show any emotions whatsoever. That makes me lonely, because I don't feel like I'm talking with human beings, but mostly a robot, that goes to work, do what he need to do without trying to talk to someone, ... then go home, sleep, repeat. If you want to talk to someone about your problems, they will say "I must do this;, I don't have time to talk". Most of the time, I feel lonely in the work, I feel lonely even in home, and work multiplies that loneliness even more"* Database administrator, 23 years

Self-determination theory suggests that feeling supported to act autonomously elicits positive wellbeing outcomes and motivation to pursue work goals [50]. However, our analysis suggests there is an experiential difference between acting autonomously at work and autonomous work—the latter of which can be relationally disengaging. Our data suggest that the automation and individuation of work may impact loneliness in a number of inter-related ways: through generating the conditions for less meaningful connections and therefore diminished sense of unity with others [51]; and through creating job tasks that require less human contact in the workplace. Where machines replace humans or where the worker is only required to interact with a machine, it can lessen the opportunities for forming connections with others that are the foundation for generating a sense of belonging [52].

> *"There's a pain and a hole, and a feeling of emptiness and an ache in the pit of my stomach ... a bitterness"* Product promoter, 22 years

For many organisations, the unintended consequences associated with relational dynamics are often not considered when implementing or changing systems and processes in the workplace [53]. Research on the expectations of younger workers suggests an increased desire for meaningful work [54] and a strong desire to be seen and appreciated as an individual [55]. This desire orients itself differently in mid-life where relationships are referenced as the core element of meaning [56]. In the workplace, a lack of input into decision making in one's job has been found to result in emotional distress and alienation [57]. This sense of exclusion from decision-making and agency over one's job was a cascading theme throughout our data. Extant literature suggests that a meaningful work experience is typically associated with a positive attitude towards oneself and one's role in the organisation, having a sense of identity and purpose, utilising talents and skills or at least developing them, and having some degree of fulfilling social relationships [51]. Our data suggest that when these factors are missing in young adults' day-to-day work experiences, and the individual desires for them to be part of their working experience, loneliness can creep into their lives.

The job characteristics model focusses on job content leading to three critical psychological states necessary for emotional health at work: (a) a feeling of personal responsibility for one's work, (b) experiencing one's work as meaningful, and (c) having knowledge of the results of one's performance [58]. Skill variety, task identity, task significance, feedback from the job, and autonomy all feed into the development of these psychological states. As we learn more about how work practices and job tasks affect relational dynamics, we can see an emphasis—building on a long history of organizational and leadership research that highlights the importance of workplace relationships vis à vis a strictly task orientation that dates back to the Hawthorne Studies—towards considering relationships as the bedrock of one's job rather than the traditional focus on task structures. This emphasis warrants further research on the relational aspects of contemporary jobs and the provision of "relational architecture" in organisations [59]. Without forethought on how work tasks are designed in organisations that considers the relational experience, we might find increasing numbers of young workers lonely in their work.

> *"There is an absence of humanity here ... I spoke about it with my mum because they really knew who they worked with but I don't see that happening for our generation"*
> Recruitment coordinator, 23 years

In summary, we identified three themes in our research that contributed to participants' feelings of loneliness: feeling unheard or unseen in their work environment, experiencing a diminished sense of belonging to the organization, and automated and individualized work leading to social disconnection. Many participants experienced work environments that emphasise individual work input/output, interpersonal emotional volatility, and systems and processes that result in limited and limiting social relationships. Such alienating values can hinder the development of any kind of desired social relationships and contribute to feelings of loneliness. Because our sample were all employees who worked onsite under supervision with others in an organisational setting, the sense of hopelessness felt in some of the participants' narratives cannot be attributed to the often alienating working conditions associated with precarious 'gig' or contractor-based work [60].

4. Conclusions

The aim of this research was to gain some insight into the experiences and consequences of young adult workers who are lonely at work. Traditionally, the opportunity for workplace social relationships could provide companionship for individuals who may not find it elsewhere. Although work is largely a social institution, our data support the notion that merely being in a social environment is not sufficient to conquer feelings of loneliness. Although the sample is small, we have identified some of the distinctive work-related challenges and conditions that contribute to work loneliness in this cohort. Our data goes some way to support the process model of loneliness [10], in that the distress of work-related loneliness is created through a relational deficiency and the deficiency stems from individual and contextual components. Our research reinforces the notion that workers are not immune to loneliness, and supports other research indicating that workers showed more psychological distress compared to the elderly during the COVID-19 pandemic and its associated isolation requirements [61].

It is tempting to place the burden of socialising and relational fulfilment on the individuals and consider how the personal characteristics of the individual may be inhibiting the quality of their social relationships. However, given the rise of loneliness in young adults it is important to consider the ways in which the work environment operates on the individual, either causing or perpetuating loneliness. Our data support the notion that loneliness at work is not simply a personal failure, but rather can be understood as a consequence of individual, social, organisational, and economic circumstances often outside of the individual's control. The nature of the work, and the work environment itself, might therefore be considered "loneliness-provoking factors" [62] (p. 127). An important contribution of this research is that loneliness is not simply about feeling socially isolated or lacking connection, it also encompasses not being seen, heard or understood, and feeling disconnected and marginalised from groups and institutions.

Limitations and Future Research

This study presents a within-person analysis of the experiences of those young workers who feel lonely at work to understand what might be contributing to, and emanating from their loneliness. Future research on the relational behaviours of lonely versus non-lonely young adult workers would make for an interesting study and extend some of the ideas presented in this research on the social cognition of emerging adults in the workplace. Additionally, all of the respondents in this study were articulate in English, technically literate, and comfortable with detailing their varied experiences through a text medium. Expanding the sample would help develop the emerging themes identified in this paper. Conducting face-to-face interviews might allow for deeper exploration of participant's experiences, which we could not explore with an anonymous survey.

Future research should increase the breadth and depth of the qualitative study with a greater number of employees from diverse organisational contexts and cultures. The participants in this study are from European countries. However, the antecedents and experiences of loneliness differ cross-culturally. For example, deficiencies with personal confidants is a stronger predictor of loneliness in individualistic societies [63], whereas lack of interactions with family are a strong predictor of loneliness in collectivist societies [64]. Future research could help understand the extent to which cultural interdependence affects the experiences of loneliness in organisations. Studying the effects of interventions is also a valuable avenue for future research: e.g., addressing maladaptive social cognitions (which has the strongest evidence of effectiveness on general loneliness; [65]; developing socialisation/on boarding processes that focus on relational aspects of work; increasing opportunities for social contact; and increasing social support.

We could end this paper on a depressing (but realistic) note about the state of loneliness in young workers, but we choose to offer an alternative view. Evidenced in the participant's quotes is the extraordinary power and possibility of harnessing social connection within organisations to improve young workers experiences of their work and their work place/space. Individuals would not experience loneliness if they did not yearn for fulfilling social connections. Simple shifts in work practices or the way we interact with others can make meaningful differences to our experiences of work.

Author Contributions: Conceptualization, S.L.W.; Data curation, S.L.W.; Formal analysis, S.L.W. and A.G.S.; Writing—original draft, S.L.W.; Writing—review and editing, S.L.W. and A.G.S. All authors have read and agreed to the published version of the manuscript.

Funding: This research received no external funding.

Institutional Review Board Statement: The study was approved by the Human Ethics Committee of The University of Canterbury, New Zealand, HEC 2020/113.

Informed Consent Statement: Informed consent was obtained from all subjects involved in the study.

Data Availability Statement: Not applicable.

Conflicts of Interest: The authors declare no conflict of interest.

References

1. Victor, C.R.; Yang, K. The Prevalence of Loneliness Among Adults: A Case Study of the United Kingdom. *J. Psychol.* **2012**, *146*, 85–104. [CrossRef] [PubMed]
2. Baarck, J.; Balahur, A.; Cassio, L.; d'Hombres, B.; Pásztor, Z.; Tintori, G. Insights from surveys and online media data, EUR 30765 EN. In *Loneliness in the EU*; Publications Office of the European Union: Luxembourg, 2021; ISBN 978-92-76-40247-3.
3. Hawkins-Elder, H.; Milfont, T.L.; Hammond, M.D.; Sibley, C.G. Who are the lonely? A typology of loneliness in New Zealand. *Aust. N. Z. J. Psychiatry* **2018**, *52*, 357–364. [CrossRef] [PubMed]
4. Franklin, A.S.; Tranter, B. *Loneliness in Australia*; Occasional Paper 13; Housing and Community Research Unit, University of Tasmania: Hobart, Australia, 2008.

5. Department for Digital, Culture, Media and Sport. *A Connected Society: A Strategy for Tackling Loneliness—Laying the Foundations for Change*; Department for Digital, Culture, Media and Sport, UK Government: London, UK, 2018.
6. Child, S.; Lawton, L. Loneliness and social isolation among young and late middle-age adults: Associations with personal networks and social participation. *Aging Ment. Health* **2019**, *23*, 196–204. [CrossRef]
7. Cigna. Loneliness in the Workplace: 2020 U.S. Report. 2020. Available online: https://www.cigna.com/static/www-cigna-com/docs/about-us/newsroom/studies-and-reports/combatting-loneliness/cigna-2020-loneliness-report.pdf (accessed on 7 December 2021).
8. Ozcelik, H.; Barsade, S.G. No employee an island: Workplace loneliness and job performance. *Acad. Manag. J.* **2018**, *61*, 2343–2366. [CrossRef]
9. Wingard, J. Loneliness Is Crippling Workplace Productivity: Here's The Leadership Prescription. 2020. Available online: https://www.forbes.com/sites/jasonwingard/2020/02/14/loneliness-is-crippling-workplace-productivity-heres-the-leadership-prescription/?sh=4f3ad2248f6f (accessed on 3 August 2022).
10. Wright, S.; Silard, A. Unravelling the antecedents of loneliness in the workplace. *Hum. Relat.* **2021**, *74*, 1060–1081. [CrossRef]
11. Hawkley, L.C.; Cacioppo, J.T. Loneliness matters: A theoretical and empirical review of consequences and mechanisms. *Ann. Behav. Med.* **2010**, *40*, 218–227. [CrossRef] [PubMed]
12. Holt-Lunstad, J.; Smith, T.B.; Baker, M.; Harris, T.; Stephenson, D. Loneliness and social isolation as risk factors for mortality: A meta-analytic review. *Perspect. Psychol. Sci.* **2015**, *10*, 227–237. [CrossRef]
13. Howard, M.C.; Follmer, K.B.; Smith, M.B.; Tucker, R.P.; Van Zandt, E.C. Work and suicide: An interdisciplinary systematic literature review. *J. Organ. Behav.* **2021**, *43*, 260–285. [CrossRef]
14. Stravynski, A.; Boyer, R. Loneliness in relation to suicide ideation and parasuicide: A population-wide study. *Suicide Life-Threat. Behav.* **2001**, *31*, 32–40. [CrossRef]
15. Achterbergh, L.; Pitman, A.; Birken, M. The experience of loneliness among young people with depression: A qualitative meta-synthesis of the literature. *BMC Psychiatry* **2020**, *20*, 415. [CrossRef]
16. Twenge, J.; Catanese, K.; Baumeister, R. Social Exclusion Causes Self-Defeating Behavior. *J. Personal. Soc. Psychol.* **2002**, *83*, 606–615. [CrossRef]
17. Stillman, T.; Baumeister, R.; Lambert, N.; Crescioni, C.; DeWall, N.; Fincham, F. Alone and without Purpose: Life Loses Meaning Following Social Exclusion. *J. Exp. Soc. Psychol.* **2009**, *45*, 211–217. [CrossRef]
18. Gonsalkorale, K.; Williams, K. The KKK Won't Let Me Play: Ostracism Even by a Despised Outgroup Hurts. *Eur. J. Soc. Psychol.* **2007**, *37*, 1176–1186. [CrossRef]
19. Silard, A. Screened. In *The Art of Living Free in the Digital Age*; Inner Leadership Press: Claremont, CA, USA, 2020.
20. Allen, K.A.; Lim, M.H.; Rodebaugh, T.L.; Eres, R.; Long, K.; Penn, D.L.; Gleeson, J.F. A pilot digital intervention targeting loneliness in youth mental health. *Front. Psychiatry* **2019**, *10*, 604. [CrossRef] [PubMed]
21. Blustein, D.L.; Kenny, M.E.; Autin, K.; Duffy, R. The psychology of working in practice: A theory of change for a new era. *Career Dev. Q.* **2019**, *67*, 236–254. [CrossRef]
22. Konno, Y.; Nagata, M.; Hino, A.; Tateishi, S.; Tsuji, M.; Ogami, A.; Yoshimura, R.; Matsuda, S.; Fujino, Y. Association between loneliness and psychological distress: A cross-sectional study among Japanese workers during the COVID-19 pandemic. *Prev. Med. Rep.* **2021**, *2*, 101621. [CrossRef] [PubMed]
23. Wilkin, C.L.; de Jong, J.P.; Rubino, C. Teaming up with temps: The impact of temporary workers on team social networks and effectiveness. *Eur. J. Work Organ. Psychol.* **2018**, *27*, 204–218. [CrossRef]
24. Nowland, R. Social Media: Is It Really to Blame for Young People Being Lonelier than Any Other Age Group? 2018. Available online: http://theconversation.com/social-media-is-it-really-to-blame-for-young-people-being-lonelier-than-any-other-age-group-104292 (accessed on 7 December 2021).
25. Insights team. Over Half of Brits Suffer from Loneliness in the Workplace. 2019. Available online: https://www.cv-library.co.uk/recruitment-insight/brits-suffer-loneliness-workplace/ (accessed on 7 December 2021).
26. Perna, M. Employees Want More Friends At Work. Why Aren't They Finding Them? Available online: https://www.forbes.com/sites/markcperna/2022/07/19/employees-want-more-friends-at-work-why-arent-they-finding-them/?sh=503f69d319ab (accessed on 3 August 2022).
27. Doumen, S.; Smits, I.; Luyckx, K.; Duriez, B.; Vanhalst, J.; Verschueren, K.; Goossens, L. Identity and perceived peer relationship quality in emerging adulthood: The mediating role of attachment-related emotions. *J. Adolesc.* **2012**, *35*, 1417–1425. [CrossRef]
28. Rook, K.S. The negative side of social interaction: Impact on psychological well-being. *J. Personal. Soc. Psychol.* **1984**, *46*, 1097. [CrossRef]
29. Amarat, M.; Akbolat, M.; Ünal, Ö.; Güneş Karakaya, B. The mediating role of work alienation in the effect of workplace loneliness on nurses' performance. *J. Nurs. Manag.* **2019**, *27*, 553–559. [CrossRef]
30. Anand, P.; Mishra, S.K. Linking core self-evaluation and emotional exhaustion with workplace loneliness: Does high LMX make the consequence worse? *Int. J. Hum. Resour. Manag.* **2021**, *32*, 2124–2149. [CrossRef]
31. Jung, H.S.; Song, M.K.; Yoon, H.H. The effects of workplace loneliness on work engagement and organizational commitment: Moderating roles of leader-member exchange and coworker exchange. *Sustainability* **2021**, *13*, 948. [CrossRef]
32. Özturk Ciftci, D. Emotional exhaustion as a mediator among workplace loneliness, work alienation and turnover intention. *Int. J. Organ. Theory Behav.* **2021**, *24*, 93–106. [CrossRef]

33. Öge, E.; Çetin, M.; Top, S. The effects of paternalistic leadership on workplace loneliness, work family conflict and work engagement among air traffic controllers in turkey. *J. Air Transp. Manag.* **2018**, *66*, 25–35. [CrossRef]
34. Uslu, O. Being alone is more painful than getting hurt: The moderating role of workplace loneliness in the association between workplace ostracism and job performance. *Cent. Eur. Bus. Rev.* **2021**, *10*, 19–37. [CrossRef]
35. Peer, E.; Brandimarte, L.; Samat, S.; Acquisti, A. Beyond the turk: Alternative platforms for crowdsourcing behavioral research. *J. Exp. Soc. Psychol.* **2017**, *70*, 153–163. [CrossRef]
36. Braun, V.; Clarke, V.; Boulton, E.; Davey, L.; McEvoy, C. The online survey as a qualitative research tool. *Int. J. Soc. Res. Methodol.* **2020**, *24*, 641–654. [CrossRef]
37. Braun, V.; Clarke, V. Using thematic analysis in psychology. *Qual. Res. Psychol.* **2006**, *3*, 77–101. [CrossRef]
38. Settles, I.H.; Buchanan, N.T.; Dotson, K. Scrutinized but not recognized:(In) visibility and hypervisibility experiences of faculty of color. *J. Vocat. Behav.* **2019**, *113*, 62–74. [CrossRef]
39. Buber, M. *I and Thou*; Scribner: New York, NY, USA, 1985.
40. Jung, C.G. *Memories, Dreams, Reflections*; Random House: New York, NY, USA, 1963.
41. Meng, J.; Wang, X.; Wei, D.; Qiu, J. State loneliness is associated with emotional hypervigilance in daily life: A network analysis. *Personal. Individ. Differ.* **2020**, *165*, 110154. [CrossRef]
42. Cacioppo, J.T.; Hawkley, L.C. People thinking about people: The vicious cycle of being a social outcast in one's own mind. In *The Social Outcast: Ostracism, Social Exclusion, Rejection, and Bullying*; Williams, K., Forgas, J., von Hippel, W., Eds.; Psychology Press: New York, NY, USA, 2005; pp. 91–108.
43. Van Orden, K.A.; Cukrowicz, K.C.; Witte, T.K.; Joiner, T.E., Jr. Thwarted belongingness and perceived burdensomeness: Construct validity and psychometric properties of the Interpersonal Needs Questionnaire. *Psychol. Assess.* **2012**, *24*, 197. [CrossRef] [PubMed]
44. Thau, S.; Aquino, K.; Poortvliet, P.M. Self-defeating behaviors in organizations: The relationship between thwarted belonging and interpersonal work behaviors. *J. Appl. Psychol.* **2007**, *92*, 840. [CrossRef]
45. Blackhart, G.C.; Baumeister, R.F.; Twenge, J.M. Rejection's Impact on Self-Defeating, Prosocial, Antisocial, and Self-Regulatory Behaviors. In *Self and Relationships: Connecting Intrapersonal and Interpersonal Processes*; Vohs, K., Finkel, E., Eds.; Guilford Press: New York, NY, USA, 2006.
46. Hagerty BM, K.; Lynch-Sauer, J.; Patusky, K.L.; Bouwsema, M.; Collier, P. Sense of belonging: A vital mental health concept. *Arch. Psychiatr. Nurs.* **1992**, *6*, 172–177. [CrossRef]
47. Walseth, K. Sport and belonging. *Int. Rev. Sociol. Sport* **2006**, *41*, 447–464. [CrossRef]
48. Gersick, C.J.; Dutton, J.E.; Bartunek, J.M. Learning from academia: The importance of relationships in professional life. *Acad. Manag. J.* **2000**, *43*, 1026–1044. [CrossRef]
49. Methot, J.R.; Rosado-Solomon, E.H.; Downes, P.E.; Gabriel, A.S. Office chitchat as a social ritual: The uplifting yet distracting effects of daily small talk at work. *Acad. Manag. J.* **2021**, *64*, 1445–1471. [CrossRef]
50. Deci, E.L.; Ryan, R.M. *Intrinsic Motivation and Self-Determination in Human Behavior*; Springer Science & Business Media: Berlin/Heidelberg, Germany, 2013.
51. Lips-Wiersma, M.; Wright, S. Measuring the meaning of meaningful work: Development and validation of the Comprehensive Meaningful Work Scale (CMWS). *Group Organ. Manag.* **2012**, *37*, 655–685. [CrossRef]
52. Seppala ERossomando, T.; Doty, J. Social connection and compassion. *Soc. Res.* **2013**, *80*, 410–430.
53. Thomas, N.K.; Sugiyama, K.; Rochford, K.C.; Stephens, J.P.; Kanov, J. Experiential organizing: Pursuing relational and bureaucratic goals through symbolically and experientially oriented work. *Acad. Manag. Rev.* **2018**, *43*, 749–771. [CrossRef]
54. Brack, J.; Kelly, K. Maximizing millennials in the workplace. *UNC Exec. Dev.* **2012**, *22*, 2–14.
55. Kultalahti, S.; Viitala, R.L. Sufficient challenges and a weekend ahead–Generation Y describing motivation at work. *J. Organ. Change Manag.* **2014**, *27*, 569–582. [CrossRef]
56. O'Connor, K.; Chamberlain, K. Dimensions of life meaning: A qualitative investigation at mid-life. *Br. J. Psychol.* **1996**, *87*, 461–477. [CrossRef] [PubMed]
57. Wall, T.D.; Corbett, J.M.; Martin, R.; Clegg, C.W.; Jackson, P.R. Advanced manufacturing technology, work design, and performance: A change study. *J. Appl. Psychol.* **1990**, *75*, 691. [CrossRef]
58. Hackman, J.R. Work redesign and motivation. *Prof. Psychol.* **1980**, *11*, 445. [CrossRef]
59. Grant, A.M. Relational job design and the motivation to make a prosocial difference. *Acad. Manag. Rev.* **2007**, *32*, 393–417. [CrossRef]
60. Caza, B.B.; Reid, E.M.; Ashford, S.; Granger, S. Working on my own: Measuring the challenges of gig work. *Hum. Relat.* **2021**, *75*, 2122–2159. [CrossRef]
61. Andreassi, S.; Monaco, S.; Salvatore, S.; Sciabica, G.M.; De Felice, G.; Petrovska, E.; Mariani, R. To work or not to work, that is the question: The psychological impact of the first COVID-19 lockdown on the elderly, healthcare workers, and virtual workers. *Healthcare* **2021**, *9*, 1754. [CrossRef]
62. de Jong-Gierveld, J. Developing and testing a model of loneliness. *J. Personal. Soc. Psychol.* **1987**, *53*, 119. [CrossRef]
63. McPherson, M.; Smith-Lovin, L.; Brashears, M.E. Social Isolation in America: Changes in Core Discussion Networks over Two Decades. *Am. Sociol. Rev.* **2006**, *71*, 353–375. [CrossRef]

64. Lykes, V.; Kemmelmeier, M. What predicts loneliness? Cultural difference between individuals and collectivist societies in Europe. *J. Cross Cult. Psychol.* **2014**, *45*, 468–490. [CrossRef]
65. Masi, C.M.; Chen, H.; Hawkley, L.C.; Cacioppo, J.T. A meta-analysis of interventions to reduce loneliness. *Personal. Soc. Psychol. Rev.* **2011**, *15*, 219–266. [CrossRef] [PubMed]

International Journal of
Environmental Research and Public Health

MDPI

Article

Relationships between Interpersonal Goals and Loneliness in Older Adults: A Cross-Sectional Study

Francesca C. Ezeokonkwo [1,*], Kathleen L. Sekula [2], Jeffrey E. Stokes [3], Laurie A. Theeke [4], Rick Zoucha [2], Meredith Troutman-Jordan [5] and Dinesh Sharma [6]

1 School of Nursing, James Madison University, Harrisonburg, VA 22807, USA
2 School of Nursing, Duquesne University, Pittsburgh, PA 15282, USA
3 Department of Gerontology, McCormack Graduate School of Policy and Global Studies, University of Massachusetts, Boston, MA 02125, USA
4 School of Nursing, George Washington University, Washington, DC 20006, USA
5 School of Nursing, University of North Carolina Charlotte, Charlotte, NC 28223, USA
6 Department of Mathematics and Statistics, James Madison University, Harrisonburg, VA 22807, USA
* Correspondence: ezeokofc@jmu.edu

Abstract: Loneliness is linked to many physiological and psychological issues and disproportionately affects older adults. Interpersonal goals (compassion and self-image) are essential to interpersonal relationships; however, how they relate to loneliness in older adults is unknown. We investigated the impact of interpersonal goals on loneliness using the Ecosystem–Egosystem Theory of Social Motivation. This study, adopting a descriptive cross-sectional correlational design, used data from the 2016 Health and Retirement Study. Participants (n = 3212) included people aged >65 years (mean age: 75; female: 60.1%). We performed exploratory factor analysis with principal axis factoring and varimax rotation to examine the suitability of compassionate and self-image goals as separate factors. The complex samples general linear model was used to assess the relationship between loneliness and interpersonal goals. Interpersonal goals were significantly negatively associated with loneliness. Respondents with higher compassion and self-image goals reported lower loneliness levels. Our results contribute to understanding how interpersonal goals relate to loneliness in older adults. These initial findings warrant further investigation.

Keywords: loneliness; interpersonal goals; compassionate and self-image goals; older adults

1. Introduction

Loneliness—operationally defined as a negative subjective experience resulting from discrepancies between individuals' desired and perceived number and closeness or quality of social relationships—is conceptualized as a psychological state simultaneously constituting a yearning for human contact as well as a feeling of aloneness [1]. Although loneliness affects people across all developmental stages, older adults are at great risk of loneliness [2] due to physical health deterioration and the loss of family and friends [3,4], as well as a lack of social resources to initiate new relationships to compensate for such losses, particularly among the oldest old [4].

Loneliness among older adults substantially impacts their quality of life [5,6]. Compared to those not experiencing loneliness, older adults exhibiting chronic loneliness report less exercise, greater tobacco use, a greater number and severity of chronic illnesses, higher depression levels, and a greater average number of nursing home stays [7].

Loneliness precipitates diminished sleep quality, shorter sleep duration, lower sleep efficiency, greater daytime fatigue in later adulthood, and reduced subjective sleep quality [8]. A 2022 study by Bogart et al. examined the cross-sectional associations between loneliness and inflammatory markers among older adults and found that higher trait loneliness and aggregated momentary measures of loneliness were associated with higher levels of C-reactive protein (CRP) [9].

The incidence of loneliness among U.S. older adults varies across studies and has been estimated to be as high as 60% in older frail adults [10]. Theeke [5] documented that 19.3% of community-dwelling older adults reported feeling lonely. In a 2015 survey of older Americans, nearly 55% of the study sample reported feeling some level of loneliness, with 27% reporting moderate and 28% reporting severe loneliness [11]. Perissinotto et al. [12] documented a 30–43% prevalence of loneliness among older community adults, whereas data from a survey by the American Association of Retired Persons (AARP) estimated that 25% of community-dwelling U.S. respondents over the age of 70 years were lonely [13].

Previous research has documented the following loneliness predictors in older adults: female sex, living alone, low income, low economic status, and age (older than 65 [14]). Older adults are at increased risk for loneliness due to physical health deterioration, retirement, relocation, and loss of family and friends through death or separation [2,3,15]. In older adults, studies have demonstrated that loneliness elicits both physiological and emotional stress responses that are linked to morbidity and mortality [16–18]. It is critical to understand the influence of loneliness on health and aging as it is known that lonely older people do utilize healthcare resources more frequently [19].

As loneliness—although an individual emotional experience—is inherently linked with one's social context and relationships, the importance of adults' own social desires and goals should be considered when assessing loneliness in later life. Foremost among these are interpersonal goals, which include compassion and self-image goals—the primary constructs of the Ecosystem–Egosystem Theory of Social Motivation. Compassionate goals involve focusing on supporting others rather than personal self-gain with the intention of facilitating others' well-being. Self-image goals involve constructing, maintaining, and defending a desired public or private image of the self to pursue one's own interests [20]. These contrasting social goals represent distinct motivational perspectives on the relationship between the self and others and have strong implications for promoting or undermining interpersonal relationships, respectively [21,22]. Compassionate goals relate to feelings of clarity, connectedness, and closeness to others, fewer interpersonal conflicts, and high positive emotions, thereby mitigating feelings of loneliness. By contrast, self-image goals relate to feelings of fear and confusion, greater loneliness, interpersonal conflicts, and low positive emotions [22]. Compassionate goals foster social support and trust, while self-image goals undermine them [20]. Interpersonal goals may offer a new perspective to examine loneliness in older adults.

Numerous studies have elucidated the prevalence of loneliness among older adults [15,23]. Studies have also explored the effect of interpersonal goals on loneliness in young populations [22,24]. However, research has not yet established the relationship between interpersonal goals and loneliness among older adults. This is an important gap in current literature, not only because loneliness increases in later life but also because older adults exhibit distinct social and emotional goals in comparison with younger and midlife adults [25]. Our study fills this knowledge gap by examining the direct relationship between loneliness and compassion and self-image goals in older adults. Understanding how interpersonal goals relate to loneliness might aid healthcare providers in developing targeted interventions that mitigate loneliness in older adults.

Theoretical Framework

This study was guided by the Ecosystem–Egosystem Theory of Social Motivation [20]. Ecosystem motivation promotes close and mutually supportive relationships through behaviors that are intended to be constructive and supportive. People with an ecosystem motivational perspective perceive others as connected with them, show concern about others' well-being, and treat their own and others' needs and desires equally, with an understanding that they are part of a larger whole. People with ecosystem motivation tend to adopt compassionate goals [26]. Egosystem motivation focuses on proving and validating self-worth. demonstrating desired qualities, and involves concerns regarding others' impressions, thereby precipitating self-consciousness and social anxiety [26]. People with an egosystem motivational perspective show greater concern regarding the fulfillment of their own needs and desires but fail to exhibit concern for others' well-being. They perceive the relationship between the self and the other as competitive; therefore, they do not regard others' needs and desires as equally important. People with egosystem motivation primarily focus on themselves and adopt self-image goals, which may diminish the social support received from others and, therefore, result in loneliness [20,26].

As hypothesized by the ecosystem–egosystem theoretical framework, compassionate and self-image goals reflect distinct ways of thinking or perspectives. Altruistic motivation (for others' benefit) and egoistic motivation (for self-benefit) represent contrasting goals and feelings. People for whom others' well-being is genuinely significant adopt compassionate goals and, consequently, exhibit a positive affect, a sense of clarity, and interpersonal closeness. When people aim to benefit or protect themselves and consider the relationship between themselves and others an egosystem, they adopt self-image goals and, consequently, exhibit fearful feelings, confusion, and interpersonal conflict [18]. Evidently, compassionate and self-image goals prevail at opposite ends. However, people occasionally exhibit overlaps between these two perspectives for short periods [27]. People exhibit self-image goals from an ecosystem perspective and compassionate goals from an egosystem perspective. Distress and interpersonal goals are mutually reinforcing–greater distress may discourage compassionate goals and encourage self-image goals [20].

This study's objective was to investigate interpersonal goals' (compassionate and self-image goals) impact on loneliness in older adults.

This study incorporated a descriptive cross-sectional, correlational secondary data analysis. The primary research question in this regard was, "How is loneliness in older adults associated with interpersonal goals (compassionate and self-image)?" Loneliness was the outcome variable, whereas compassionate goals and self-image goals were the predictor variables. Note that where mentioned below, "loneliness" refers to "loneliness in adults". The two hypotheses of the study were as follows:

Hypothesis 1 (H1). *Compassionate goals will be associated with lower loneliness.*

Hypothesis 2 (H2). *Self-image goals will be associated with greater loneliness.*

2. Materials and Methods

Study data were derived from the following two components of the Health and Retirement Study (HRS) data file (publicly available data): the 2016 HRS core dataset of the public biennial survey data (https://hrs.isr.umich.edu/about (accessed on 6 November 2020)), the RAND, and the Psychosocial and Lifestyle Questionnaire. As this study applied secondary data analysis using de-identified data, IRB approval was not required. Our analyses used data from 2016 when interpersonal goal measures were introduced in the HRS survey. The response rate for the HRS is high—typically 85–90% [28], and somewhat lower for the Psychosocial and Lifestyle Questionnaire—generally 73–88% [29]. Inclusion criteria were community-dwelling older adults aged 65 years and older who completed the HRS survey and Psychosocial and Lifestyle Questionnaire without needing a proxy. In 2016, the HRS included 20,912 participants. The following respondents were excluded: individuals under the age of 65 (n = 10,940), participants living in the nursing home (n = 429), and those who completed the survey by proxy (n = 450). Further, because HRS administers the Leave Behind Questionnaire (LBQ) to a random 50% subset of HRS households at alternating waves, we also excluded participants who were either not eligible for the LBQ in 2016 (n = 4683) or did not complete it (n = 998). Of the 3412 participants fulfilling the inclusion criteria, 200 (6%) respondents with missing values for items corresponding to the research variables were excluded. Thus, the final sample comprised 3212 cases.

A power analysis was conducted using the G*Power 3.1 software [30], which indicated that 159 participants were required to obtain a medium effect size of f = 0.25—with standard power and standard alpha of 0.80 and 0.05, respectively.

The revised 11-item UCLA Loneliness Scale [31] was used by the HRS to measure participants' loneliness within the past week. After reverse-coding four negatively worded items, the overall loneliness score was computed as the 11 items' average. Higher scores indicated greater loneliness. The internal reliability of the 11-item UCLA exhibits a Cronbach's α value of 0.87 [31].

A modified six-item measure of interpersonal goals was used to assess compassionate and self-image goals [20,32]. Three items assessed compassionate goals: "compassion for others", "supportive of others", and "avoid being selfish". Three items assessed self-image goals: "get others to see your positive qualities", "get others to respect you", and "avoid appearing unattractive". The six items were reverse-coded, and the scores ranged from 1 (not at all) to 5 (extremely) [29]. In the original study of the 13-item scale, Cronbach's alpha was 0.90 for compassionate goals and 0.83 for self-image goals [24].

We computed Cronbach's alpha reliability coefficients for the scales of loneliness, compassionate goals, and self-image goals. For this current study, reliability for loneliness was high ($\alpha = 0.87$), which was the same as documented by previous research [31], but lower for compassionate goals ($\alpha = 0.68$) and self-image goals ($\alpha = 0.60$). We also performed exploratory factor analysis to examine the suitability of compassionate and self-image goals as separate factors [20,29,32]. In this analysis, two factors were forced with principal axis factoring as the extraction method and a varimax rotation. Table 1 displays the rotated factor loadings. All compassionate goal items loaded strongly (>0.52) on Factor 1 and weakly (<0.40) on Factor 2, supporting compassionate goals as a distinct factor. Two items of self-image goals loaded strongly (>0.61) on Factor 2 and weakly (<0.40) on Factor 1. The remaining item of self-image goals (avoid appearing unattractive) did not load strongly on either factor (<0.40), potentially indicating a difference in the salience of "appearing unattractive, unlovable, or undesirable to others" among older vs. younger adults [25]. Conforming to both prior research using these scales [20,32] and HRS guidelines for variable construction [29], the "appearing unattractive" item was retained in the self-image goals scale used in the present analyses.

Table 1. Varimax Rotated Factor Loadings for Compassionate and Self-Image Goals Items.

Item	Factor	
	1	2
Compassion for others	0.60	0.13
Supportive of others	0.75	0.23
Avoid being selfish	0.52	0.31
Avoid appearing unattractive	0.34	0.24
Get others to see your positive qualities	0.37	0.61
Get others to respect you	0.16	0.82

Further, we included sociodemographic (age, sex, race, ethnicity, functional impairment, homecare utilization) and socioeconomic (education, income, employment status, household size) covariates based on a review of prior literature. The reference categories selected included male sex, an educational level lower than high school, retired or not in the labor force for employment status, no functional impairment, and home care utilization.

We performed linear regressions using the complex samples general linear model command in SPSS. The complex samples analysis procedure used the PLBWGTR variable as the sampling weight, the SECU variable as the primary sampling unit, and the STRATUM variable as the sampling strata [33,34]. We computed three sets of complex sample linear regression: (1) regression with compassionate goals predicting loneliness, (2) self-image goals predicting loneliness, and (3) the full model with compassionate and self-image predicting loneliness. In all three sets of analyses, we controlled for the aforementioned sociodemographic and socioeconomic variables.

3. Results

Table 2 presents the descriptive statistics. Participant ages ranged from 65 to 99 years (mean 75.7), predominantly in the 65–74 years age group (44.9%); Female (60.1%); White (81.0%), non-Hispanic (90.6%); the most common level of education among participants was high school graduate (31.0%); and 80.0% were retired or not in the labor force. Most participants (89.6%) had not utilized home care in the previous two years; 83.5% exhibited no functional impairment. On average, participants' income was $14,458.34, and the number of people in the household was two.

Table 2. Frequencies and Percentages for Categorical Variables.

Variable	Frequency	Percent
Age (years)		
65–74	1442	44.9
75–84	1358	42.3
≥85	412	12.9
Gender		
Male	1281	39.9
Female	1931	60.1
Ethnicity		
Not Hispanic	2909	90.6
Hispanic	303	9.4
Race		
White/Caucasian	2599	81.0
Black/African American	455	14.2
Other	155	4.8
Education		
Less than high school	488	15.2
GED	143	4.5
High-school graduate	995	31.0
Some college	790	24.6
College and above	795	24.8
Employment		
Employed	613	19.1
Unemployed	28	0.9
Retired or not in labor force	2571	80.0
Home health care		
No	2877	89.6
Yes	335	10.4
Functional impairment		
No	2683	83.5
Yes	529	16.5

Hypothesis 1: As hypothesized, compassionate goals were a significant negative predictor in both the separate model (B = −0.16, p < 0.001) and the combined model (B = −0.14, p < 0.001). This result indicates that those with a higher level of compassionate goals exhibited lower loneliness after controlling for other factors (Tables 3 and 4).

Hypothesis 2: We found that self-image goals were a significant negative predictor in the separate model (B = −0.09, p < 0.001) and combined model (B = −0.03, p = 0.015), indicating that those with higher levels of self-image goals exhibited lower loneliness after controlling for other factors (Tables 4 and 5). Thus, our second hypothesis was not supported.

Table 4 displays the parameter estimates for the regression with compassionate goals, self-image goals, and the control variables predicting loneliness. Compassionate goals (B = −0.14, p < 0.001) and self-image goals (B = −0.03, p = 0.015) were significant negative predictors. Having a college or higher degree, functional impairment, and healthcare utilization all correlate with loneliness (Tables 3–5).

Table 3. Complex Samples General Linear Model with Compassionate Goals Predicting Loneliness.

	B	SE	95% CI B Lower	95% CI B Upper	t	df	p-Value
(Intercept)	2.27	0.12	2.04	2.51	19.27	56	<0.001
Compassionate goals	−0.16	0.01	−0.19	−0.13	−11.93	56	<0.001
Age	0.00	0.00	−0.01	0.00	−1.08	56	0.286
Sex [Female]	0.01	0.02	−0.03	0.05	0.60	56	0.551
Race [White/Caucasian]	−0.03	0.04	−0.11	0.04	−0.95	56	0.348
Race [Black/African American]	−0.04	0.04	−0.13	0.04	−1.10	56	0.277
Race [Hispanic]	0.01	0.04	−0.06	0.09	0.35	56	0.730
Education [GED]	0.05	0.05	−0.05	0.14	0.97	56	0.336
Education [High school graduate]	−0.02	0.03	−0.08	0.04	−0.79	56	0.433
Education [Some college]	0.01	0.03	−0.05	0.07	0.27	56	0.792
Education [College and above]	−0.09	0.03	−0.14	−0.03	−3.11	56	0.003
Income	0.00	0.00	0.00	0.00	−2.95	56	0.005
Number of people in household	0.00	0.01	−0.02	0.02	−0.09	56	0.929
Employment [Employed]	−0.04	0.02	−0.09	0.01	−1.67	56	0.100
Employment [Unemployed]	0.19	0.12	−0.06	0.43	1.52	56	0.135
Functional impairment [Yes]	0.12	0.03	0.05	0.18	3.79	56	<0.001
Home health care [Yes]	0.08	0.03	0.02	0.13	2.59	56	0.012

Table 4. Complex Samples General Linear Model Predicting Loneliness (Full Model).

	B	SE	95% CI B Lower	95% CI B Upper	t	df	p-Value
(Intercept)	2.30	0.12	2.07	2.53	19.83	56	<0.001
Compassionate goals	−0.14	0.02	−0.17	−0.11	−9.19	56	<0.001
Self-image goals	−0.03	0.01	−0.06	−0.01	−2.50	56	0.015
Age	0.00	0.00	0.00	0.00	−1.00	56	0.320
Sex [Female]	0.01	0.02	−0.03	0.05	0.66	56	0.513
Race [White/Caucasian]	−0.03	0.04	−0.11	0.04	−0.94	56	0.352
Race [Black/African American]	−0.05	0.04	−0.13	0.03	−1.17	56	0.247
Race [Hispanic]	0.01	0.04	−0.07	0.09	0.29	56	0.776
Education [GED]	0.05	0.05	−0.05	0.14	0.99	56	0.328
Education [High school graduate]	−0.02	0.03	−0.08	0.04	−0.71	56	0.483
Education [Some college]	0.02	0.03	−0.05	0.08	0.48	56	0.635
Education [College and above]	−0.08	0.03	−0.13	−0.02	−2.85	56	0.006
Income	0.00	0.00	0.00	0.00	−2.92	56	0.005
Number of people in household	0.00	0.01	−0.02	0.02	−0.13	56	0.897
Employment [Employed]	−0.04	0.03	−0.09	0.01	−1.49	56	0.142
Employment [Unemployed]	0.19	0.12	−0.06	0.43	1.54	56	0.130
Functional impairment [Yes]	0.11	0.03	0.05	0.17	3.70	56	<0.001
Home health care [Yes]	0.08	0.03	0.02	0.14	2.72	56	0.009

Table 5. Complex Samples General Linear Model with Self-Image Goals Predicting Loneliness.

	B	SE	95% CI B Lower	95% CI B Upper	t	df	p-Value
(Intercept)	1.97	0.12	1.74	2.21	16.83	56	<0.001
Self-image goals	−0.09	0.01	−0.12	−0.07	−7.96	56	<0.001
Age	0.00	0.00	0.00	0.00	−0.62	56	0.538
Sex [Female]	−0.02	0.02	−0.06	0.02	−0.95	56	0.347
Race [White/Caucasian]	−0.04	0.04	−0.12	0.04	−1.01	56	0.317
Race [Black/African American]	−0.05	0.04	−0.14	0.03	−1.29	56	0.203
Race [Hispanic]	0.04	0.04	−0.04	0.12	0.96	56	0.342

Table 5. *Cont.*

	B	SE	95% CI B Lower	95% CI B Upper	t	df	p-Value
Education [GED]	0.01	0.05	−0.09	0.10	0.13	56	0.895
Education [High school graduate]	−0.05	0.03	−0.11	0.01	−1.71	56	0.094
Education [Some college]	−0.02	0.03	−0.08	0.04	−0.67	56	0.506
Education [College and above]	−0.12	0.03	−0.17	−0.06	−4.29	56	<0.001
Income	0.00	0.00	0.00	0.00	−2.63	56	0.011
Number of people in household	0.00	0.01	−0.02	0.02	−0.11	56	0.911
Employment [Employed]	−0.04	0.03	−0.09	0.02	−1.33	56	0.188
Employment [Unemployed]	0.17	0.12	−0.07	0.41	1.45	56	0.152
Functional impairment [Yes]	0.11	0.03	0.05	0.17	3.78	56	<0.001
Home health care [Yes]	0.08	0.03	0.02	0.14	2.85	56	0.006

4. Discussion

This secondary data analysis is the first study to explore the relationship between interpersonal goals and loneliness among older adults. To the best of our knowledge, these factors have not been previously examined in relation to loneliness in older adults. The research findings demonstrate that loneliness decreases as interpersonal compassion and self-image goals increase. This study is rooted in the study by Crocker and Canevello [20], which introduced interpersonal goals through their Ecosystem–Egosystem Theory of Social Motivation.

Per this study's results, one hypothesis was supported and one was not. The first hypothesis was confirmed, indicating that loneliness was lower among those with greater compassionate goals. These findings are consistent with prior studies' findings [20,22,24]. In previous studies, having more compassionate goals has also been linked to decreased symptoms of anxiety and depression [24], increased self-esteem [35], feeling more peaceful and less isolated [34], increased constructive approaches to interpersonal problems [36], and increased satisfaction with life [37].

The second hypothesis, that is, self-image goals would be associated with greater loneliness, was not supported. Indeed, we found a significant *negative* association between self-image goals and loneliness, contradicting previous studies: As self-image goals increase, loneliness increases among college students [20,22,24]. As the comparative study participants were from a younger population, these contradictions could be because of the different priorities of college students and older adults. In particular, as older adults age, they become less focused on fostering larger social networks or initiating new social relationships and instead focus more heavily on their closest and most rewarding relationships [25]. Therefore, self-image goals may provoke loneliness among younger adults aiming to impress new people and grow their social networks but play an entirely different role among an older population seeking *quality* rather than *quantity* in their social relationships.

No definitive data explain the difference between younger and older adults regarding self-image goals. However, consistent with Erikson's psychological development stages [38], college students are preoccupied with the self-image-driven, egocentric, and competitive establishment of role/career identity and intimate partnerships—based on a perceived fear of scarcity and inexperience with the value of collaborative effort. However, older adults, who may exhibit relatively greater satisfaction with their lifelong accomplishments, would have arrived at an appreciation of the importance of collective—and perhaps growing—dependency on cooperative effort, thus adopting a more altruistic and compassionate perspective. Consequently, we determined that differentiating between young and older adults is important.

In the full linear regression model, higher scores on both compassionate and self-image goals were significantly related to decreased loneliness. Participants with higher levels of compassion and self-image goals reported lower loneliness levels. Previous studies have found that females and older individuals are more likely to experience elevated loneliness [39–41]. However, like the findings of the HRS secondary analysis by Theeke [5], the meta-analysis by Maes et al. [42], and another study by Sunwoo [43], this study found no significant sex- and age-related differences in loneliness. As documented previously [44,45], our study found a strong positive correlation between functional impairment and loneliness. A lower educational level is also correlated with greater loneliness [45]. Similar to Theeke [5], our study found no association between the frequency of home care utilization and loneliness. Further, race, ethnicity, income, household size, and employment status were not significant loneliness predictors.

A key strength of this study is the use of a large population-based, nationally representative survey. This study can be replicated using international-level data to provide a meaningful comparison from a multicultural perspective. The study focused on interpersonal goals and advanced frontiers for researchers to further explore how interpersonal goals relate to loneliness in older adults. Finally, this study's results contribute to the growing body of knowledge regarding loneliness in older adults and can act as a valuable reference for examining post-COVID-19 loneliness in older adults.

This study exhibited some limitations. Data were obtained from a secondary source; therefore, only the variables available in the dataset were used. Second, verifying cause and effect was impossible owing to the study's cross-sectional nature. Third, the study primarily focused on providing a broad overview of interpersonal goals' effect on loneliness among older adults; thus, additional longitudinal and experimental research is required to inform our understanding in this area. While most findings were consistent with those of previous studies, this was the first exploration of interpersonal goals' effect on older adults; therefore, these results cannot be compared to those of previous studies. Fourth, Blacks and Hispanics were underrepresented in the study sample. Thus, the results cannot be generalized beyond the races and ethnicities included. Finally, the HRS survey comprises self-reported data, which are subject to response bias that may directly or indirectly influence the study's outcomes.

Despite the study's limitations, our findings are meaningful and provide a satisfactory foundation for future research. This study advances our understanding of the benefits of genuinely caring for—and extending support to—others. Further, this study opens novel avenues for the development of psychological interventions to mitigate loneliness. Disseminating these findings may aid public health policymakers and healthcare workers. The role of interpersonal goals in loneliness among older adults is under-researched.

This study's results have implications for future research and practice. In the present study, individuals' compassion and self-image goals were both associated with reduced loneliness among older adults. First, these results underline the differences between older and younger adults concerning their social goals and behaviors. Second, the findings elucidate the importance of identifying personal perspectives or resources that may be targeted in interventions aimed at reducing loneliness and preventing its adverse effects on the health and longevity of older adults.

In particular, healthcare providers play a pivotal role in assessing and recognizing loneliness and ensuring that patients receive appropriate care and treatment. Therefore, healthcare practitioners should assess loneliness in older adults; this is especially important for community and home healthcare practitioners providing home care to older adults. Healthcare providers should particularly focus on and conduct extensive loneliness assessments using standardized tools. If the indicators of loneliness are detected, practitioners should document them and facilitate follow-up evaluations and treatment accordingly. It is suggested that healthcare providers should actively schedule and promote activities that would promote interpersonal goals with more opportunities given to older adults with functional impairment. Future research could benefit from considering interpersonal goals' effect on loneliness among older adults from varied cultural and religious backgrounds.

5. Conclusions

The findings of this study can help us to better understand the relationship between loneliness and interpersonal goals in older adults. Further, the findings highlight that interpersonal goals are significantly related to loneliness. Loneliness exhibits significant detrimental effects on individuals' health. Healthcare practitioners who work with older adults should take measures to enhance their interpersonal goals, with special attention given to those with functional impairment. Further, mitigating loneliness among older adults is not only beneficial for their life satisfaction and well-being but may also provide a psychosocial resource to help them better confront the challenges of aging.

Author Contributions: Conceptualization, F.C.E. and K.L.S.; methodology, J.E.S., L.A.T. and M.T.-J.; software, F.C.E. and D.S.; formal analysis, F.C.E. and D.S.; investigation, F.C.E., K.L.S., J.E.S., L.A.T., M.T.-J. and R.Z.; data curation, F.C.E., K.L.S. and J.E.S.; writing original draft preparation, F.C.E. and K.L.S.; writing—review and editing, J.E.S., L.A.T., M.T.-J. and R.Z.; visualization, F.C.E. and D.S.; supervision, K.L.S.; project administration F.C.E.; funding acquisition, F.C.E. All authors have read and agreed to the published version of the manuscript.

Funding: The study was supported by a grant from the Epsilon Phi Chapter of SIGMA, Duquesne University School of Nursing awarded to F.C.E. The HRS (Health and Retirement Study) is sponsored by the National Institute on Aging (grant number NIA U01AG009740) and is conducted by the University of Michigan.

Institutional Review Board Statement: Not applicable.

Informed Consent Statement: Not applicable.

Data Availability Statement: The study data were derived from the 2016 HRS core dataset of the public biennial survey available at https://hrs.isr.umich.edu/about (accessed on 6 November 2020).

Acknowledgments: The authors thank Gary Yu, Associate Research Scientist, New York University Rory Meyers College of Nursing, New York, for his initial assistance with statistical analysis.

Conflicts of Interest: The authors declare no conflict of interest.

References

1. Gierveld, J.D.J. A review of loneliness: Concept and definitions, determinants and consequences. *Rev. Clin. Gerontol.* **1998**, *8*, 73–80. [CrossRef]
2. Luhmann, M.; Hawkley, L.C. Age differences in loneliness from late adolescence to oldest old age. *Dev. Psychol.* **2016**, *52*, 943–959. [CrossRef] [PubMed]
3. Lee, E.E.; Depp, C.; Palmer, B.W.; Glorioso, D.; Daly, R.; Liu, J.; Tu, X.M.; Kim, H.-C.; Tarr, P.; Yamada, Y.; et al. High prevalence and adverse health effects of loneliness in community-dwelling adults across the lifespan: Role of wisdom as a protective factor. *Int. Psychogeriatr.* **2018**, *31*, 1447–1462. [CrossRef] [PubMed]
4. Dykstra, P.A.; van Tilburg, T.; Gierveld, J.D.J. Changes in Older Adult Loneliness: Results from a seven-year longitudinal study. *Res. Aging* **2005**, *27*, 725–747. [CrossRef]
5. Theeke, L.A. Predictors of Loneliness in U.S. Adults Over Age Sixty-Five. *Arch. Psychiatr. Nurs.* **2009**, *23*, 387–396. [CrossRef]
6. Theeke, L.A.; Mallow, J. Loneliness and quality of life in chronically ill rural older adults. *Am. J. Nurs.* **2013**, *113*, 28–37. [CrossRef]
7. Theeke, L.A. Sociodemographic and Health-Related Risks for Loneliness and Outcome Differences by Loneliness Status in a Sample of U.S. Older Adults. *Res. Gerontol. Nurs.* **2010**, *3*, 113–125. [CrossRef]
8. Hawkley, L.C.; Preacher, K.J.; Cacioppo, J.T. Loneliness impairs daytime functioning but not sleep duration. *Heal. Psychol.* **2010**, *29*, 124–129. [CrossRef]
9. Van Bogart, K.; Engeland, C.G.; Sliwinski, M.J.; Harrington, K.D.; Knight, E.L.; Zhaoyang, R.; Scott, S.B.; Graham-Engeland, J.E. The Association between Loneliness and Inflammation: Findings from an Older Adult Sample. *Front. Behav. Neurosci.* **2022**, *15*, 801746. [CrossRef]
10. Taube, E.; Kristensson, J.; Sandberg, M.; Midlöv, P.; Jakobsson, U. Loneliness and health care consumption among older people. *Scand. J. Caring Sci.* **2015**, *29*, 435–443. [CrossRef]
11. Musich, S.; Wang, S.S.; Hawkins, K.; Yeh, C.S. The Impact of Loneliness on Quality of Life and Patient Satisfaction Among Older, Sicker Adults. *Gerontol. Geriatr. Med.* **2015**, *1*, 2333721415582119. [CrossRef] [PubMed]
12. Perissinotto, C.M.; Stijacic Cenzer, I.; Covinsky, K.E. Loneliness in older persons: A predictor of functional decline and death. *Arch. Intern. Med.* **2012**, *172*, 1078–1083. [CrossRef]
13. Wilson, C.; Moulton, B. *Loneliness among Older Adults: A National Survey of Adults 45+. Prepared by Knowledge Networks and Insight Policy Research*; AARP: Washington, DC, USA, 2010. [CrossRef]

14. Victor, C.R.; Yang, K. The Prevalence of Loneliness Among Adults: A Case Study of the United Kingdom. *J. Psychol.* **2012**, *146*, 85–104. [CrossRef]
15. Kemperman, A.; Van den Berg, P.; Weijs-Perrée, M.; Uijtdewillegen, K. Loneliness of Older Adults: Social Network and the Living Environment. *Int. J. Environ. Res. Public Health* **2019**, *16*, 406. [CrossRef] [PubMed]
16. Holt-Lunstad, J.; Smith, T.B.; Baker, M.; Harris, T.; Stephenson, D. Loneliness and Social Isolation as Risk Factors for Mortality: A Meta-Analytic Review. *Perspect. Psychol. Sci.* **2015**, *10*, 227–237. [CrossRef] [PubMed]
17. Rico-Uribe, L.A.; Caballero, F.F.; Martín-María, N.; Cabello, M.; Ayuso-Mateos, J.L.; Miret, M. Association of loneliness with all-cause mortality: A meta-analysis. *PLoS ONE* **2018**, *13*, e0190033. [CrossRef]
18. Yanguas, J.; Pinazo-Henandis, S.; Tarazona-Santabalbina, F.J. The complexity of loneliness. *Acta Biomed.* **2018**, *89*, 302–314. [CrossRef]
19. Gerst-Emerson, K.; Jayawardhana, J. Loneliness as a Public Health Issue: The Impact of Loneliness on Health Care Utilization Among Older Adults. *Am. J. Public Health* **2015**, *105*, 1013–1019. [CrossRef]
20. Crocker, J.; Canevello, A. Creating and undermining social support in communal relationships: The role of compassionate and self-image goals. *J. Pers. Soc. Psychol.* **2008**, *95*, 555–575. [CrossRef]
21. Canevello, A.; Crocker, J. Compassionate goals and affect in social situations. *Motiv. Emot.* **2017**, *41*, 158–179. [CrossRef]
22. Duarte, J.; Pinto-Gouveia, J. Focusing on Self or Others Has Different Consequences for Psychological Well-Being: A Longitudinal Study of the Effects of Distinct Interpersonal Goals. *J. Soc. Clin. Psychol.* **2015**, *34*, 809–825. [CrossRef]
23. Cohen-Mansfield, J.; Hazan, H.; Lerman, Y.; Shalom, V. Correlates and predictors of loneliness in older-adults: A review of quantitative results informed by qualitative insights. *Int. Psychogeriatr.* **2015**, *28*, 557–576. [CrossRef] [PubMed]
24. Crocker, J.; Canevello, A.; Breines, J.G.; Flynn, H. Interpersonal goals and change in anxiety and dysphoria in first-semester college students. *J. Pers. Soc. Psychol.* **2010**, *98*, 1009–1024. [CrossRef] [PubMed]
25. Lang, F.R.; Carstensen, L.L. Time counts: Future time perspective, goals, and social relationships. *Psychol. Aging* **2002**, *17*, 125–139. [CrossRef] [PubMed]
26. Crocker, J.; Canevello, A. Relationships and the self: Egosystem and ecosystem. In *APA Handbook of Personality and Social Psychology*; Mikulincer, M., Shaver, P.R., Simpson, J.A., Dovidio, J.F., Eds.; American Psychological Association: Washington, DC, USA, 2015; Volume 3. [CrossRef]
27. Crocker, J.; Olivier, M.-A.; Nuer, N. Self-image Goals and Compassionate Goals: Costs and Benefits. *Self Identity* **2009**, *8*, 251–269. [CrossRef]
28. HRS. Sample Sizes and Response Rates. Available online: https://hrs.isr.umich.edu/sites/default/files/biblio/ResponseRates_2017.pdf (accessed on 7 November 2020).
29. Smith, J.; Ryan, L.; Fisher, G.; Sonnega, A.; Weir, D. *Psychosocial and Lifestyle Questionnaire 2006–2016: Documentation Report*; Survey Research Center, Institute for Social Research, University of Michigan: Ann Arbor, MI, USA, 2017.
30. Faul, F.; Erdfelder, E.; Buchner, A.; Lang, A.-G. Statistical power analyses using G*Power 3.1: Tests for correlation and regression analyses. *Behav. Res. Methods* **2009**, *41*, 1149–1160. [CrossRef]
31. Lee, J.; Cagle, J.G. Validating the 11-Item Revised University of California Los Angeles Scale to Assess Loneliness Among Older Adults: An Evaluation of Factor Structure and Other Measurement Properties. *Am. J. Geriatr. Psychiatry* **2017**, *25*, 1173–1183. [CrossRef]
32. Canevello, A.; Crocker, J. Creating good relationships: Responsiveness, relationship quality, and interpersonal goals. *J. Pers. Soc. Psychol.* **2010**, *99*, 78–106. [CrossRef]
33. HRS. *Health and Retirement Study 2020 Tracker Early*; Version 1.0; HRS: Ann Arbor, MI, USA, 2022.
34. Sonnega, A.; Faul, J.D.; Ofstedal, M.B.; Langa, K.M.; Phillips, J.W.; Weir, D.R. Cohort Profile: The Health and Retirement Study (HRS). *Int. J. Epidemiol.* **2014**, *43*, 576–585. [CrossRef]
35. Canevello, A.; Crocker, J. Interpersonal goals, othersc regard for the self, and self-esteem: The paradoxical consequences of self-image and compassionate goals. *Eur. J. Soc. Psychol.* **2011**, *41*, 422–434. [CrossRef]
36. Canevello, A.; Crocker, J. How Self-Image and Compassionate Goals Shape Intrapsychic Experiences. *Soc. Pers. Psychol. Compass* **2015**, *9*, 620–629. [CrossRef]
37. Roper, M.; Tobin, S.J. Compassionate Goals, Facebook Use, and Subjective Well-Being: Examining the Roles of Relationship Maintenance and Connectedness. *Cyberpsychol. Behav. Soc. Netw.* **2022**, *25*, 527–533. [CrossRef] [PubMed]
38. Orenstein, G.A.; Lewis, L. Eriksons stages of psychosocial development. In *StatPearls*; StatPearls Publishing: Treasure Island, FL, USA, 2021. Available online: https://www.ncbi.nlm.nih.gov/books/NBK556096/ (accessed on 25 October 2021).
39. Ayalon, L.; Shiovitz-Ezra, S. The relationship between loneliness and passive death wishes in the second half of life. *Int. Psychogeriatr.* **2011**, *23*, 1677–1685. [CrossRef] [PubMed]
40. Pinquart, M.; Sorensen, S. Influences on Loneliness in Older Adults: A Meta-Analysis. *Basic Appl. Soc. Psychol.* **2001**, *23*, 245–266. [CrossRef]
41. Vozikaki, M.; Papadaki, A.; Linardakis, M.; Philalithis, A. Loneliness among older European adults: Results from the survey of health, aging and retirement in Europe. *J. Public Heal.* **2018**, *26*, 613–624. [CrossRef]
42. Maes, M.; Qualter, P.; Vanhalst, J.; Noortgate, W.V.D.; Goossens, L. Gender Differences in Loneliness across the Lifespan: A Meta–Analysis. *Eur. J. Pers.* **2019**, *33*, 642–654. [CrossRef]

43. Sunwoo, L. Loneliness among older adults in the Czech Republic: A socio-demographic, health, and psychosocial profile. *Arch. Gerontol. Geriatr.* **2020**, *90*, 104068. [CrossRef]
44. Gyasi, R.M.; Peprah, P.; Abass, K.; Siaw, L.P.; Adjakloe, Y.D.A.; Garsonu, E.K.; Phillips, D.R. Loneliness and physical function impairment: Perceived health status as an effect modifier in community-dwelling older adults in Ghana. *Prev. Med. Rep.* **2022**, *26*, 101721. [CrossRef]
45. Tough, H.; Gross-Hemmi, M.; Stringhini, S.; Eriks-Hoogland, I.; Fekete, C. Who is at Risk of Loneliness? A Cross-sectional Recursive Partitioning Approach in a Population-based Cohort of Persons with Spinal Cord Injury. *Arch. Phys. Med. Rehabil.* **2021**, *103*, 305–312. [CrossRef]

International Journal of
Environmental Research and Public Health

MDPI

Article

The Role of Functional Deficits, Depression, and Cognitive Symptoms in the Perceived Loneliness of Older Adults in Mexico City

Ana Belén Ramírez López [1], Yaneth Rodríguez-Agudelo [2], Francisco Paz-Rodríguez [2], Silvia Aracely Tafoya [3], Benjamín Guerrero López [3] and Claudia Diaz Olavarrieta [3,*]

[1] Mexican Institute of Social Security, Morelos Psychiatry Hospital, San Pedro el Chico, Gustavo A. Madero, Mexico City 07450, Mexico; anabelen.ramlo@comunidad.unam.mx

[2] Research Division, National Institute of Neurology and Neurosurgery MVS, Mexico City 14269, Mexico; jrodriguez@innn.edu.mx (Y.R.-A.); fpaz@innn.edu.mx (F.P.-R.)

[3] Department of Psychiatry and Mental Health, Faculty of Medicine, National Autonomous University of Mexico, Mexico City 04510, Mexico; stafoya@unam.mx (S.A.T.); dr.bguerrero@unam.mx (B.G.L.)

* Correspondence: cdiazolavarrieta@unam.mx; Tel.: +52-(55)-55-80-60-46-00

Abstract: The world is aging and experiencing loneliness. Functional impairment in instrumental activities of daily living (IADL) in older people (OP) with mild neurocognitive disorder (MNCD) predicts loneliness. After the pandemic, there was an increase in perceived loneliness. We explored the association between loneliness, depression, deficits in IADL, and cognitive symptoms among OP. From February to December 2023, using a cross-sectional design, we interviewed probable cases with mild cognitive impairment and caregivers in two public facilities. We administered the UCLA Loneliness Scale v3, Lawton IADL Scale, Mini-Mental State Examination (MMSE), and Yesavage's Geriatric Depression Scale. Samples were matched: 85 per group, 82.4% were women, married (52.95%), and mean age of 69.17 (±6.93) years. In our study, 30% displayed moderate to high levels of perceived loneliness. Multivariate analysis showed loneliness was associated with depression, low levels of IADL, and older age, but not with cognitive symptoms, which explained 22% of the total variance (F 165) = 16.99, ($p < 0.001$). Targeting symptoms and behaviors that could be modified (i.e., depression and functionality) can improve feelings of perceived loneliness and have an impact on morbidity and mortality with which it is associated.

Keywords: loneliness; functionality; mild neurocognitive disorder

1. Introduction

The aging of the world population constitutes a significant public health concern, as the percentage of people over 60 years old will double between 2015 and 2050 [1]. Mexico's official statistics estimate that between 2020 to 2025, this age group (60+ years) will grow by 3.5% and, according to data from the United Nation's Economic Commission for Latin America and the Caribbean (ECLAC), the regional growth between 2010 and 2060 will reach 10% [2,3].

According to the World Health Organization (WHO), the experience of loneliness among older people (OP) is a widespread condition; between 20% and 34% of OP in China, Europe, Latin America, and the United States feel lonely [4]. Research comparing global prevalences display significant variability, with prevalences ranging from 2% to 50% [5]. Prior to the start of the COVID-19 pandemic, the National Study of Health and Aging in Mexico reported that most of the elderly population had social and family networks, with only 9.5% of those aged 60–79 years and 15.1% aged $\geq$ 80 years living alone. In this same age group, 91.3% and 90.8% were in touch with their children; in addition, 58.9% and 56.2% reported receiving support from neighbors. However, the percentage mentioning feelings of loneliness was high for both groups, at 41.8% and 43.6%, respectively [6]. After the start of the pandemic, Mexico's National Health and Nutrition Survey noted that 12.3% of people aged ≥ 65 were living alone (vs 11.4% before the pandemic), with a high prevalence of social isolation (participants who were not in contact with others via mobile phones or electronic devices, 45.3%) and loneliness (almost 50%) reported among people living alone; however, the survey did not explore the perception of loneliness among those not living alone [7]. Age and social isolation, the new "geriatric giants", are associated with the perception of loneliness [8,9].

Loneliness, defined as the quality of a person's relationships with others, is a "distressing feeling that accompanies the perception that one's social needs are not being met by the quantity or especially the quality of one's social relationships" [10]. Loneliness is a complex and multifactorial experience, currently considered an index of quality of life and health, which can increase the risk of mortality from any cause by up to 45% among people aged ≥ 60 years, and it can also significantly increase the risk of developing diseases including cardiovascular disease, cognitive impairment, functional impairment, and psychiatric disorders [11–15].

The SARS-CoV-2 pandemic abruptly imposed restrictive and isolation measures on the world's social interaction [16,17]. After countries adopted these measures, an increase in loneliness was observed among up to one third (33.7%) of the elderly for whom this was an entirely novel and disquieting experience. Furthermore, the probability of experiencing loneliness showed a twofold increase among those who lived alone compared to those who lived as a couple [18].

Limited functionality in instrumental activities of daily living (IADL) has been considered a predictor of loneliness and social isolation; as the limitations increase, there is a greater experience of loneliness and greater distance from others. Research among OP, including those more at risk of developing dementia and those with limitations to carry out IADL, have shown they have less social support, a decreased social network size, and lower participation in social activities than those without such deficits or limitations [19,20]. Functionality is a complex condition influenced by cognitive, psychological, physical, and environmental factors [21]. Previously it was believed that people with mild neurocognitive disorder (MNCD) would not display significant functional deficits; however, deficits in at least one instrumental life activity daily have shown prevalences of up to 80% among subjects with MNCD [22,23]. Depending on which domains are involved, different cognitive functions will also be compromised; in addition, limitations in activities of daily living have also been shown to be a statistically significant predictor of incident dementia [24]. Regarding functional limitations in IADL in Mexican OP, in 2015 14.6% of the population > 60 years displayed some type of deficit or limitation, with differences according to sex: it was found in 18.5% of women and 10% of men [25]. A study in the U.S. showed IADL impairments in 31.3% of people ≥ 65 years, women with impaired IADL had a prevalence of 29.8%, and men had a prevalence of impairment of 20.2%. The degree of impairment found in Mexican women was similar to that of other countries [26,27].

Studying the association between loneliness, depression, functionality, and outcomes in social resources among OP in Mexico, controlling for participants with probable mild neurocognitive disorder and healthy senior citizens, is of paramount importance. The elderly, especially those with neurocognitive symptoms, are highly susceptible and more at risk of experiencing loneliness [28]. Exploring its impact on this age group using standardized measuring instruments that are easy to administer could allow us to characterize this phenomenon more thoroughly. It will permit a more multifaceted understanding of the ways in which these variables interact, and we will be able to draft a comprehensive assessment protocol that will lead to multidisciplinary interventions with the aim of strengthening the elderly's social support networks and improving the physical and mental health of patients seeking care at a public tertiary reference center for neurological diseases (National Institute of Neurology and Neurosurgery, NINN) and those treated in the psychogeriatric clinic of third-level care at a public psychiatric hospital in Mexico City.

The present study is based on two hypotheses: (1) we will observe a high prevalence of loneliness among older people; and (2) the extent of loneliness will be more significant in participants displaying a greater number of depressive symptoms, a higher prevalence of cognitive impairment, lower levels of functioning in daily activities, advanced age, and a lack of a partner (i.e., living alone).

2. Materials and Methods

2.1. Participants and Procedure

Ours was a cross-sectional study carried out in two public third-level-of-care facilities. We invited older people seen in the outpatient clinic of a psychogeriatric clinic for suspected cognitive impairment, patients with probable neurological deficits, and elderly caregivers of neurological patients treated in a neuropsychology clinical laboratory during February–December 2023. We did not establish other inclusion or exclusion criteria; all patients and caregivers were aged $\geq$ 60 years. Once they agreed to participate, they signed informed consent forms. A member of the study team then confirmed they were able to answer the study surveys, and they were recruited as participants.

The study was approved by the bioethics and research committees of both study sites. Once we obtained the informed consent of each participant, we collected sociodemographic data, and the study instruments were administered during the consultation hour assigned to each participant.

For both groups, the UCLA Loneliness Scale and the PHQ-9 questionnaire were self-administered, while the Yesavage Geriatric Depression Scale, the Lawton Index, and the Mini-Mental State Examination (MMSE) were administered by a trained researcher. A total of 86 patients were invited to participate from the psychogeriatric clinic, one participant was excluded due to missing data, and the final sample size included 85 patients.

Because our samples were recruited from two study sites and showed disparate sociodemographic characteristics, we needed to ensure both samples were appropriately matched by sex, age, and marital status. This was done to prevent any potential confounding effects associated with these variables, allowing for a more nuanced examination of our primary independent variables, including probable depression, MMSE scores, and functional capacity. We thus obtained a total of 85 participants in each group (those with probable neurological deficits and healthy subjects). Lastly, the groups were treated as a single entity to analyze the impact of the primary independent variables.

2.2. Measurements

2.2.1. Loneliness

The University of California Los Angeles (UCLA) Loneliness Scale version 3 [29], includes 20 items with four response options that are rated on a Likert-type scale ranging from 1 = "Never" to 4 = "Always". The UCLA Loneliness Scale includes eleven items that indicate the presence of loneliness and nine referring to its absence (they are calculated in reverse); the total score is made by adding the scores of each item. This scale is widely used in research to evaluate the degree of loneliness, and it does not establish a clinical cut-off point that indicates significant levels of loneliness. However, the following cut-off points have been proposed: scores of 20 to 34 indicate a low degree of loneliness; scores of 35 to 49 indicate a moderate degree of loneliness; scores of 50 to 64 indicate a moderately high degree of loneliness; and scores of 65 to 80 points indicate a high degree of loneliness [30,31]. For this study, we administered the Loneliness Scale v3 in Spanish for Mexico. The instrument has shown high internal consistency (alpha coefficient = 0.96) and a test–retest correlation over a two-month period of 0.73 [32].

2.2.2. Functionality

The Lawton Instrumental Activities of Daily Living Scale, developed at the Philadelphia Geriatric Center, was used to assess physical autonomy and IADL in inpatient or outpatient settings [33]. The index is used to identify the degree of independence of OP in carrying out IADL, and it assesses eight activities: using the telephone, cooking, washing clothes, doing housework, using transportation, managing finances, making purchases, and managing medications. Each item is assigned a numerical value, 1 = "independent" or 0 = "dependent", and the final score is obtained from the sum of the values of all the responses, ranging between 0 and 8, where 0 indicates maximum dependence and 8 total independence. In the Spanish population, it showed a Cronbach's alpha coefficient of 0.94 and factor loadings of 0.67 to 0.90, confirming the homogeneity of the construct [34].

2.2.3. Cognitive Impairment

To detect the presence of probable cognitive impairment, we used the Mini-Mental State Examination (MMSE), a screening test for neurocognitive disorders [35]. The test includes 19 items that assesses six cognitive domains: spatial and temporal orientation, fixation memory, evocation memory, attention, calculation, and language. To obtain a rating, the number of correct answers in the tests is counted and a higher score indicates an unimpaired cognitive state. The MMSE is also used to detect cognitive decline, determine the severity of cognitive decline if this is present, and monitor a person's cognitive changes. We used the version adapted and validated into Spanish [36], which considers sociodemographic variables such as age and level of educational attainment. A sensitivity of 97% and specificity of 88%, with an area under the curve of 0.85, has been reported to identify cognitive impairment. In our study, the MMSE cut-off score to determine cognitive decline was 24.

2.2.4. Confounding Variables

Considering sociodemographic characteristics, we enquired about sex, age, level of education, and marital status.

2.2.5. Probable or Confirmed Current Major Depressive Episodes

In the psychogeriatric clinic participants, the diagnosis of current depression was based on the psychiatric interview of the Diagnostic and Statistical Manual of Mental Disorders, Fifth Edition (DSM 5-TR) [37] and Yesavage's 15-item Geriatric Depression Scale (GDS-15) criteria [38]. Among the participants who were caretakers of neurological patients and were included in the study, the probable presence of current depression was evaluated using the Patient Health Questionnaire (PHQ-9), which is a self-administered questionnaire with nine items that provides a quantitative assessment of the severity of depressive symptoms at the time it is administered. Its score is obtained by adding the responses of each item [39]. Traditionally, a score ≥ 10 is considered to indicate a probable episode of major depression [40]. Although we used two different measuring instruments to evaluate the presence of depressive symptomatology, research has confirmed both are comparable. The GDS-15 and PHQ-9 have comparable diagnostic accuracy in classifying older adults with depressive episodes [41,42].

2.3. Data Analysis

The data was analyzed using the SPSS statistical program, v.23.0 (IBM Corp. Armonk, NY, USA). An $\alpha < 0.05$ was considered statistically significant. The Kolmogorov–Smirnov test was applied to verify the normality of the data. In addition, the omega coefficient of the instruments was calculated with the JASP 14.0.01 statistical package [43]. Descriptive statistics were used to characterize the sample, and bivariate analysis was performed to compare the groups: chi-squared or Fisher test for qualitative variables; *t* test or Mann–Whitney U test for quantitative variables. To assess the association between the study variables, we used Spearman correlation analysis. Lastly, we used multiple linear regression analysis to determine the predictors of loneliness, including depression and MMSE and IADL scores as independent variables, and the demographic characteristics of the study participants were also included: sex, marital status, whether they had a partner or not, study group (those with probable neurological deficits and healthy subjects), and level of schooling. We performed the regression model only with predictors that correlate with the dependent variable. We assumed no collinearity when the values of the variance inflation factors were less than 4.0 and the tolerance factors were greater than 0.2, and a Durbin–Watson residual close to 2 was observed to consider that no autocorrelation occurred (Hair et al., 2006] [44]. Outliers were determined with a z score greater than 3 or less than −3 (see Figure 1). The alpha–omega value for the loneliness scale was 0.924 and the alpha–omega value for the IADL scale was 0.940.

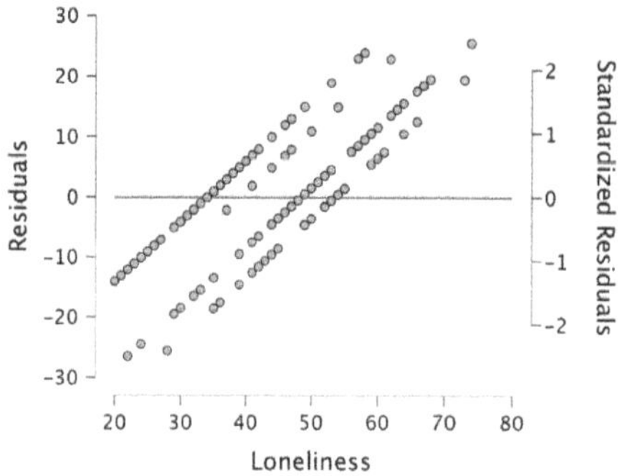

Figure 1. Loneliness vs. standardized residuals. Information on possible outliers.

3. Results

3.1. Characteristics of Study Participants

The samples were matched according to some of their demographic characteristics (sex, age, and marital status), resulting in a total of 85 participants in each group (Table 1). In general, there was a higher proportion of women (82.4%), a higher proportion of married participants (52.95%), and a mean age of 69.17 years. The following differences were observed between the groups, the sample treated in the psychiatric hospital and the one seen at the clinical neuropsychology laboratory (NINN), respectively: the frequency of cases with depression was 35.3% and 10.6%; the level of schooling had an average of 6.75 and 8.74 years; the degree of cognitive impairment showed a score of 23.87 and 25.74 in the MMSE; the functionality in IADL was 5.88 and 7.51 points; and finally, for the degree of loneliness the scores were 50.27 and 34.55 points. We noted that 68% of all participants displayed some degree of loneliness, but 30% of the total sample had a moderately high to high degree of perceived loneliness.

Table 1. Characteristics of study participants.

	Group		Total	p
	Participants with Probable Neurological Deficits	Healthy Participants (Caregivers)		
	n (%)	n (%)	n (%)	
Sex				
Women	70 (82.4)	70 (82.4)	140 (82.3)	
Men	15 (17.6)	15 (17.6)	30 (17.7)	1.000
Marital status				
Married/common law	40 (47.1)	50 (58.8)	90 (52.9)	
Widowed	29 (34.1)	24 (28.2)	53 (31.2)	
Divorced	8 (9.4)	2 (2.4)	10 (5.9)	
Single	8 (9.4)	9 (10.6)	17 (10.0)	0.155
Depression				
Yes	30 (35.3)	9 (10.6)	39 (22.9)	
No	55 (64.7)	76 (89.4)	131 (77.1)	<0.001

Table 1. *Cont.*

	Group		Total	p
	Participants with Probable Neurological Deficits	Healthy Participants (Caregivers)		
	n (%)	n (%)	n (%)	
Degree of perceived loneliness				
Low	9 (10.6)	45 (52.9)	54 (31.8)	
Moderate	31 (36.5)	34 (40.0)	65 (38.2)	
Moderately high	38 (44.7)	6 (7.1)	44 (25.9)	
High	7 (8.2)	0 (0)	7 (4.1)	<0.001
	Mean ± SD	Mean ± SD	Mean ± SD	
Age (years)	71.47 ± 7.53	70.27 ± 6.92	69.17 ± 6.93	0.340
Level of schooling (years)	6.75 ± 3.59	8.74 ± 4.84	9.02 ± 5.07	0.009
MMSE (score)	23.87 ± 2.72	25.74 ± 2.73	25.28 ± 2.83	<0.001
IADL (score)	5.88 ± 2.15	7.51 ± 1.11	7.06 ± 1.67	<0.001
Loneliness (score)	50.27 ± 11.86	34.55 ± 9.59	38.82 ± 12.72	<0.001

Note: Comparisons were made using chi-squared/Fisher test and Mann–Whitney U test. IADL, Instrumental activities of daily living. MMSE, Mini-Mental State Exam.

3.2. Spearman Correlations

When analyzing correlations (Table 2), we noted a statistically significant, low, and negative correlation between loneliness and level of schooling, sex (being female), group (probable neurological deficits), and MMSE and IADL scores. Furthermore, as expected we also observed a low significant and directly proportional correlation between perceived loneliness and depression. We also found a moderate negative correlation between age and IADL. Depression showed a low negative correlation with MMSE and IADL scores.

Table 2. Spearman correlations.

Variable	1	2	3	4	5	6	7	8
1. Perceived loneliness	—							
2. Age	0.109	—						
3. Level of schooling	−0.273 **	−0.279 **	—					
4. Depression	0.311 **	0.076	−0.122	—				
5. Sex	−0.292 **	−0.080	0.209 **	−0.115	—			
6. Group	0.594 **	0.073	−0.201 *	0.294 **	0.000			
7. MMSE	−0.286 **	−0.207 **	0.335 **	−0.194 **	0.148 *	0.355 **		
8. IADL	−0.396 **	−0.421 **	0.298 **	−0.185 **	0.125 *	0.460 **	0.382 **	—

Notes: IADL, Instrumental activities of daily living. MMSE, Mini-Mental State Exam. ** The correlation was significant at alpha level of 0.01; * The correlation was significant at alpha level of 0.05.

3.3. Multiple Regression Model for Perceived Loneliness in Older Adults and Association between Model Variables

Lastly, Table 3 shows the multiple linear regression analysis where the predictor variable of perceived loneliness was associated with the group they were recruited into (probable neurological deficits) and symptoms of depression. The adjusted R2 coefficient indicates our model explained 36% of the total loneliness variance. The F value in the analysis of variance (F 166) = 48.94, ($p < 0.001$) shows the existence of a significant linear association between group (probable neurological deficits) and depression as the main variables of the model.

Table 3. Multiple regression model for loneliness in older adults (n = 166).

Variable	Unstandardized	Standard Error	B	*T*	*p*	95% CI
(Intercept)	62.90	2.86		22.02	<0.001	60.76, 71.13
Group (probable neurological deficits)	14.43	1.71	0.54	8.43	<0.001	11.05, 17.81
Depression	5.08	2.03	0.16	2.502	0.013	1.07, 9.10
F	48.94					
Adjusted R^2	0.36					
Durbin–Watson	1.72					

Note. The following covariates were considered but not included: level of schooling, sex, does not live with a partner, and MMSE scores.

4. Discussion

Ours was a cross-sectional study carried out in two public third-level-of-care facilities among 85 older adults who were seen in the outpatient clinics of a psychogeriatric clinic for suspected cognitive impairment and 85 participants who were caregivers of neurologic patients (older adults), all seen during February–December 2023. We explored the association between perceived loneliness, depression, deficits in daily functioning, and cognitive symptoms among OP, hypothesizing that all of these would be predictors of a greater perception of loneliness. Our results indicate a high prevalence of loneliness among participants, as well as a greater perception of it among those with depressive symptoms, decreased degree of daily functioning and being older; however, the perception of loneliness was not associated with cognitive symptoms. To our knowledge, this is the first attempt at studying the effects of depression and level of functionality on older adults' perception of loneliness post COVID-19 among this age group in Mexico City.

Regarding our first hypothesis, we found that a third of the study participants surveyed displayed levels of perceived loneliness in the moderate to high range. Previous studies worldwide, reported through a systematic review, showed higher prevalences of loneliness in OP compared to younger ones. The prevalence of loneliness in groups of OP in European countries fluctuated between 4.2% and 24.2%, with lower levels of loneliness found among those with higher socioeconomic status, improved health status, greater welfare generosity, and high social participation [45]; challenging conditions that are often not met in low- or middle-income countries such as Mexico. The level of perceived loneliness observed in our study was like that reported during the COVID-19 pandemic [18]; however, it was also similar to the level reported in people over 50 years of age in the US [13].

The second hypothesis proposed several factors that may be associated with the experience of loneliness. In our study, we observed higher levels of loneliness associated with greater difficulties in functioning and greater affective (depressive) symptoms, and a slight association with the presence of cognitive symptoms, in accordance with criteria suggested by Surkalim et al., 2022 [45]. We also believe that the sudden confinement imposed by the pandemic may have increased the participants' perception of loneliness, since health and isolation conditions may not have returned to their pre-pandemic levels, an area that merits further research.

It is worth noting that the association found between deficits in daily functioning and loneliness has been previously reported. One study indicates that perceived loneliness can be associated with a decrease in physical activity mediated by marital status, since widowed people with higher rates of loneliness seem to exhibit decreased functioning more than those who are married or separated [46]. While other studies point out that these findings depend on sex, it is an association observed only in women, but not in men [11,13].

These studies indicate a directionality that ranges from loneliness to functioning, but a systematic review pointed out that this relationship can also be bidirectional [12]. Although our study, due to its cross-sectional nature, does not allow us to establish a causal relationship, we think there may be factors that influence each other. Regarding the association found between depression and perception of loneliness, this finding has also been reported consistently. Again, most studies point to loneliness as a precursor of depression [47,48], but there is also evidence that shows that feelings of loneliness can contribute to the presence of depression [49]. Likewise, it has been suggested that depression, when associated with cognitive symptoms, increases loneliness in OP [50]. Therefore, we can put forth a bidirectional association between these variables, which can become a vicious circle that has an increasingly negative effect and decreases the patient's sense of well-being. We also noted that the MMSE scores were correlated with loneliness, but the multiple regression model did not find a significant association. This finding is contrary to what has been reported in the literature [51]; however, we think the symptoms of depression could have explained these two variables, or the patients' symptoms could have been mild, and thus we were not able to observe its effect.

Among the study limitations, we find that our cross-sectional study design did not allow us to infer causality among study variables, and even though we were able to pair our samples (by sex, age and marital status) to make them homogeneous, we had to carry out convenience sampling. A further limitation was the use of different instruments to assess probable depression, because participants came from two disparate public institutions. While both scales are internationally recognized and have reliability, validity, and well-established cutoff points for depression in our population, their scores are not directly comparable. Consequently, they can only be considered as indicators of the presence of significant depression symptoms. A study strength was that we were able to sample patients and healthy controls from two of the most underprivileged districts of a mega-city (Mexico City), who had some of the highest COVID-19 morbidity and mortality rates and thus could be subject to experiencing higher rates of perceived loneliness due to the limited home, work, and family infrastructure imposed during confinement [18,52].

5. Conclusions

Loneliness has been shown to increase the morbidity and mortality of older adults [9]. Data mostly from industrialized countries is consistent with our study findings, so there is a pressing need to implement strategies for first-level-of-care physicians to identify lonely patients. While our study was fielded in tertiary-care public facilities, we could extrapolate and perhaps increase our prevalences when we consider the patient population normally seen in primary care. It seems that Mexico's epidemiological transition now includes frail, elderly people living in underprivileged conditions, such as our study participants, who reported a heightened perception of loneliness and mental health indicators that are consistent with the need to implement strategies to help reduce this new giant, even in countries such as ours with a myriad of competing health inequities.

Author Contributions: Oversaw fieldwork and data collection, A.B.R.L., Y.R.-A. and F.P.-R.; selected the data collection instruments in consultation with the study team, B.G.L., C.D.O., A.B.R.L., Y.R.-A., F.P.-R. and S.A.T.; oversaw the study design and data analysis, S.A.T., A.B.R.L. and F.P.-R.; wrote and edited the first drafts of the manuscript, A.B.R.L., S.A.T. and C.D.O.; oversaw project administration A.B.R.L., Y.R.-A. and F.P.-R.; all authors reviewed, edited and approved all drafts of the manuscript. All authors have read and agreed to the published version of the manuscript.

Funding: This research received no external funding.

Institutional Review Board Statement: The study was conducted in accordance with the Declaration of Helsinki and approved by Research and Ethics Commissions of two national public institutions (NINNN-IRB # 11/20 protocol approval date 23/02/23 and R-2023-3501-086 protocol approval date 13 June 2023).

Informed Consent Statement: Written informed consent was obtained from all study participants.

Data Availability Statement: The original contributions presented in this study are included in the article. Further inquiries can be directed to the corresponding author.

Acknowledgments: We thank all subjects who participated in this study.

Conflicts of Interest: The authors declare no conflicts of interest.

References

1. United Nations. *World Population Ageing 2019*; United Nations: New York, NY, USA, 2019.
2. INEGI. *Encuesta Nacional Sobre Salud y Envejecimiento en México 2018 (ENASEM)*; Instituto Nacional de Estadística y Geografía (INEGI): Aguascalientes, México, 2018.
3. CEPAL. *Envejecimiento, Personas Mayores y Agenda 2030 Para el Desarrollo Sostenible: Perspectiva Regional y de Derechos Humanos*; Naciones Unidas: Santiago, Chile, 2018; Volume N.
4. World Health Organization. *Social Isolation and Loneliness among Older People: Advocacy Brief*; World Health Organization: Geneva, Switzerland, 2021.
5. Miranda-Sánchez, B.S. *Determinantes del Sentimiento de Soledad Incidente en Adultos Mayores*; World Health Organization: Geneva, Switzerland; Universidad Nacional Autónoma de México: Ciudad de México, México, 2021.
6. Ávila, J.; Michaels-Obregón, A.; Wong, R. Envejecimiento en México: Los adultos más vulnerables. In *Boletín Informativo ENASEM*; ENASEM: Mexican Health and Aging Study: Aguascalientes, México, 2020; Volume N° 154 (LC/PUB.2018/24-P).
7. Shamah-Levy, T.; Romero-Martínez, M.; Barrientos-Gutiérrez, T.; Cuevas-Nasu, L.; Bautista-Arredondo, S.; Colchero, M.A.; GaonaPineda, E.B.; Lazcano-Ponce, E.; Martínez-Barnetche, J.; Alpuche-Arana, C.; et al. *Encuesta Nacional de Salud y Nutrición 2020 sobre COVID-19. Resultados Nacionales*; Instituto Nacional de Salud Pública, Secretaría de Salud: Cuernavaca, México, 2021.
8. Giné-Garriga, M.; Jerez-Roig, J.; Coll-Planas, L.; Skelton, D.A.; Inzitari, M.; Booth, J.; Souza, D.L.B. Is loneliness a predictor of the modern geriatric giants? Analysis from the survey of health, ageing, and retirement in Europe. *Maturitas* **2021**, *144*, 93–101. [CrossRef] [PubMed]
9. Freedman, A.; Nicolle, J. Social isolation and loneliness: The new geriatric giants: Approach for primary care. *Can. Fam. Physician* **2020**, *66*, 176–182. [PubMed]
10. Hawkley, L.C.; Cacioppo, J.T. Loneliness matters: A theoretical and empirical review of consequences and mechanisms. *Ann. Behav. Med.* **2010**, *40*, 218–227. [CrossRef] [PubMed]
11. Guo, L.; An, L.; Luo, F.; Yu, B. Social isolation, loneliness and functional disability in Chinese older women and men: A longitudinal study. *Age Ageing* **2021**, *50*, 1222–1228. [CrossRef] [PubMed]
12. Pollak, C.; Verghese, J.; Blumen, H. Loneliness and Functional Decline in Aging: A Systematic Review. *Res. Gerontol. Nurs.* **2023**, *16*, 202–212. [CrossRef] [PubMed]
13. Qi, X.; Belsky, D.W.; Yang, Y.C.; Wu, B. Association Between Types of Loneliness and Risks of Functional Disability in Older Men and Women: A Prospective Analysis. *Am. J. Geriatr. Psychiatry* **2023**, *31*, 621–632. [CrossRef]
14. Vespa, A.; Spatuzzi, R.; Fabbietti, P.; Di Rosa, M.; Bonfigli, A.R.; Corsonello, A.; Gattafoni, P.; Giulietti, M.V. Association between Sense of Loneliness and Quality of Life in Older Adults with Multimorbidity. *Int. J. Environ. Res. Public Health* **2023**, *20*, 2615. [CrossRef] [PubMed]
15. Yang, F.; Zhang, J.; Wang, J. Correlates of loneliness in older adults in Shanghai, China: Does age matter? *BMC Geriatr.* **2018**, *18*, 300. [CrossRef] [PubMed]
16. Brooks, S.K.; Webster, R.K.; Smith, L.E.; Woodland, L.; Wessely, S.; Greenberg, N.; Rubin, G.J. The psychological impact of quarantine and how to reduce it: Rapid review of the evidence. *Lancet* **2020**, *395*, 912–920. [CrossRef]
17. Wilder-Smith, A.; Freedman, D.O. Isolation, quarantine, social distancing and community containment: Pivotal role for old-style public health measures in the novel coronavirus (2019-nCoV) outbreak. *J. Travel Med.* **2020**, *27*, taaa020. [CrossRef] [PubMed]
18. Vlachantoni, A.; Evandrou, M.; Falkingham, J.; Qin, M. The Impact of Changing Social Support on Older Persons' Onset of Loneliness During the COVID-19 Pandemic in the United Kingdom. *Gerontologist* **2022**, *62*, 1147–1159. [CrossRef] [PubMed]
19. Kim, S.; Choe, K.; Lee, K. Depression, Loneliness, Social Support, Activities of Daily Living, and Life Satisfaction in Older Adults at High-Risk of Dementia. *Int. J. Environ. Res. Public Health* **2020**, *17*, 9448. [CrossRef]
20. Tomioka, K.; Kurumatani, N.; Hosoi, H. Association between Social Participation and Instrumental Activities of Daily Living Among Community-Dwelling Older Adults. *J. Epidemiol.* **2016**, *26*, 553–561. [CrossRef] [PubMed]
21. Salvador-Carulla, L.; Gasca, V.I. Defining disability, functioning, autonomy and dependency in person-centered medicine and integrated care. *Int. J. Integr. Care* **2010**, *10*, e025. [CrossRef] [PubMed]
22. Mcalister, C.; Schmitter-Edgecombe, M.; Lamb, R. Examination of Variables That May Affect the Relationship between Cognition and Functional Status in Individuals with Mild Cognitive Impairment: A Meta-Analysis. *Arch. Clin. Neuropsychol.* **2016**, *31*, 123–147. [CrossRef]
23. Brown, P.J.; Devanand, D.P.; Liu, X.; Caccappolo, E.; Alzheimer's Disease Neuroimaging Initiative. Functional impairment in elderly patients with mild cognitive impairment and mild Alzheimer disease. *Arch. Gen. Psychiatry* **2011**, *68*, 617–626. [CrossRef] [PubMed]
24. Fieo, R.; Zahodne, L.; Tang, M.; Manly, J.; Cohen, R.; Stern, Y. The Historical Progression from ADL Scrutiny to IADL to Advanced ADL. Assessing Functional Status in the Earliest Stages of Dementia. *J. Gerontol. Ser. A-Biol. Sci. Med. Sci.* **2018**, *73*, 1695–1700. [CrossRef] [PubMed]
25. Barreto-Anaya, A.I. *Análisis de la Autonomía Física de las Personas de 75 Años y Más: Aproximación a Partir del Estudio Nacional de Salud y Envejecimiento en México (ENASEM) 2018*; Facultad Latinoamericana de Ciencias Sociales: Aguascalientes, México, 2021.
26. Knoll, K.; Rhee, Y.; Hamm, J.M.; Hammer, K.D.P.; Heimbuch, H.; Holloway, J.; Jurivich, D.; Lahr, P.; McGrath, B.; Parker, K.; et al. The Prevalence and Trends of Instrumental Activities of Daily Living Impairments in the United States from 2008–2018. *J. Alzheimers Dis. Rep.* **2023**, *7*, 271–278. [CrossRef] [PubMed]

27. Gómez, F.; Osorio-García, D.; Panesso, L.; Curcio, C.L. Healthy aging determinants and disability among older adults: SABE Colombia. *Rev. Panam. Salud Publica* **2021**, *45*, e98. [CrossRef]
28. Yu, J.; Lam, C.L.; Lee, T.M. Perceived loneliness among older adults with mild cognitive impairment. *Int. Psychogeriatr.* **2016**, *28*, 1681–1685. [CrossRef]
29. Russell, D.W. UCLA Loneliness Scale (Version 3): Reliability, validity, and factor structure. *J. Pers. Assess.* **1996**, *66*, 20–40. [CrossRef] [PubMed]
30. Deckx, L.; van den Akker, M.; Buntinx, F. Risk factors for loneliness in patients with cancer: A systematic literature review and meta-analysis. *Eur. J. Oncol. Nurs.* **2014**, *18*, 466–477. [CrossRef] [PubMed]
31. Valdelamar, A.; Parra, A.M.; Sánchez, R.; De La Hoz, F. Adaptación transcultural de la versión colombiana de la Escala de Soledad de UCLA en pacientes con diagnóstico de cáncer. *Rev. Colomb. Cancerol.* **2022**, *26*, 97–110. [CrossRef]
32. Serrano-Gonzalez, R. *Adaptación de la Escala de Soledad -Loneliness Scale UCLA-en Mujeres en Situación de Violencia del Estado de México*; Universidad Autónoma del Estado de México: México, México, 2018.
33. Lawton, M.P.; Brody, E.M. Assessment of older people: Self-maintaining and instrumental activities of daily living. *Gerontologist* **1969**, *9*, 179–186. [CrossRef] [PubMed]
34. Vergara, I.; Bilbao, A.; Orive, M.; Garcia-Gutierrez, S.; Navarro, G.; Quintana, J.M. Validation of the Spanish version of the Lawton IADL Scale for its application in elderly people. *Health Qual Life Outcomes* **2012**, *10*, 130. [CrossRef] [PubMed]
35. Folstein, M.; Folstein, S.E.; McHugh, P. "Mini-mental state": A practical method for grading the cognitive state of patients for the clinician. *J. Psychiatr. Res.* **1975**, *12*, 189–198. [CrossRef] [PubMed]
36. Beaman, S.R.D.; Beaman, P.E.; Garcia-Peña, C.; Villa, M.A.; Heres, J.; Córdova, A.; Jagger, C. Validation of a Modified Version of the Mini-Mental State Examination (MMSE) in Spanish. *Aging Neuropsychol. Cogn.* **2004**, *11*, 1–11. [CrossRef]
37. American Psychiatric Association. *Manual Diagnóstico Y Estadístico de los Trastornos Mentales*, 5th ed.; Panamericana: Ciudad de México, México, 2013.
38. Martínez-de-la-Iglesia, J.; Onís-Vilches, M.C.; Dueñas Herrero, R.; Albert-Colomer, C.; Aguado-Taberné, C.; Luque-Luque, R. Versión española del cuestionario de Yesavage abreviado (GDS) para el despistaje de depresión en mayores de 65 años: Adaptación y validación. *Medifam* **2002**, *12*, 26–40. [CrossRef]
39. Kroenke, K.; Spitzer, R.L.; Williams, J.B. The PHQ-9: Validity of a brief depression severity measure. *J. Gen. Intern. Med.* **2001**, *16*, 606–613. [CrossRef]
40. Levis, B.; Benedetti, A.; Thombs, B.D.; Collaboration, D.S.D.D. Accuracy of Patient Health Questionnaire-9 (PHQ-9) for screening to detect major depression: Individual participant data meta-analysis. *BMJ* **2019**, *365*, l1476. [CrossRef]
41. Pellas, J.; Damberg, M. Accuracy in detecting major depressive episodes in older adults using the Swedish versions of the GDS-15 and PHQ-9. *Upsala J. Med. Sci.* **2021**, *20*, 126. [CrossRef]
42. Zhang, H.; Wang, S.; Wang, L.; Yi, X.; Jia, X.; Jia, C. Comparison of the Geriatric Depression Scale-15 and the Patient Health Questionnaire-9 for screening depression in older adults. *Geriatr. Gerontol. Int.* **2020**, *20*, 138–143. [CrossRef]
43. Navarro, D.J.; Foxcroft, D.R.; Faulkenberry, T.J. *Learning Statistics with JASP: A Tutorial for Psychology Students and Other Beginners (0.7)*; University of Amsterdam: Sydney, NSW, Australia, 2019.
44. Hair, J.F.; Anderson, R.E.; Tatham, R.L.; Black, W.C. *Multivariate Data Analysis with Readings*; Pearson Prentice Hall: New York, NY, USA, 2006; Volume 6.
45. Surkalim, D.L.; Luo, M.; Eres, R.; Gebel, K.; van Buskirk, J.; Bauman, A.; Ding, D. The prevalence of loneliness across 113 countries: Systematic review and meta-analysis. *BMJ* **2022**, *376*, e067068. [CrossRef]
46. Pollak, C.; Verghese, J.; Buchman, A.S.; Jin, Y.; Blumen, H.M. Loneliness Predicts Progression of Frailty in Married and Widowed, but Not Unmarried Community Dwelling Older Adults. *J. Frailty Aging* **2024**, *13*, 163–171. [CrossRef]
47. Erzen, E.; Çikrikci, Ö. The effect of loneliness on depression: A meta-analysis. *Int. J. Soc. Psychiatry* **2018**, *64*, 427–435. [CrossRef]
48. Zhang, Y.; Kuang, J.; Xin, Z.; Fang, J.; Song, R.; Yang, Y.; Song, P.; Wang, Y.; Wang, J. Loneliness, social isolation, depression and anxiety among the elderly in Shanghai: Findings from a longitudinal study. *Arch. Gerontol. Geriatr.* **2023**, *110*, 104980. [CrossRef]
49. Drageset, J.; Espehaug, B.; Kirkevold, M. The impact of depression and sense of coherence on emotional and social loneliness among nursing home residents without cognitive impairment—A questionnaire survey. *J. Clin. Nurs.* **2012**, *21*, 965–974. [CrossRef]
50. Brush, C.J.; Kallen, A.M.; Meynadasy, M.A.; King, T.; Hajcak, G.; Sheffler, J.L. The P300, loneliness, and depression in older adults. *Biol. Psychol.* **2022**, *171*, 108339. [CrossRef]
51. Karska, J.; Pszczołowska, M.; Gładka, A.; Leszek, J. Correlations between Dementia and Loneliness. *Int. J. Mol. Sci.* **2023**, *25*, 271. [CrossRef]
52. Baarck, J.; d'Hombres, B.; Tintori, G. Loneliness in Europe before and during the COVID-19 pandemic. *Health Policy* **2022**, *126*, 1124–1129. [CrossRef]

International Journal of
Environmental Research and Public Health

MDPI

Article

Association of Loneliness and Mindfulness in Substance Use Treatment Retention

Johnathan M. Herczyk [1,*], Keith J. Zullig [1], Stephen M. Davis [2], Jennifer Mallow [3], Gerald R. Hobbs [4], Danielle M. Davidov [1], Laura R. Lander [5] and Laurie Theeke [6]

1 Department of Social and Behavioral Sciences, School of Public Health, West Virginia University, Morgantown, WV 26506, USA
2 Department of Health Policy, Management and Leadership, School of Public Health, West Virginia University, Morgantown, WV 26506, USA
3 School of Nursing, West Virginia University, Morgantown, WV 26506, USA
4 Department of Statistics, West Virginia University, Morgantown, WV 26506, USA
5 Department of Behavioral Medicine and Psychiatry, Rockefeller Neurosciences Institute, School of Medicine, West Virginia University, Morgantown, WV 26506, USA
6 School of Nursing, The George Washington University, Washington, DC 20052, USA
* Correspondence: jmherczyk@hsc.wvu.edu

Abstract: Background: Elevated mental illness prevalence complicates efforts designed to address the opioid crisis in Appalachia. The recovery community acknowledges that loneliness impacts mood and engagement in care factors; however, the predictive relationship between loneliness and retention in medication-assisted outpatient treatment programs has not been explored. Our objectives were to identify associations between mental health factors and retention in treatment and elucidate treatment retention odds. Data were collected from eighty participants (n = 57 retained, n = 23 not retained) of a mindfulness-based relapse prevention (MBRP) intervention for individuals receiving medication for opioid use disorder (MOUD) in Appalachia. Loneliness, depression, and anxiety did not differ between the retained and not retained, nor did they predict not being retained; however, mindfulness was significantly lower among those not retained in treatment compared to those retained (OR = 0.956, 95% CI (0.912–1.00), and $p < 0.05$). Preliminary findings provide evidence for mindfulness training integration as part of effective treatment, with aims to further elucidate the effectiveness of mindfulness therapies on symptom reduction in co-occurring mental health disorders, loneliness, and MOUD treatment retention.

Keywords: loneliness; mindfulness; mental health; MOUD; retention; intervention strategies

1. Introduction

The widespread distribution and misuse of opioids have resulted in the opioid crisis in the United States, which has been linked to nearly 1 million fatal overdoses since 1999 [1]. Despite consistent decreases in opioid prescribing patterns since 2012 [2] and the implementation of evidence-based strategies provided by the Centers for Disease Control and Prevention (CDC) to impede the continued escalation in overdose fatalities [3], increases in mortality persist. The U.S. recorded 105,800 fatal overdoses during the COVID-19 pandemic in 2021 [4], a 15% increase from the year prior [1].

Elevated rates of mental illness are complicating efforts to adequately address this dire public health issue. In 2021, 19.4 million U.S. adults had a co-occurring mental, behavioral, or emotional disorder with a substance use disorder [5]. A recent meta-analysis reports that 36.1% (95% CI 32.4–39.7%) of individuals with opioid use disorder (OUD) concurrently experienced depression, and 29.1% (95% CI 24.0–33.3%) experienced anxiety [6]. Loneliness, the perceived lack of social connections, is also significant to the experience of substance use and mental illness, owing to its influence on mood, motivation, and decision making [7].

1.1. Loneliness

Although frequently used interchangeably, social isolation and loneliness are two distinct, yet related, components of social connections. Social isolation is a deficiency in physical interactions between an individual and persons or systems in their social network [8,9]. On the other hand, loneliness is a discrepancy between the actual and perceived quality as well as availability of support from one's relationships. Individuals may experience loneliness intermittently or chronically throughout their lives [8]; however, regardless of the experiential frequency, loneliness is detrimental to the health and survival of populations. The experience of loneliness is profound and prevalent throughout the United States, with a recent Surgeon General report highlighting the topic and providing a call to action. Loneliness and social isolation both impact and increase the risk of cardiovascular disease, stroke, dementia, and even premature death [10]. Evidence supports the idea that loneliness increases the risk of mood and anxiety disorders [10,11]. A systematic review into predictors of loneliness within SUD populations reports that people with substance use issues are lonelier than those without, and women as well as younger people with substance use issues may be lonelier than their peers [12]. A cross-sectional study on New England and Pacific Northwest opioid treatment programs found inverse relationships between men and women: Men with little to no loneliness were more likely to use illicit opioids than their severely lonely counterparts (OR = 2.86, 95% CI 1.15–7.14) [13]. In contrast, severely lonely women were more likely to use illicit opioids when compared to those with little to no loneliness (OR = 3.00, 95% CI 1.19–7.57) [13].

Mindfulness is a mental state of being fully present in the moment without judgment in addition to being aware of one's surroundings and actions. This meditative practice has garnered credibility as a component of relapse prevention and treatment programs for substance use disorders because of the influence that mindfulness has on decision making, similar to loneliness. Mindfulness improves an individual's awareness of internal and external stimuli that influence substance use behaviors; for populations with substance use disorders, this is focused on drug use triggers. Mindfulness-based relapse prevention (MBRP) interventions focus on improving individuals' awareness to the current moment (e.g., drug use triggers) and adapting to recognize as well as control outcomes. Within populations with substance use disorders, MBRP has been shown to reduce depression, anxiety, and drug craving symptoms, as well as improve tolerance of challenging physical and emotional situations [14]. This supports the importance of considering mindfulness when assessing loneliness in substance-using populations. One such MBRP intervention within the Appalachian region has supported these notions [15] as well as identified an inverse correlation between mindfulness and loneliness among individuals diagnosed with OUD [16].

1.2. Mental Health in Central Appalachia

Appalachia is a region of the Eastern United States, marked by the Appalachian Mountains, which stretch from southern New York to northern Mississippi. Although Appalachia is comprised of 13 states in total, West Virginia is uniquely situated in Central Appalachia and is the only state fully within the region. Overall, the Central Appalachian region suffers from poor social determinants of health (e.g., income, education, and employment), and this is amplified for the 35.5% of the population living in rural areas of the state [17].

Overall mental health quality is lower among Central Appalachians. Extensive research has found loneliness to be pervasive and detrimental to quality of life among middle-aged [18] and older, chronically ill, Appalachians [19]. Moderate loneliness is hypothesized to be widespread yet under-reported by adults living in the region due to the Appalachian cultural value of self-reliance [20] as well as the isolating geography of the region [21]. Physical barriers and rurality limit access to care and opportunities for social connections [21], thus contributing to the prevalence of loneliness in Central Appalachia. Furthermore, rates of depression are 17% higher [22]. Surveillance data continue to report that West Virginia has the highest age-adjusted opioid overdose mortality rate of 90.9 per

100,000 people in 2021, an increase of nearly 40 points compared to prepandemic rates [23]; however, the region remains underserved by mental health providers and designated as a health professional shortage area [24], with additional access barriers being introduced by state legislation, such as prohibitions on new methadone treatment programs [25].

The recovery community has long noted the influence that loneliness has on mood, motivation [7], and decision making, as well as engagement in managing one's health [11]. A recent intervention has shown promise for reducing loneliness by employing mindfulness techniques [26], a concept that has also shown promise for reducing drug craving, depression, and anxiety among individuals receiving medication for opioid use disorder (MOUD) [15]. Although loneliness has been associated with an increased likelihood of using illicit opioids [13] and, thus, subsequently experiencing a period of relapse, the predictive relationship between loneliness and retention in MOUD outpatient treatment has not been explored, particularly in Appalachian populations.

Because the initial services are difficult to access, retaining individuals in MOUD treatment is critical to improve outcomes within the region. Retention in treatment is essential to avoiding relapse, overdose, and death, with longer retention improving mortality rates [27–30]. The prevalence of retention in treatment is considerably variable in the recent literature, ranging from 19% to 91% over twelve months [27,28]. Consistent definitions of retention are uncommon [31], making it difficult to compare findings across interventions; therefore, no best practice has been reported to increase retention in MOUD [28,31], despite multiple attempts to address known barriers to retention [32–34]. No study has been found to have investigated the influence of loneliness on retention in treatment within Appalachia.

Therefore, the current study's objectives were as follows: (1) identify associations between mental health factors and demographics with retention in MOUD treatment, and (2) elucidate the odds of retention in MOUD treatment due to perceived loneliness and other mental health diagnoses. It was hypothesized that higher perceptions of loneliness would decrease the odds of retention.

2. Materials and Methods

This secondary analysis utilized data obtained from participants at the start of their participation in an MBRP intervention at an outpatient comprehensive opioid addiction treatment (COAT) program at a large university located in the Central Appalachian region. Biweekly medication management and group therapy are included in the COAT program model, as is weekly attendance at community-based self-help meetings (e.g., Narcotics Anonymous). The COAT program combines cognitive behavioral therapy with MOUD, as appropriate. Medication management relies on the use of Suboxone®, or buprenorphine, which is a safe and effective partial agonist prescribed by physicians to control drug cravings and withdrawal symptoms, with a lower potential for misuse or abuse by an individual with OUD [35]. Individuals were recruited from the COAT program during the intermediate stage (at least 90 consecutive days of sobriety) and required to be 18 years or older, have received a diagnosis of opioid use disorder over the past year (using DSM-5 criteria), obtained a 12-step sponsor, and comprehend as well as communicate in English. Conversely, exclusion criteria for the MBRP intervention included risk of suicide, risk of incarceration, and/or having a psychotic disorder or comorbid diagnosis that prevented engagement in a mindfulness intervention. All of the exclusion criteria were assessed by the treating physician through the COAT program.

At the time of recruitment, individuals were provided the option of receiving MBRP plus MOUD or continuing cognitive behavioral therapy treatment as usual (TAU) plus MOUD for a 24-week intervention conducted between September 2017 and December 2019. MBRP is a noninvasive and nonpharmacologic 8-week treatment that targets an array of factors (e.g., awareness of triggers and cravings, mindfulness in high-risk situations and daily life, acceptance, self-care, etc.) For a complete description of the recruitment procedures and the MBRP intervention, see Zullig et al. [15].

2.1. Measures and Data Collection

All of the individuals that contributed self-reported demographic and mental health data at the time of enrollment (baseline) were included in this investigation. Mental health data were also collected after 12 weeks, 24 weeks, and 36 weeks postintervention using the following measures but were unused in the current study. Loneliness was assessed using the 20-item Revised UCLA Loneliness Scale (R-UCLA), which consists of Likert scale questions (11 negative and 9 positive statements that are reverse-coded). The R-UCLA has established validity, with Cronbach's alpha estimates ranging from 0.89 to 0.94, and an average test–retest reliability estimate ($r = 0.73$) [36]. Participants respond to each item to describe their feelings; the available responses are 1 = Never, 2 = Rarely, 3 = Sometimes, or 4 = Often. The range of possible scores is 20–80; higher scores indicate greater loneliness. Sample statements include "I am unhappy doing so many things alone" and "I have nobody to talk to." The baseline internal consistency estimate for the R-UCLA in this study was 0.92.

Depression was assessed using the 5-item Overall Depression Severity and Impairment Scale (ODSIS), and anxiety was assessed with the 5-item Overall Anxiety Severity and Impairment Scale (OASIS). For the ODSIS, summing each item score produces a total score, with potential scores ranging from 0 to 20; scores greater than or equal to 8 are used to determine a diagnosis of depression. The ODSIS demonstrates good estimates of convergent and discriminant validity across clinical and nonclinical samples [37]. The OASIS is scored similarly, with the sum of each item and total potential score ranging from 0 to 20. On the OASIS, scores ≥ 8 are also used to determine a diagnosis of anxiety [37]. The scale demonstrates excellent reliability and convergent as well as divergent validity ($\alpha = 0.80$) in both clinical and nonclinical samples [38]. The baseline internal consistency estimates for the ODSIS and OASIS in this study were 0.89 and 0.92, respectively.

Mindfulness was operationalized using the Five-Facet Mindfulness Questionnaire (FFMQ). The FFMQ contains 39 items across five subscales (observing, describing, acting with awareness, accepting without judgment, and nonreactivity). It has demonstrated evidence of good internal consistency, with alpha values from 0.76 to 0.91 [39]. The response options for each item are 1 = Never or very rarely true, 2 = Rarely true, 3 = Sometimes true, 4 = Often true, or 5 = Very often or always true. The FFMQ is scored by summing each subscale score into a total score; values for the total score range from 39 to 195, with higher scores indicating greater mindfulness. The baseline internal consistency estimate for the FFMQ total scale in this study was 0.89 [39].

Retention in treatment was defined as remaining in either TAU or MBRP throughout the 36-week data collection period. As part of COAT clinic standards at the time of this study, individuals who missed two consecutive sessions were considered not retained and subsequently dismissed. Demographic variables included age at baseline, gender (male/female), marital status (single, married, and divorced or separating), education (non-high school, high school or GED, and any college), employment (full-time, part-time, and unemployed), and insurance coverage (Medicaid, Medicare, private insurance, and no insurance). *Race* was dichotomized as either white or other to mirror the results of the most recent United States census for West Virginia, where 93.5% of the state's population was Non-Hispanic White [40]. The study from which deidentified data were obtained for secondary analysis was approved by the Institutional Review Board of West Virginia University.

2.2. Analysis

Data were analyzed using JMP® 16 (SAS Institute Inc., Cary, NC, USA). Descriptive statistics were calculated for all of the demographic and mental health variables. Fisher's exact tests were used to explore associations between demographic variables and retention in treatment. Pearson and point biserial correlation analyses were used to identify correlations between retention in treatment and each mental health variable. Two sample t-tests were employed to identify differences in mean age, and mental health scores between those retained and not retained were investigated with Student's *t*-tests. The significance level for all of the analyses was set at $\alpha \leq 0.05$.

Multiple logistic regression was used to elucidate the odds of dropping out or being dismissed from treatment and an individual's loneliness after adjustment for potential confounders at any point during the 36-week data collection period. The small sample size constrained the number of predictors that could be reliably considered in the final model, with the least frequent event, termination of treatment, observed 22 times [41]. Relaxing the 10 events per predictor norm to 5–9 events per predictor has been supported for use in logistic regression; therefore, 4 predictors were included in the model [42]. The inclusion of predictors was driven by the hypothesis, with loneliness automatically being included. The inclusion of depression and anxiety [7,19], as well as mindfulness [15], was informed by the currently available literature as well as the identified associations between the psychometric variables measured.

3. Results

3.1. Sample Demographics

A total sample of 89 individuals contributed data at the baseline; however, nine participants were excluded from the current analyses due to not meeting the inclusion criteria set forth for the larger MBRP intervention. Therefore, eighty individuals were included in the current analysis, where 57.5% (n = 46) identified as female. The mean age of the participant population was 36 years (SD: 8.9 years), and most of the participants identified as white (n = 75, 94%). Over half (57%) of the participants were either employed full-time (n = 31) or part-time (n = 15). Bivariate analyses (Table 1) showed that there was a statistically significant association between retention and gender ($p < 0.001$), education ($p < 0.001$), employment status ($p < 0.001$), insurance provider ($p < 0.001$), and race ($p < 0.001$). Despite these associations, none of these variables were significantly predictive of retention in MOUD when logistically modeled and, thus, were not considered for inclusion.

Table 1. Demographic associations with, differences between, and predictability of retention.

Variable	Total (n = 80)	Retained (n = 57)	Not Retained (n = 22)	Bivariate p-Value	Regression p-Value
‡ Age				0.836	0.859
Mean (SD)	36 (8.9)	36 (10)	35 (5.4)		
Range	23–67	23–67	23–45		
† Gender				*<0.001*	0.159
Male	37	27 (47%)	10 (45%)		
Female	41	29 (50%)	12 (55%)		
Other	2	2 (3%)			
† Education				*<0.001*	0.559
Non-high school	6	5 (9%)	1 (5%)		
High school or GED	47	35 (61%)	12 (54%)		
Any college	26	17 (30%)	9 (41%)		
† Employment				*<0.001*	0.416
Full-time	31	21 (36%)	10 (45%)		
Part-time	15	10 (17%)	5 (23%)		
Not employed	34	27 (47%)	7 (32%)		
† Insurance				*<0.001*	0.140
Medicaid	64	45 (79%)	19 (86%)		
Medicare	5	5 (9%)	-		
Other	10	7 (12%)	3 (14%)		

Table 1. *Cont.*

Variable	Total (*n* = 80)	Retained (*n* = 57)	Not Retained (*n* = 22)	Bivariate *p*-Value	Regression *p*-Value
† Marital Status				*<0.001*	0.601
Single	46	33 (57%)	13 (59%)		
Married	16	11 (19%)	5 (23%)		
Divorced or separating	18	14 (24%)	4 (18%)		
† Race				*<0.001*	0.120
White	75	54 (96%)	21 (95%)		
Other	3	2 (4%)	1 (5%)		

† Fisher's exact test; ‡ two-tailed *t*-test. Italic is to denote statistical significance.

Moderate to severe loneliness was highly prevalent (R-UCLA ≥ 40) within the study population at the baseline, with a mean score of 49 (SD: 5.1, range of 36 to 64). Fifty-one of the participants (89%) that were retained in treatment were classified as lonely, and 21 (95%) of those that were not retained in MOUD were lonely. The mean depression score within the population was 5.9 (SD: 4.4), with 33 (41%) of the total participants having an ODSIS score greater than or equal to eight, indicative of depression. Severe anxiety (OASIS ≥ 10) was prevalent in 32 (40%) of the enrolled population. Bivariate analyses (Table 2) showed no differences ($p > 0.05$) in mean loneliness, depression, nor anxiety between those that were retained and those that discontinued treatment; however, mean mindfulness was significantly higher ($p = 0.018$) among those retained in treatment (mean: 125, SD: 12) than among individuals that discontinued treatment (mean: 117, SD: 14).

Table 2. Mean (SD) scores and bivariate results of mental health variables.

Mental Health Variable	Total	Retained (*n* = 57)	Not Retained (*n* = 22)	*p*-Value
Anxiety (OASIS)				
‡ Mean (SD) score	7.7 (4.4)	7.6 (4.2)	7.9 (5.1)	0.812
Range	0–19	0–15	0–19	
Depression (ODSIS)				
‡ Mean (SD) score	5.9 (4.4)	5.9 (4.1)	5.7 (5.2)	0.843
Range	0–18	0–16	0–18	
Loneliness (R-UCLA)				
† Mean (SD) score	49 (5.1)	49 (5.4)	48 (4.5)	0.609
Range	36–64	36–64	38–56	
* Mindfulness (FFMQ)				
‡ Mean (SD) score	123 (13)	125 (12)	117 (14)	*0.018*
Range	78–147	86–147	78–146	

† One-tailed *t*-test; ‡ two-tailed *t*-test; and * $p < 0.05$.

3.2. *Correlations between Mental Health Variables and Retention*

Pearson correlations were computed to identify relationships among the mental health predictor variables measured at the baseline. Statistically significant positive correlations between all of the predictors ($p < 0.05$) were observed, with the largest positive correlation observed between anxiety and depression, r (65) = 0.72, $p < 0.001$. Point biserial correlations revealed no statistical correlation between retention in MOUD and loneliness ($r_{pb} = 0.059$, $p = 0.599$), anxiety ($r_{pb} = -0.027$, $p = 0.811$), nor depression ($r_{pb} = 0.022$, $p = 0.843$); however, these calculations did reveal a statistically significant, yet small, positive association between retention in MOUD and mindfulness ($r_{pb} = 0.28$, $p = 0.012$).

3.3. Logistic Regression

The predictor variable loneliness was found to not statistically contribute to the model (β = 0.0237, SE = 0.045, L-R χ^2 = 0.27, and p = 0.601). Likewise, anxiety (β = 0.0209, SE = 0.052, L-R χ^2 = 0.16, and p = 0.685), depression (β = −0.0245, SE = 0.052, L-R χ^2 = 0.22, and p = 0.637), and mindfulness (β = 0.0237, SE = 0.045, L-R χ^2 = 0.27, and p = 0.601) were not individually correlated with retention in treatment. Results from the adjusted model are reported in Table 3. A lack of fit analysis (χ^2 = 73 (62), p = 0.153) suggests that the model fit the data well. The results of the regression analysis revealed that, while holding other predictors constant, the odds of not being retained in MOUD were not statistically influenced by loneliness (OR = 0.926, 95% CI (0.792–1.08), and p = 0.333), depression (OR = 1.01, 95% CI (0.836–1.22), p = 0.921), or anxiety (OR = 1.07, 95% CI (0.887–1.29), p = 0.476).

Table 3. Adjusted logistic regression results.

Predictor	β	Std Error	L-R χ^2	p-Value	OR	95% CI
Anxiety	0.0681	0.095	0.51	0.476	1.07	0.887–1.29
Depression	0.0096	0.096	0.01	0.921	1.01	0.836–1.22
Loneliness	−0.0773	0.079	0.94	0.333	0.926	0.792–1.08
* Mindfulness	−0.0451	0.024	3.6	0.047	0.956	0.912–1.00

* $p < 0.05$.

However, there was a marginally significant difference in the odds of not being retained in MOUD between individuals who reported greater perceived mindfulness compared to individuals who reported reduced perceived mindfulness. Specifically, individuals who reported greater perceived mindfulness (as measured by the FFMQ scores) were 4% less likely to discontinue MOUD than their counterparts who reported reduced perceived mindfulness (OR = 0.956, 95% CI (0.912–1.00), and $p < 0.05$) after accounting for other mental health constructs.

4. Discussion

The current analysis investigating the capabilities of loneliness perceived by individuals prior to participating in an MBRP intervention and the intermediate stage of treatment to predict the cessation of treatment did not yield statistically significant results; however, promising findings indicate that greater mindfulness increased retention in MOUD treatment and may present a treatment option to be incorporated into standard-of-care pharmacological interventions.

Perceived loneliness did not differ between those that were retained in MOUD compared to those that were not. Likewise, when accounting for depression and anxiety, two co-occurring mental health issues shown to be correlated with loneliness [19], the odds of treatment cessation were not statistically significant. Therefore, loneliness was not found to be a predictor of retention in the current model. Despite the nonsignificant findings related to loneliness, additional, longitudinal, and randomized investigations should incorporate and re-evaluate the influence of this perception on retention in treatment. Loneliness is recognized to be directly related to substance abuse [12,13] and drug craving [16]. It is important to distinguish between loneliness and social support or isolation; inconsistent definitions of loneliness have conflated these two concepts [12], making it more difficult to detect the true influence of this perception of the availability and quality of relationships. Regardless of the null results of loneliness to predict retention in treatment, loneliness was clinically prevalent in this population and aligns with the increased national prevalence observed over the same period.

A national survey conducted in July 2019 found the prevalence of loneliness to be 61% among Americans aged ≥ 18 years [43], a 7% increase from the previous year [44]. This was exacerbated postpandemic. Further surveillance conducted in 2021 reported young adults feeling lonely and left out 2.5 times (46%, 18 years–34 years) more than older adults (16%, $\geq$ 55 years) [45]. These recent estimations not only exemplify that loneliness is prevalent [43], but also that it is increasing postpandemic [44]. Recognizing the prevalence of loneliness and the numerous influences that it has on physical and chronic disease [7,8,19,46], mental health [10,11,18,20], and substance misuse [12,13] supports the need for further investigations into interventions addressing loneliness. Additional investigations should further focus on loneliness among Appalachians, particularly those receiving MOUD, with the aim of developing interventions for incorporation into OUD treatment programs.

Statistically, mindfulness marginally demonstrated the capacity to predict retention in treatment in our sample. In the current study, more mindful individuals were 4% less likely to not be retained in MOUD treatment. This observation may be due to participants' resiliency, or the ability to manage challenging thoughts, feelings, situations, and overall adversity. Resiliency plays a critical protective role for individuals during the treatment and recovery process; however, it is highly influenced by a person's own experiences. Mindfulness has been shown to promote resiliency and reduce maladaptive coping within college-aged students [47]. Becoming more mindful indicates one's awareness and ability to focus on internal as well as external triggers [14]; this may subsequently increase one's ability to adapt and enhance inherent resiliency, ultimately leading to retention in treatment. Although resiliency was not measured and considered in the current work, the relationship between it and mindfulness among individuals receiving MOUD should be further explored and considered, with a focus on effective mindfulness-based interventions.

Even though there is support for joint MOUD, counseling, and behavioral therapies [48], there remains no recommendation for the most effective therapy combination for individuals with OUD. Zullig et al. [15] supports the notion that mindfulness-based therapy can be effectively integrated into MOUD and successfully reduce drug craving, depression, and anxiety. This aligns with previous work conducted on a second model of mindfulness-based therapy, mindfulness-oriented recovery enhancement (MORE) [49]. Additionally, MBRP has shown potential to reduce loneliness among individuals in the intermediate stage of MOUD [16]. The current study provides additional evidence to also suggest that MBRP may improve OUD treatment retention. Retaining individuals in MOUD treatment programs is vital to reduce relapse and, subsequently, prevent overdoses as well as death [27]. Preliminary findings from the current study suggest that mindfulness may serve as a predictive indicator of discontinuing treatment.

Uniform definitions of retention are uncommon, making it difficult to compare findings across interventions; therefore, no best practice has been reported to increase retention in MOUD [28,31]. Integrating mindfulness-based therapies and actively monitoring this practice may prove effective at improving retention and reducing overdoses as well as mortality in OUD populations. This notion is supported by the American Society of Addiction Medicine, whose updated practice guidance encourages the integration of psychosocial and environmental assessments in conjunction with pharmacotherapies in treatment programs [50]. The current results provide preliminary evidence for mindfulness training integration as a component of effective treatment; however, since there is still not evidence to support the most effective behavioral therapy, it is recommended that future endeavors elucidate the effectiveness of MBRP versus MORE therapies with regard to reductions in co-occurring mental health disorder symptoms, loneliness, and influence on retention in treatment.

Consistent with a recent meta-analysis [51], no gender differences were observed between the retention groups, although significant ($p < 0.001$) associations were noted between retention in MOUD and gender, education, employment, insurance, marital status, and race; however, these social determinants of health and demographics were not statistically significant in predicting individuals not being retained in treatment. Future studies may wish to further explore, with an adequate sample size, the impact of social determinants of health, loneliness, and mindfulness on retention in MOUD.

Limitations

Findings from the current study are subject to certain limitations. A small sample size in the total enrolled population ultimately limited the number of individuals discontinuing treatment, thus reducing the potential generalizability. This also narrowed the ability to truly understand the impact of loneliness on retention and treatment, which bears the need for further investigation. Although predictors in the logistic regression model were selected based on theoretical considerations from previous work and clinical relevance, high correlations between some predictors suggest collinearity, which may have diluted the effect of each predictor on the outcome. Additionally, although only a single adjusted regression model was tested, conducting a Bonferroni correction for multiple comparisons would show marginally significant results for mindfulness; however, this does not negate the clinical importance of mindfulness and the role it plays during the treatment and recovery process; thus, further investigation is warranted. Additionally, participants in the MBRP intervention were not randomized into groups, and the intervention itself was quasi-experimental. Hence, selection bias cannot be discredited. Finally, nearly 94% of the participants identified as white, therefore limiting its generalizability to ethnically diverse populations and regions; however, this is representative of the Appalachian region.

5. Conclusions

Recognizing the prevalence of loneliness and the health outcomes associated with its perception [19,46] is an important consideration in the treatment of Appalachian adults receiving MOUD treatment. Assessments of loneliness in the current study were conducted pre-COVID-19. Estimates of loneliness in the general population increased 2.5 times in 2021 compared to 2019 [43,45]; therefore, it is assumed that perceptions of loneliness also worsened within MOUD populations. Furthermore, although loneliness was not significantly predictive of retention in treatment, moderate loneliness was still observed within this population of patients in the intermediate stage of outpatient MOUD treatment, thus supporting a further need to investigate this discrepancy between the actual and perceived quality as well as availability of support from one's relationships.

Moreover, acknowledging that mindfulness may offer a broad array of benefits, including increasing retention in MOUD, reducing co-occurring mental health issues [15,16,49], improving resiliency [47], and decreasing loneliness [16] further provides evidence of the potential benefits that mindfulness-based therapies offer adults in MOUD. Incorporating mindfulness-based therapies into treatment programs may address the prevalence of loneliness, reduce relapsing as well as overdosing, and ultimately save lives. Further investigation to explore barriers to access and retention in treatment experienced by individuals with OUD is warranted.

Author Contributions: Conceptualization, K.J.Z., J.M.H. and L.T.; methodology, J.M.H., G.R.H. and K.J.Z.; software, J.M.H.; validation, S.M.D., K.J.Z., G.R.H. and L.T.; formal analysis, J.M.H., S.M.D. and K.J.Z.; investigation, K.J.Z. and L.R.L.; resources, K.J.Z. and L.R.L.; data curation, K.J.Z. and L.R.L.; writing—original draft preparation, J.M.H., S.M.D. and K.J.Z.; writing—review and editing, J.M.H., S.M.D., K.J.Z., J.M., L.T., G.R.H., D.M.D. and L.R.L.; visualization, J.M.H.; supervision, S.M.D. and K.J.Z.; project administration, K.J.Z. and L.R.L.; funding acquisition, K.J.Z. and L.R.L. All authors have read and agreed to the published version of the manuscript.

Funding: This research was supported in part by grant number 6R49CE002109–05-06, funded by the US Centers for Disease Control and Prevention. Its contents are solely the responsibility of the authors and do not necessarily represent the official views of the Centers for Disease Control and Prevention or the Department of Health and Human Services.

Institutional Review Board Statement: The study was conducted in accordance with the Declaration of Helsinki and approved by the Institutional Review Board of West Virginia University (protocol # 1708720058, approved on 26 August 2017).

Informed Consent Statement: Informed consent was obtained from all of the subjects involved in the study from which these data were obtained for secondary analysis.

Data Availability Statement: The datasets used and/or analyzed during the current study are available from the corresponding author upon reasonable request.

Conflicts of Interest: The authors declare no conflict of interest.

References

1. CDC National Center for Health Statistics. Wide-Ranging Online Data for Epidemiologic Research (WONDER) 2021. Available online: http://wonder.cdc.gov/ (accessed on 6 August 2021).
2. Guy, G.P., Jr.; Zhang, K.; Bohm, M.K.; Losby, J.; Lewis, B.; Young, R.; Murphy, L.B.; Dowell, D. Morbidity and Mortality Weekly Report Vital Signs: Changes in Opioid Prescribing in the United States, 2006–2015. *Morb. Mortal. Wkly. Rep.* **2015**, *66*, 697–704. [CrossRef]
3. CDC National Center for Injury Prevention and Control. Strategies and Partnerships. Available online: https://www.cdc.gov/drugoverdose/strategies/index.html (accessed on 26 June 2022).
4. CDC National Center for Health Statistics. U.S. Overdose Deaths in 2021 Increased Half as Much as in 2020—But Are Still Up 15%. Available online: https://www.cdc.gov/nchs/pressroom/nchs_press_releases/2022/202205.htm (accessed on 27 June 2022).
5. *Substance Abuse and Mental Health Services Administration Key Substance Use and Mental Health Indicators in the United States: Results from the 2021 National Survey on Drug Use and Health*; HHS Publication No. PEP22-07-01-005, NSDUH Series H-57; (Department of Health and Human Services) HHS: Washington, DC, USA, 2022.
6. Santo, T.J.; Campbell, G.; Gisev, N.; Martino-Burke, D.; Wilson, J.; Colledge-Frisby, S.; Clark, B.; Tran, L.T.; Degenhardt, L. Prevalence of Mental Disorders among People with Opioid Use Disorder: A Systematic Review and Meta-Analysis. *Drug Alcohol Depend.* **2022**, *238*, 109551. [CrossRef] [PubMed]
7. Steptoe, A.; Shankar, A.; Demakakos, P.; Wardle, J. Social Isolation, Loneliness, and All-Cause Mortality in Older Men and Women. *Proc. Natl. Acad. Sci. USA* **2013**, *110*, 5797–5801. [CrossRef]
8. National Academy of Sciences, Engineering, and Medicine. *Social Isolation and Loneliness in Older Adults*; The National Academies Press: Washington, DC, USA, 2020; ISBN 9780309671002.
9. Mahar, A.L.; Cobigo, V.; Stuart, H. Conceptualizing Belonging. *Disabil. Rehabil.* **2013**, *35*, 1026–1032. [CrossRef] [PubMed]
10. Office of the U.S. Surgeon General. *Our Epidemic of Loneliness and Isolation: The U.S. Surgeon General's Advisory on the Healing Effects of Social Connection and Community*; Department of Health and Human Services: Washington, DC, USA, 2023.
11. Beutel, M.E.; Klein, E.M.; Brähler, E.; Reiner, I.; Jünger, C.; Michal, M.; Wiltink, J.; Wild, P.S.; Münzel, T.; Lackner, K.J.; et al. Loneliness in the General Population: Prevalence, Determinants and Relations to Mental Health. *BMC Psychiatry* **2017**, *17*, 97. [CrossRef]
12. Ingram, I.; Kelly, P.J.; Deane, F.P.; Baker, A.L.; Goh, M.C.; Raftery, D.K.; Dingle, G.A. Loneliness among People with Substance Use Problems: A Narrative Systematic Review. *Drug Alcohol Rev.* **2020**, *39*, 447–483. [CrossRef]
13. Polenick, C.A.; Cotton, B.P.; Bryson, W.C.; Birditt, K.S. Loneliness and Illicit Opioid Use Among Methadone Maintenance Treatment Patients. *Subst. Use Misuse* **2019**, *54*, 2089–2098. [CrossRef]
14. Ramadas, E.; Lima, M.P.; Caetano, T.; Lopes, J.; Dixe, M.D. Effectiveness of Mindfulness-Based Relapse Prevention in Individuals with Substance Use Disorders: A Systematic Review. *Behav. Sci.* **2021**, *11*, 133. [CrossRef]
15. Zullig, K.J.; Lander, L.R.; Tuscano, M.; Garland, M.; Hobbs, G.R. Faulkenberry, Laurel Testing Mindfulness-Based Relapse Prevention with Medications for Opioid Use Disorder Among Adults in Outpatient Therapy: A Quasi-Experimental Study. *Mindfulness* **2021**, *12*, 3036–3046. [CrossRef]
16. Mills, R.; Zullig, K.J.; Theeke, L.A.; Lander, L.R.; Hobbs, G.R.; Herczyk, J.; Davis, S.M. Assessing Loneliness among Adults Receiving Outpatient Treatment with Medication for Opioid Use Disorder (MOUD). *Int. J. Environ. Res. Public Health* **2022**, *19*, 13481. [CrossRef]
17. Rural Health Information Hub. West Virginia. Available online: https://www.ruralhealthinfo.org/states/west-virginia (accessed on 8 January 2023).
18. Theeke, L.; Carpenter, R.D.; Mallow, J.; Theeke, E. Gender Differences in Loneliness, Anger, Depression, Self-Management Ability and Biomarkers of Chronic Illness in Chronically Ill Mid-Life Adults in Appalachia. *Appl. Nurs. Res.* **2019**, *45*, 55–62. [CrossRef]
19. Theeke, L.A.; Mallow, J. Loneliness and Quality of Life in Chronically Ill Rural Older Adults. *Am. J. Nurs.* **2013**, *113*, 28–37. [CrossRef]
20. Theeke, L.A.; Goins, R.T.; Moore, J.; Campbell, H. Loneliness, Depression, Social Support, and Quality of Life in Older Chronically Ill Appalachians. *J. Psychol. Interdiscip. Appl.* **2012**, *146*, 155–171. [CrossRef] [PubMed]
21. Appalachian Regional Commission. *Communicating about Opioids in Appalachia: Challenges, Opportunities, and Best Practices*; Appalachian Regional Commission: Washington, DC, USA, 2018.
22. Marshall, J.L.; Thomas, L.; Lane, N.M.; Holmes, G.M.; Arcury, T.A.; Randolph, R.; Silberman, P.; Holding, W.; Villamil, L.; Thomas, S.; et al. *Creating a Culture of Health in Appalachia: Health Disparities in Appalachia*; Appalachian Regional Commission: Washington, DC, USA, 2017; pp. 117–122.
23. CDC National Center for Health Statistics. Drug Overdose Mortality by State. Available online: https://www.cdc.gov/nchs/pressroom/sosmap/drug_poisoning_mortality/drug_poisoning.htm (accessed on 7 May 2023).

24. Health Resources & Services Administration. HPSA Find. Available online: https://data.hrsa.gov/tools/shortage-area/hpsa-find (accessed on 5 July 2023).
25. Winstanley, E.L.; Lander, L.R.; Berry, J.H.; Mahoney, J.J.; Zheng, W.; Herschler, J.; Marshalek, P.; Sayres, S.; Mason, J.; Haut, M.W. West Virginia's Model of Buprenorphine Expansion: Preliminary Results. *J. Subst. Abus. Treat.* **2020**, *108*, 40–47. [CrossRef]
26. Lindsay, E.K.; Young, S.; Brown, K.W.; Smyth, J.M.; Creswell, J.D. Mindfulness Training Reduces Loneliness and Increases Social Contact in a Randomized Controlled Trial. *Proc. Natl. Acad. Sci. USA* **2019**, *116*, 3488–3493. [CrossRef]
27. Biondi, B.E.; Vander Wyk, B.; Schlossberg, E.F.; Shaw, A.; Springer, S.A. Factors Associated with Retention on Medications for Opioid Use Disorder among a Cohort of Adults Seeking Treatment in the Community. *Addict. Sci. Clin. Pract.* **2022**, *17*, 15. [CrossRef]
28. Timko, C.; Schultz, N.R.; Cucciare, M.A.; Vittorio, L.; Sciences, B.; Arkansas, C.; Affairs, V.; Rock, N.L.; Rock, N.L.; Rock, L.; et al. Retention in Medication-Assisted Treatment for Opiate Dependence: A Systematic Review. *J. Addict. Dis.* **2016**, *35*, 22–35. [CrossRef] [PubMed]
29. Klimas, J.; Hamilton, M.A.; Gorfinkel, L.; Adam, A.; Cullen, W.; Wood, E. Retention in Opioid Agonist Treatment: A Rapid Review and Meta-Analysis Comparing Observational Studies and Randomized Controlled Trials. *Syst. Rev.* **2021**, *10*, 216. [CrossRef] [PubMed]
30. Chan, B.; Gean, E.; Arkhipova-Jenkins, I.; Gilbert, J.; Hilgart, J.; Fiordalisi, C.; Hubbard, K.; Brandt, I.; Stoeger, E.; Paynter, R.; et al. Retention Strategies for Medications for Opioid Use Disorder in Adults: A Rapid Evidence Review. *J. Addict. Med.* **2021**, *15*, 74–84. [CrossRef]
31. Chan, B.; Gean, E.; Arkhipova-Jenkins, I.; Gilbert, J.; Hilgart, J.; Fiordalisi, C.; Hubbard, K.; Brandt, I.; Stoeger, E.; Paynter, R.; et al. *Retention Strategies for Medications for Addiction Treatment in Adults with Opioid Use Disorder: A Rapid Evidence Review*; AHRQ Publication No 20-EHC012; Agency for Healthcare Research and Quality: Rockville, MD, USA, 2020.
32. Zemore, S.E.; Ware, O.D.; Gilbert, P.A.; Pinedo, M. Barriers to Retention in Substance Use Treatment: Validation of a New, Theory-Based Scale. *J. Subst. Abus. Treat.* **2021**, *131*, 108422. [CrossRef]
33. Acevedo, A.; Harvey, N.; Kamanu, M.; Tendulkar, S.; Fleary, S. Barriers, Facilitators, and Disparities in Retention for Adolescents in Treatment for Substance Use Disorders: A Qualitative Study with Treatment Providers. *Subst. Abus. Treat. Prev. Policy* **2020**, *15*, 42. [CrossRef]
34. Greene, J.A.; Bina, R.; Gum, A.M. Interventions to Increase Retention in Mental Health Services: A Systematic Review. *Psychiatr. Serv.* **2016**, *67*, 485–495. [CrossRef] [PubMed]
35. Substance Abuse and Mental Health Services Administration. Buprenorphine. Available online: https://www.samhsa.gov/medications-substance-use-disorders/medications-counseling-related-conditions/buprenorphine (accessed on 8 January 2023).
36. Russell, D.W. UCLA Loneliness Scale (Version 3): Reliability, Validity, and Factor Structure. *J. Personal. Assess.* **1996**, *66*, 20–40. [CrossRef] [PubMed]
37. Bentley, K.H.; Gallagher, M.W.; Carl, J.R.; Barlow, D.H. Development and Validation of the Overall Depression Severity and Impairment Scale. *Psychol. Assess.* **2014**, *26*, 815–830. [CrossRef] [PubMed]
38. Norman, S.B.; Cissell, S.H.; Means-Christensen, A.J.; Stein, M.B. Development and Validation of an Overall Anxiety Severity and Impairment Scale (OASIS). *Depress. Anxiety* **2006**, *23*, 245–249. [CrossRef]
39. Baer, R.A.; Smith, G.T.; Hopkins, J.; Krietemeyer, J.; Toney, L. Using Self-Report Assessment Methods to Explore Facets of Mindfulness. *Assessment* **2006**, *13*, 27–45. [CrossRef]
40. United States Census Bureau. U.S. Census Bureau QuickFacts: West Virginia. Available online: https://www.census.gov/quickfacts/WV (accessed on 28 September 2022).
41. Stokes, M.E.; Davis, C.S.; Koch, G.G. *Categorical Data Analysis Using SAS®*, 3rd ed.; SAS Institute Inc.: Cary, NC, USA, 2012; pp. 190–253. ISBN 978-1-60764-664-8.
42. Vittinghoff, E.; McCulloch, C.E. Relaxing the Rule of Ten Events per Variable in Logistic and Cox Regression. *Am. J. Epidemiol.* **2007**, *165*, 710–718. [CrossRef]
43. Cigna. *Loneliness and the Workplace: A 2020 U.S. Report*; Cigna Healthcare: Bloomfield, CT, USA, 2020.
44. Cigna. *Cigna U.S. Loneliness Index*; Cigna Healthcare: Bloomfield, CT, USA, 2018.
45. Cigna/Ipsos. The Loneliness Epidemic Persists: A Post-Pandemic Look at the State of Loneliness among U.S. Adults | Cigna Newsroom. Available online: https://newsroom.cigna.com/loneliness-epidemic-persists-post-pandemic-look (accessed on 26 July 2022).
46. Cacioppo, S.; Grippo, A.J.; London, S.; Goossens, L.; Cacioppo, J.T. Loneliness: Clinical Import and Interventions. *Perspect. Psychol. Sci.* **2015**, *10*, 238–249. [CrossRef]
47. Pidgeon, A.M.; Pickett, L. Examining the Differences between University Students' Levels of Resilience on Mindfulness, Psychological Distress and Coping Strategies. *Eur. Sci. J.* **2017**, *13*, 103–113.
48. Santucci, K. Psychiatric Disease and Drug Abuse. *Curr. Opin. Pediatr.* **2012**, *24*, 233–237. [CrossRef]
49. Garland, E.L.; Roberts-Lewis, A.; Tronnier, C.D.; Graves, R.; Kelley, K. Mindfulness-Oriented Recovery Enhancement versus CBT for Co-Occurring Substance Dependence, Traumatic Stress, and Psychiatric Disorders: Proximal Outcomes from a Pragmatic Randomized Trial. *Behav. Res. Ther.* **2016**, *77*, 7–16. [CrossRef] [PubMed]

50. American Society of Addiction Medicine. *The ASAM National Practice Guideline for the Treatment of Opioid Use Disorder: 2020 Focused Update*; American Society of Addiction Medicine: Rockville, MD, USA, 2020; p. 95.
51. Hochheimer, M.; Unick, G.J. Systematic Review and Meta-Analysis of Retention in Treatment Using Medications for Opioid Use Disorder by Medication, Race/Ethnicity, and Gender in the United States. *Addict. Behav.* **2022**, *124*, 107113. [CrossRef] [PubMed]

International Journal of
Environmental Research and Public Health

MDPI

Review

Love and Infidelity: Causes and Consequences

Ami Rokach [1,*] and Sybil H. Chan [2]

[1] Department of Psychology, York University, Toronto, ON M3J 1P3, Canada
[2] Faculty of Education, Western University, London, ON N6A 3K7, Canada
* Correspondence: rokach@yorku.ca

Abstract: This is a narrative review addressing the topic of romantic infidelity, its causes and its consequences. Love is commonly a source of much pleasure and fulfillment. However, as this review points out, it can also cause stress, heartache and may even be traumatic in some circumstances. Infidelity, which is relatively common in Western culture, can damage a loving, romantic relationship to the point of its demise. However, by highlighting this phenomenon, its causes and its consequences, we hope to provide useful insight for both researchers and clinicians who may be assisting couples facing these issues. We begin by defining infidelity and illustrating the various ways in which one may become unfaithful to their partner. We explore the personal and relational factors that enhance an individual's tendency to betray their partner, the various reactions related to a discovered affair and the challenges related to the nosological categorization of infidelity-based trauma, and conclude by reviewing the effects of COVID-19 on unfaithful behavior, as well as clinical implications related to infidelity-based treatment. Ultimately, we hope to provide a road map, for academicians and clinicians alike, of what some couples may experience in their relationships and how can they be helped.

Keywords: love; infidelity; affairs; attachment injury; trauma; COVID; healing

1. Love and Infidelity: Causes and Consequences

Grøntvedt et al., opined that "it is hard to imagine romantic and committed relationships devoid of transgressions of some kind. Despite the best intentions not to cause any harm or disappointment to one's partner, breaking rules and promises are largely inevitable in long-term relationships" [1]. While some transgressions may be trivial and easily forgiven and forgotten, those involving betrayal may have significant effects on the relationship. It seems that any form of infidelity from either party may have potential to instigate a breakup [2]. In fact, research across 160 cultures revealed that spousal infidelity is the most common reason for a breakup [1]. Infidelity may not only have a destructive impact on the relationship, which may lead to separation or divorce, but may negatively affect the partners' overall emotional wellbeing, leading to enhanced depressive symptoms andlowered self-esteem [3]. However, comprehensive reviews encompassing many aspects of infidelity (e.g., distinctions between emotional and sexual affairs, gender differences to extradyadic behaviors, the impacts of infidelity-based trauma) are sparse in the literature. As such, the following paper presents a "narrative review" of research related to the causes, consequences and reasonings of infidelity in adult romantic relationships.

2. Methods

We chose to include a mixture of qualitative and quantitative peer-reviewed research that directly addressed the subject of sexual and emotional infidelity, as well as infidelity-based trauma, as major variables of investigation for the purposes of this review. We focused on including work from a diverse collection of scholarly journals ranging from notable to lesser-known databases. We began our research by examining current issues from highly ranked journals in the fields of marriage and family therapy, sex therapy and couples counseling from the past 10 to 12 years. These journals included *Sexual and Relationship Therapy, Journal of Marital and Family Therapy, Journal of Family Psychology, Journal of Marriage and Family, Journal of Couple and Relationship Therapy, Journal of Sex and Marital Therapy* and the *Journal of Sex Research*. Following this, we reviewed several major social science databases, including ERIC, PsycINFO, PubMED and Google Scholar, using the following terms: "emotional infidelity", "sexual infidelity", "relationship trauma", "extradyadic relationships", "extradyadic behaviors", "infidelity-based trauma", "extramarital affairs" and "romantic betrayal". We also examined the references of these articles and selected those that fit the criteria described above.

3. Defining Infidelity

While considerable research has been carried out on the topic of infidelity, little agreement exists regarding its definition. Drigotas opined that infidelity occurs when a person feels that their partner has violated the relationship norm by interacting with someone who is not a part of their relationship [4]. However, Blow and Hartnett defined infidelity as " ... a sexual and/or emotional act engaged in by one person within a committed relationship, where such an act occurs outside of the primary relationship, and constitutes a breach of trust and/or violation of agreed upon norms (overt and covert) by one or both individuals in that relationship in relation to romantic, emotional or sexual exclusivity" [5]. Reviewing both definitions, a distinction needs to be made between sexual and emotional infidelity and its newer concepts related to inappropriate online and offline behavior, which we will address later [6].

Generally, infidelity is defined as any type of secret emotional, sexual or romantic behavior that violates the exclusivity that romantic relationships have by definition. However, there are varied definitions of infidelity, which can be divided into subtypes of sexual, emotional, combined (sexual and emotional) and internet infidelity [7]. Examples of the various (and sometimes contradictory) definitions, can be gleaned from Bernard who believed that partners who failed to love, honor and support their partners were engaging in infidelity, since they did not honor their vows to remain with their romantic partner [8]. In contrast, Pittman and Wagers held a different position and maintained that the hallmark of infidelity involves the secrecy and concealment of behaviors with an individual outside of the committed relationship [9]. Thompson had a more comprehensive view of infidelity, and postulated that infidelity occurs if: (a) the extradyadic behavior is not condoned by one's romantic partner, (b) that behavior occurs outside of the primary relationship and (c) the behavior can be described, such as intercourse, flirting, etc. [10].

Sexual infidelity was defined by Leeker and Carlozzi as "the occurrence of sexual involvement with a third party that violates the ground rules established by the couple (e.g., kissing, fondling, oral sex, vaginal sex, anal sex)" [11].

Emotional infidelity was seen as "the occurrence of emotional involvement with a third party that violates the ground rules established by the couple (e.g., trusting another, sharing your deepest thoughts with another, falling in love in another, being vulnerable with another, being more committed to another, spending more money on another)" [11].

Research that explored which type of infidelity, sexual or emotional, would be more upsetting found that men were more distressed by sexual infidelity, while women were more upset by emotional infidelity [12,13] Research which addressed the reactions of lesbian and heterosexual women and gay and heterosexual men to infidelity found that for all four groups, emotional infidelity was more distressing than sexual infidelity [11]. Cramer et al., fund that women perceived emotional infidelity as more upsetting than men did, and the explanation provided by them was that women believe that men are not able to maintain sexual faithfulness in their relationships, but will still remain emotionally loyal to their spouses regardless [14].

Leeker and Carluzzi explored how sexual orientation, love and infidelity expectations might affect the reaction towards emotional and sexual infidelity [11]. Their study involved 296 individuals: 72 lesbians, 114 heterosexual women, 53 gay men and 57 heterosexual men, who were older than 18 years of age and who indicated that they were currently involved in a committed romantic relationship. They found that sex and sexual orientation were significant predictors of general distress, anger, anxiety, jealousy, humiliation, in response to both emotional and sexual infidelity. Commitment was predictive of distress and anger in response to emotional infidelity, while sexual infidelity aroused distress and anxiety.

Addressing the various types of infidelity, emotional infidelity includes the development of deep, intimate feelings for an extradyadic partner, while sexual infidelity refers to engaging in sexual behavior with that person. Those who engage in both emotional and sexual behavior are said to be involved with composite infidelity, while internet infidelity is carried out (at least initially) virtually/online [7]. Other researchers have employed even narrower definitions of infidelity by focusing on specific behaviors such as spending time with another individual and going on romantic dates, engaging in kissing, fondling, or even sexual intercourse, suggesting that they all constitute unfaithful behaviour [5,15].

Differences between the various types of infidelity were also observed in the work of Guitar et al., who reported that emotional infidelity is more complex than sexual infidelity [16]. Three hundred and seventy-nine undergraduate students provided their interpretations of emotional and sexual infidelity, which were later categorized into themes for content analysis. Participants' responses indicated that emotional infidelity included themes such as love and betrayal along with sexual infidelity and/or intentions to have sexual relations with someone outside the pair bond. Particularly, women saw emotional infidelity as carrying the potential of later sexual betrayal in such partnerships. This suggests that the nuances involved with conceptualizing emotional infidelity may surpass the conditions needed to fulfill sexual infidelity, and that these differences may be most salient when observing differences across genders.

In fact, research has shown that men appear to hold more permissive attitudes towards extramarital sex than women do [17]. They also reported experiencing greater levels of stress related to the sexual infidelity of their partner, whereas women react more negatively to emotional infidelity than men [3]. However, women also seem to consider more behaviors as infidelity compared to men in both offline and online spaces [3].

Moreover, shared opinions regarding what specific behaviors are considered as unfaithful in nature have also been identified in the literature. For example, work by Bozoyan and Schmiedeberg found that extradyadic intercourse was regarded as infidelity [3]. Kissing someone who is not one's partner was also reported as infidelity, especially if emotional involvement was part of it. The results of their research point to a perception of sexual infidelity as more distressing than emotional infidelity. However, women tended to judge behaviors as being unfaithful slightly more strictly than men, which is in line with other research in the existing literature [17]. Despite this, it appears that overall gender differences regarding the prevalence of infidelity have been shrinking over the past few decades [18].

3.1. Measuring Infidelity

Whitty and Quigley constructed a survey which aimed to explore what would upset participants from a list of several described situations [19]. Next, drawing from Harris and Christenfeld's work, participants were then asked how they would feel if their partner was unfaithful and was in love with someone else [20]. Sabini and Green relied on Buss et al.'s much-utilized approach and described a situation where the partner of the participant was having deep emotional or sexual involvement with someone else [21,22]. Participants were asked to describe how they would feel in such a situation. They found that both, men and women, saw a partner's emotional involvement as a more threatening sign of their partners' leaving than when there was only sexual involvement.

In their study on infidelity, Leeker and Carlozzi utilized Cramer et al.'squestionnaire, in which participants rated the likelihood of their partner engaging in each item with a third party, on a seven-point Likert scale, aiming to identify their reactions to emotional vs. sexual intimacy [11,14]. Another measure which was utilized in Leeker and Carlozzi's study was continuous emotion ratings [13]. These ratings served as the dependent variable in their study, assessing how angry, anxious, jealous and humiliated each participant felt in response to infidelity in their romantic relationship.

3.2. Perspectives on Infidelity

Symons and Buss were the first to view infidelity from an evolutionary perspective [23]. They opined that women are more likely to be affected by emotional infidelity rather than by sexual infidelity due to the fact that women carry the fetus and give birth. Thus, they are more threatened by the emotional betrayal of their romantic partner, for whom they count on to provide for the developing family unit. Men on the other hand are more threatened by sexual infidelity. Fisher et al., observed that for thousands of years, women depended on men to provide their food, shelter and safety, and this is the reason why they are more hurt by emotional infidelity which may threaten the partner's commitment [24]. Men, however, are more threatened by sexual infidelity, as evolutionarily, they were not sure whether the child was theirs (versus the mother who carries her own child) and did not want to protect, feed and care for someone else's offspring. This was referred to as jealousy as a specific innate module (JSIM). While the evolutionary perspective is the most accepted one, the social-cognitive perspective was proposed as an alternative to JSIM, and maintained that jealousy is not a simple module but includes several different feelings, each triggered by a different aspect of the jealousy-provoking situation. Anger was identified as a major component of the response to infidelity [25,26].

4. Distress Related to Emotional and Sexual Infidelity

4.1. The Role of Adult Attachment on Infidelity-Based Trauma

Colloquially dubbed as a "theory of trauma", attachment theory was originally developed by John Bowlby to describe the different forms of emotional attachment (i.e., secure, anxious–ambivalent, avoidant, disorganized) and subsequent attachment behaviors that exist between a mother and infant [27]. As the child's cognition begins to mature, they begin to develop internalized expectations, or internal working models, about how they should behave with their caregivers and how their caregivers should comfort them during times of distress or separation [27]. Overtime, the child learns how to perceive, process and resolve stressful events that involve their caregiver which ultimately inform their early understandings of attachment and later romantic relationships in adulthood [28].

However, parallels to this evolutionary behavioral system from infancy become prevalent as early styles and characteristics of attachment emerge in response to an unfaithful, romantic affair amongst committed partners [29]. Johnson et al., compares the harsh emotional pain experienced by victims of infidelity to the same attachment injuries as an infant separated from their mother [28]. Attachment injuries refer to traumatic interpersonal experiences which violate an individual's internal representation of another as a trustworthy and reliable base for support [29]. The traumatic reactions caused by infidelity emulate behaviors and attitudes seen in a disorganized attachment style as immense emotional, psychological and cognitive dysregulation is evident amongst these afflicted romantic partners [5,30]. This includes reports of developing lower self-esteem, self-confidence, a lack of trust in others and a strong fear of abandonment in future romantic relationships [31]. Hazan and Shaver conclude that the subversive impact of infidelity harms the individual's ability to be open to future romantic pursuits as the betrayal of a loving, secure partner is everlasting [29].

Reactions to infidelity vary significantly according to each person. Interpretations of infidelity are often based on an individual's perspective of what they want to perceive from the event. The unfaithful affair may be interpreted as a threatening message or a conciliatory one; a process that is commonly referred to as causal attribution [32]. It would, consequently, be beneficial to enlighten couples prior to their long-term commitment—especially those whose attachment is not secure—that infidelity need not to "destroy" their trust in their partner, and that healing may occur, despite the traumatic event. Relationship satisfaction may also affect how people process and interpret these transgressions. Although, less satisfied partners may perceive infidelity as more threatening to the relationship, which may enhance the chances of relational dissolution. Others, on the other hand, may forgive the transgression and continue with their relationship [1].

4.2. Emotional Reactions to Infidelity

Infidelity can lead to emotional dysregulation for both victims and perpetrators of extradyadic behaviors. Specific emotional manifestations of infidelity-based trauma include feelings of extreme anger, betrayal, insecurity, rage, shame, guilt, jealousy and sadness [24,31,33–40].

Depressive symptoms following the disclosure of an affair are commonplace for victims of infidelity [30,33,38,41]. Women who had experienced threats of marital dissolution or of their husband's infidelity were six times more likely to be diagnosed with a major depressive episode than those who had not experienced either of those events [42]. These women were also more likely to report heightened symptoms of nonspecific depression and anxiety [42]. Research by Lonergan et al., further supports these findings, as their participants demonstrated clinically significant scores of psychological distress which was associated with intrusive images, memories and rumination about their previous unfaithful relationship(s) [38].

Jealousy is the most frequently experienced emotion in response to discovering spousal infidelity. This mechanism was acquired by humans thousands of years ago and often occurs in combination with anger, insecurity, rejection, fear, betrayal, paranoia, depression, loneliness, confusion, envy and resentment, as well as PTSD [21,30]. Intense feelings, such as the ones mentioned, may trigger aggressive behavior, which may be expressed towards one's spouse; this is the leading cause of homicide in the United States according to Leeker and Carlozzi [11]. It is evident that the impact of infidelity can have dangerous outcomes for those afflicted by this type of betrayal.

Future research may address the issue of intense emotions in light of romantic betrayal, aiming to find a method that the betrayed could employ to control those negative feelings. Thus, preventing that distress from overcoming their wishes regarding the union (assuming that they would want the union to continue).

4.3. Predictors of Emotional Reactions to Infidelity

Sex and sexual orientation were shown to be significant predictors of general distress, anger, anxiety, jealousy and humiliation in response to both emotional and sexual infidelity. Commitment was predictive of distress and anger in response to emotional infidelity, while sexual infidelity aroused distress and anxiety. Interestingly, Leeker and Carlozzi did not find an association between the influence of the three components of love on emotional responses [11]. Interestingly, neither passion or expectations about the likelihood of a partner committing sexual or emotional infidelity were able to predict emotional responses to either emotional or sexual infidelity. Generally, they concluded that women and heterosexuals are significantly more distressed by a current partner's sexual or emotional infidelity in comparison with their male, lesbian and gay counterparts. As is intuitively apparent, those with greater commitment to their partners are more likely to be distressed and angered by a partner's emotional infidelity, while those who feel that their union connection is less intimate will be more distressed and anxious by a partner's sexual infidelity. Lastly, regardless of how passionate the relationship is, just imagining one's partner being involved in infidelity evokes strong, negative emotions. Another interesting finding of the study was that gender was not predictive of jealousy in response to sexual infidelity.

Heterosexual men often report more distress in response to sexual infidelity than heterosexual women, although heterosexual women, lesbian women and gay men tend to report similarly high levels of distress to emotional infidelity. Apparently, it was found that sexual orientation was a significant predictor of emotional reactions to emotional and sexual infidelity. Commitment was positively correlated with distress and anger in the face of emotional infidelity, but not the sexual type. When there was less intimacy in the relationship, it was predictive of distress and anxiety in response to sexual infidelity, but not emotional infidelity. Leeker and Carlozzi opined that it is possible that having less of an emotional bond decreases the betrayed partner's sense of safety and security when faced with a partner's sexual infidelity, which may result in lowered distress and anxiety [11]. Notably, it is difficult to speculate why these emotions were felt in response to one infidelity type and not the other.

4.4. *Effects of Sex and Sexual Orientation on Emotional Reactions to Infidelity*

In Leeker and Carlozzi's study, gender and sexual orientation did not significantly interact to elicit emotional responses to sexual and emotional infidelity. Women, regardless of their sexual orientation, reacted more strongly to both types of infidelity than men. Women's reactions to emotional infidelity were similar to those of men, while they were angrier than men in the face of sexual infidelity. When faced with sexual infidelity, women were almost as humiliated as they were anxious and jealous, whereas men were much less concerned with humiliation. Both women and men were more distressed by sexual infidelity than emotional infidelity overall [11,43,44].

In the Leeker and Carlozzi study, women and men agreed that sexual infidelity mostly elicited anger, followed by anxiety and jealousy [11]. Additionally, these researchers found that heterosexuals' scores were also significantly higher than lesbian and gay individuals' scores, but no significant sexual orientation differences were found between emotional and sexual infidelity. Evolutionary theory would explain this result by suggesting that lesbian and gay people should not be as affected by infidelity compared to heterosexuals, since infidelity by same-sex partners does not pose the evolutionary threats of raising another man's child or losing a male partner's resources to another woman [45].

4.5. *Effects of Infidelity Type on Emotional Reactions*

Among all participants of the Leeker and Carlozzi study, sexual infidelity elicited significantly more intense emotional reactions than emotional infidelity, with significant differences in distress, anger and humiliation [11]. Sexual infidelity elicited significantly more anger than the other emotions. The researchers also found that emotional infidelity elicited significantly more anxiety and jealousy than anger and humiliation. Sexual infidelity, on the other hand, elicited significantly more anger than all other emotions and may, thus, reflect the common viewpoint that sexual infidelity is preventable and intolerable, whereas emotional infidelity is perceived as less controllable [46].

Seminal research by Buss et al., asked college students to imagine their romantic partner being engaged in a deep emotional attachment with another person or imagine their partner enjoying passionate sexual intercourse with that person [21]. Participants were then asked which upset scenario them more. Results found that 60% of men believed sexual infidelity to be more stressful, whereas only 17% of women felt that way. This is in line with evolutionary theory, which state that men and women react differently to the two different transgressions as a result of sexually dimorphic selection pressures [47].

4.6. *Understanding Infidelity Victimization in the Context of Trauma and Stressor-Related Disorders*

The diagnostic category of "trauma and stressor-related disorders" is a new addition to the fifth edition of the *Diagnostic and Statistical Manual for Mental Disorders* (DSM-5) which lists external environmental stressors as an etiological factor for various mental illnesses [48]. For PTSD, the stressor must involve exposure to or experience involving actual or threatened death, serious injury or sexual violence (e.g., Criterion A) [48]. In contrast, the stressors needed to diagnose adjustment disorder [AD] can include those that fall into "everyday" normal life such as job loss, the death of a loved one or divorce [38,48]. According to Maercker and Lorenz, the similarities of both conditions can be traced back to cognitive distortions surrounding safety and trust which are developed from the maladaptive memories of a traumatic event [49]. They suggest that these memories are often combined with negative appraisals about the traumatic incident to radically impact an individual's opinion of the world and themselves as dangerous, damaging and destructive.

Several authors have cited the emotional, cognitive and behavioral reactions to infidelity as evidence to support its status as a traumatic experience that is comparable to PTSD, despite AD being a better diagnostic fit [38,50,51]. Both disorders share similar psychophysiological symptoms that are typically demonstrated in cases of infidelity, including feelings of elevated anxiety, hyperarousal, rumination, intrusive flashbacks, emotional dissociation and depression [50,52]. However, an important distinction that should be stressed is of the diagnostic criterions needed to diagnose PTSD in the DSM-5. For example, research by Steffens and Rennie and Laaser et al., found that infidelity victims met all the criteria for PTSD apart from Criterion A [41,53]. Similar results were shown in work by Roos et al. and Gordon et al., which found that victims of romantic betrayal experienced clinical levels of PTSD symptomology that included high levels of depressive symptoms and stress [51,54]. These findings suggest that victims of romantic betrayal do experience significant psychological and emotional distress, but not due to the trauma of direct or threatened exposure to deadly circumstances, as needed to fulfill Criterion A for PTSD [48]. Therefore, these symptoms may be better understood within the diagnostic context of AD, rather than in PTSD.

It is therefore suggested that attachment-based trauma, as seen in extradyadic affairs, should be regarded as a valid traumatic experience, but should also be nuanced and critically distinct to that of PTSD trauma [30,35,55]. Some clinicians argue that framing the experience of infidelity as a form of trauma may facilitate greater emotional recovery for its victims, thus, demonstrating the benefits of validating such an emotionally distressing event [56,57]. Therefore, conceptualizing infidelity as its own unique traumatic experience within the lens of AD may help to accurately capture the impact of these situations while shedding light on the potential overdiagnosis and reliance of the PTSD label [49,58,59].

4.7. *Physical Health Consequences of Infidelity-Based Trauma*

Few studies have examined the relationship between infidelity-based trauma and its subsequent physical health consequences, although immediate physical reactions shortly following the discovery of these affairs have been cited by some researchers. For example, work by Lonergan et al., found that infidelity victims reported persistent somatic symptoms such as insomnia, weight loss, difficulty with concentration and a lack of appetite and libido immediately after experiencing romantic betrayal [38]. Another study conducted by Roos et al., found that undergraduate students experiencing infidelity as victims of romantic betrayal reported having difficulty breathing, bodily trembles, extreme nervousness and a racing heart when recalling their previous relationship [51]. This is further supported by findings from Shackelford et al., which found that female participants reported greater symptoms of nausea and physical illness when asked to imagine their partner as unfaithful under experimental settings [40]. Ultimately, it is suggested that further work should be performed to examine the lasting physical effects of infidelity-based trauma to promote preventative care for those involved in these relationships.

4.8. *Suicidality and Infidelity*

Infidelity may feel like an unstoppable problem which may invoke thoughts of suicidal ideation and suicidality among vulnerable individuals [60,61]. An article by Snyder et al., described how these issues may impact both perpetrators and injured partners of an affair [62]. For the injured party, fluctuating feelings of rage, powerlessness, abandonment and victimization may leave them shaken and unable to support themselves after learning about their partner's betrayal. This may lead to suicidal ideation. However, perpetrators of infidelity may experience similar emotional reactions after the discovery of their affair, such as depression, acute anxiety and suicidality. This is believed to occur persistently following threats of divorce or marital separation following disclosure [62].

To date, only one study by Stephens has closely examined the relationship between suicidal behavior and relationship-related distress such as infidelity [63]. A community sample of 50 women with histories of previous suicide attempts were asked about their intimate relationships with men in relation to their suicidal behaviors. It was found that partner infidelity, along with battering, "smothering love" and denial of affection, were the most prominent themes that lead to suicidality and suicidal ideation. Interestingly, Stephens also asserted that age may be a confounding variable for this topic as well [63]. Younger participants reacted to specific negative events in their romantic relationships by attempting suicide, while older participants would do so in response to long-term conflicts with their partners. This may suggest that the threshold for suicidality in those afflicted by infidelity is different for individuals depending on their age and range of experiences related to love.

Similarly, research by Martin et al., further supports the relationship between infidelity and suicidal behavior in their work examining the role of marital status, life stressors and communication regarding suicidality in U.S. Air Force personnel [64]. Researchers examined 100 decedents who died by suicide and examined their social supports (e.g., communication with friends, family and coworkers), medical and fiscal records (e.g., personnel files, finances, mental health details), toxicology and autopsy reports and evidence from the death scene (e.g., suicide notes) to gather a comprehensive understanding of the conflicts that contribute to suicide. Among this sample, 9% of suicide completers were found to have experienced the infidelity of a spouse within 24 h prior to their passing. Martin et al., also observed that 5% of decedents had committed infidelity within this time frame as well [64]. Findings from this study highlight the rapid and deadly risks of infidelity disclosure in precipitating suicidal behavior for both victims and perpetrators of romantic betrayal.

These limited studies show that further research is necessary to examine specific factors that drive suicidality in certain victims of infidelity. The importance of this topic warrants greater investigation into how potential influences such as age, personality and relationship duration impact infidelity-based suicidality.

4.9. Why Do People Think They Get into Affairs?

Selterman et al., wanted to understand how those who were involved in infidelity feel, think and behave, and suggested that all of these factors are affected by their motivation to have extramarital affairs [65]. Their findings suggest that there may be meaningfully different infidelity typologies characterized by both different underlying motivations, different relational processes and different behavioral outcomes. Thompson's deficit model of infidelity suggested that relationships which are not optimal and are characterized by low satisfaction, high conflict and a lack of good communication play a significant role in the causal factors leading to infidelity [10]. Like other models and theories, this model sees infidelity as a symptom of deeper underlying relational difficulties that the couple is struggling with. In their study, Selterman et al., explored the infidelity of 495 participants, including 259 women and 213 men who had significant variability in relationship length, ranging from 1 month to 28 years [65]. Results indicated that while almost all participants engaged physically with their affair partners, only 53% had intercourse with them. Men were more likely to report engaging in these sexual behaviors. Those motivated by sexual desire, and seeking love and variety, reported greater sexual satisfaction with their affairs. On the other hand, those motivated by situational factors were less sexually satisfied with the affair, which was also short lived, in contrast with those in long-term committed relationships [66,67].

Selterman et al., found eight different variables which related to infidelity motivation. These included things such as feeling angry at a partner's behavior; wanting more sex than is available in the primary relationship; wanting more intimacy and love than is available to them; having low commitment to the relationship; wanting greater autonomy; clouded judgement due to situational factors, such as stress; feeling mistreated or neglected; and wanting a greater number of sexual partners [65]. Consistent with the deficit model of relationship infidelity, they found that motivations related to a lack of love and neglect predicted participants' reported intimacy with affair partners, such as expressing their love verbally in "I love you" statements, public displays of affection and engaging in longer affairs, while situational motivation was inversely associated with these experiences. The authors opined that when people feel emotional shortfalls in their primary relationships, they may search for a deeper quality of romantic connection which includes more intimacy in their affairs to compensate for the insufficient intimacy experienced with primary partners.

Furthermore, emotional closeness to their primary partners was negatively associated with the emotional satisfaction which people involved in affairs experienced [65]. In some instances, people become involved in affairs to hurt their partner. They are usually angry, score lower on commitment and experience a lack of love in their relationship. In light of the devastating effects of affairs, it is possible that while some participants wanted their primary partners to suffer, others had no intention to hurt their partner or terminate the relationship [68]. Commitment affected the post-affair contact that people maintained with their affair partners; those who had a higher level of commitment, versus those who did not, did not maintain contact with their affair partners. Focusing on one's partner and the relationship may enhance personal and relational growth following an affair, while if that is missing, the relationship may not survive an affair. People who lacked love, appreciation and sexual desire in their primary relationship are more liable to leave it and establish a primary relationship with their affair partner [65].

5. Infidelity in Marital Relationships

The scientific literature points to the occurrence of what is variously labeled infidelity, extradyadic involvement, unfaithfulness, affairs, stepping out, cheating or some other synonym indicative of secret romantic activity with a secondary partner while in an exclusive romantic relationship. This secretive activity can range from emotional involvement all the way to penetrative sex. Estimates suggest that infidelity occurs in about a quarter of all marriages, and at the beginning of the 21st century, a dramatic increase in infidelity of the oldest cohort of men (ages 65–90) was noted [18].

Infidelity causes grief and relational problems to the individual, the couple and even their offspring. It was found to be associated with depression, anxiety and even PTSD, leading to divorce [42,69,70]. Additionally, infidelity was linked to domestic violence and increased exposure to sexually transmitted diseases [21,71].

5.1. Factors That Increase Infidelity

5.1.1. Demographics

While early research suggested that men are more likely to commit infidelity than women recent work has suggested that the gender gap is narrowing [56,72]. A study observing the relationship between religion and infidelity found that non-religious people report more cases of infidelity than religious ones [73]. Education has also been shown to be positively associated with infidelity, in that those with higher education are more likely to engage in infidelity than the less educated, often depending on other factors in their lives. Individuals with higher incomes are also more prone to engage in infidelity, although, this may simply be because their professional and personal lives include more opportunities to engage in extradyadic relations. About half of all those who engaged in infidelity met their extradyadic partner at work [74].

5.1.2. The Individual

Personal characteristics such as neuroticism, prior history of infidelity, number of sex partners before marriage, psychological distress and an insecure attachment orientation, as well as permissive attitudes toward sex, have been positively associated with infidelity [75–77]. Coming from a family where infidelity was present also increases the risk of one being involved in infidelity [7].

When not caused by marital conflict or low marital satisfaction, infidelity may be associated with opportunity and permissive values. For instance, Treas and Giesen found an increased likelihood of sexual infidelity among men and women with stronger sexual interest levels [78]. Some research used the Big Five personality traits and found extraversion, high neuroticism, low conscientiousness and high psychoticism to be positively correlated with engaging in infidelity [76,79]. The dual control model of sexual response suggests that one's sexual behavior depends on the balance of sexual desire and inhibition; inhibition may be related to fear of performance failure or of possible consequences related to extradyadic sexual relations [80]. A number of studies have shown that the propensity for sexual excitation is related to sexual responsiveness, sexual desire levels, sexual compulsivity and a lifetime number of casual sexual partners. Sexual inhibition may be adaptive, but high levels of it may lead to sexual dysfunctions, while low levels may result in increased risky sexual behavior [81].

In their 2011 study, Mark et al., found that up to 22% of people engaged in extradyadic relationships [82]. They found that perceived sexual compatibility and happiness in a relationship were significant predictors of infidelity in women, while age, marital status and the importance of religion did not significantly affect one's proclivity for affairs. They also found that a stronger tendency to lose one's sexual arousal when facing possible risks serves as a protective effect for engaging in infidelity. Interestingly, they found that experiencing sexual problems in their extradyadic relationship was less threatening for individuals with arousal difficulties. The authors propose that perhaps these individuals are less concerned with their sexual performance with a partner to whom they are not emotionally committed to or one they have been with for a long time. As can be expected, they found that higher levels of sexual excitation were associated with increased sexual risk-taking behaviors, particularly in men. Women were found to be more likely to engage in infidelity when they were dissatisfied in their relationship or felt that they were sexually incompatible with their partner, which may point to the interconnection of sexual and relationship factors in increasing the possibility of infidelity. In other words, if a woman is unsatisfied with her current relationship, she may seek intimacy and closeness somewhere else. An interesting finding of Mark et al.'s study was that sexual excitation did not predict involvement in infidelity for women [82]. That may support the notion that women's sexual infidelity is less motivated by sexual needs, arousability or desire, while in men, this is often not the case.

5.1.3. Relationships

Decreased satisfaction in a present relationship is closely related to infidelity amongst married people [83]. When commitment is not central to the relationship, that too contributes to infidelity [4]. Interestingly, cohabitation before marriage was found to be positively associated with infidelity [84].

5.1.4. Context

The gender gap in infidelity of married couples is ascribed to women's increased presence in the working world. There, the woman spends many daily hours working closely with the opposite sex and interacting about issues and topics that they both seem to value. Moreover, when one spouse works out of the home and the other stays at home, the chances of infidelity increase [85]. In the last twenty years, the internet has provided increased opportunity for infidelity. Up to 30% of internet users go online for sexual purposes, and up to two-thirds of them engage in offline sexual intercourse with their online partner [86].

5.1.5. Marital Deception

Dew et al., explored two kinds of marital deceptions: financial marital deception (FMD) and extramarital infidelity (EMI) [87]. EMI was well researched, while MFD was much less so. Interestingly, one may bring about the other. Social exchange theory (SET), which originated in social psychology's interpersonal relationship area, and was pioneered by Thibault and Kelley, asserted the rewards, costs and expectations that partners have of their relationship, which may entice them to remain with their partner, modify the relationship or leave all together [88]. Nye observed that each spouse evaluates the "outcomes", meaning the costs and benefits entailed in their marriage [89]. Then, the spouses compare the outcomes to those to which they expect to receive in that relationship, which are termed in SET, the comparison level, or CL; this will determine whether the spouse will remain in the marriage. If a spouse finds that his or her marital outcomes exceed the CL, they will be satisfied with the relationship and remain in it. However, if a spouse's outcomes fall beneath their CL, they will become dissatisfied with the relationship and may seek to change or terminate it. This may lead to relationships out of the marital union, remaining in the relationship despite a lowered satisfaction level or leaving the relationship. Dissatisfied spouses will engage in what was termed "comparison level of the alternative" (CLalt), which may lead them to leave the relationship.

5.1.6. Moral Commitment

To remain in the marriage was found to be negatively associated with EMI and possibly MFD. Most people, at least in Western countries, want marital fidelity and plan to avoid EMI. They want to behave in a way that upholds marital norms and/or their wedding vows to their spouse, and to remain loyal to them [90]. Personal dedication to one's marriage, and the desire to make it succeed, is a type of commitment to the marriage, which is separate from moral commitment, since dedication is focused particularly on increasing the rewards and happiness of the couple [91]. Personal dedication, then, may make it less likely for marital dissatisfaction to occur when its outcomes fall below the CL. This may lead to a situation in which a spouse may be dissatisfied with the marriage, but viewing it as a long-term commitment will motivate them to invest in it and be less interested in alternative relationships, despite their present unhappiness [92]. Recent research about MFD and EMI found that personal dedication commitment (in the form of marital stability and trust of one's partner) is negatively associated with MFD [87]. Additionally, personal dedication commitment is associated with a lower level of sexually unfaithful behaviors [93]. Religiosity was also found to be associated with a better marital relationship, since most religions hold marriage to be sacred and special. This may stem from religious peoples' hesitation to violate something that they believe is sacred, particularly when they are part of a religious community which does not condone infidelity and unfaithfulness [94]. Dew et al., also found that those who engaged in minor EMI, such as flirting, had an increased likelihood of engaging in EMI with the person with whom they flirted, in addition to increased chances of engaging in MFD, since marriages that are growing in a positive direction provide less motivation to engage in EMI [93,95].

6. The Effect of Infidelity in Cyberspace

Social media sites are platforms where users generate and post their own content to create and maintain virtual relationships [96]. These platforms are very popular, as indicated by, for example, Facebook's 2.45 billion active monthly users [97]. These popular platforms contribute to increased opportunities for infidelity [98]. In her research, Adam found that flirting or sexual behavior conducted via social media is indeed perceived similarly not only to cyber-sexual behaviors but also to physical sexual infidelity, which is similarly hurtful to romantic relationships [98].

6.1. Infidelity and COVID-19

When discussing infidelity, we would be remiss if we did not review research that assessed infidelity during the pandemic that swept the world just a short time ago. Gordon and Mitchell asserted that COVID increased the chance that people would be involved in infidelity, particularly in light of the stress that was brought about by the pandemic [99]. These challenges may potentially have resulted in lower relational and sexual satisfaction, which may justify—in the eyes of a partner—becoming involved in an affair [100]. While social distancing was practiced during the pandemic, and has consequently decreased the opportunities for physical contact with affair partners, the use of virtual apps to stay connected (e.g., Face Time, Zoom, and Skype) drastically increased during this time and may be more likely to be used to contact affair partners than prior to the pandemic [101]. Dating sites have flourished, and they have also been utilized as an opportunity to get involved in affairs [102]. Infidelity may have devastating consequences for the couple, and those discovered during the pandemic may have a greater possibility to cause negative consequences [99]. Anxiety and depression, which are known to follow the discovery of an affair, may be exacerbated due to the pandemic, which by itself is liable to cause such a reaction [103]. Significant financial loss, which occurred frequently due to closures of work sites and limited operations or unemployment, may also precipitate infidelity [103].

6.2. How Does COVID-19 Impact Affair Recovery?

The pandemic may have made recovering from infidelity more complicated. During that time, the couple's access to healthcare resources and social support, such as their friends and confidants, was more restricted; thus, addressing the emotional injury that an affair caused was much more difficult [104]. Additionally, couples who focused on decreasing their anxiety and stress caused by the pandemic, dealing with financial concerns and spending their mental and emotional energies on struggling to survive during such a difficult time may have been less able to cope with difficulties caused by an affair [105]. Heightened emotional arousal resulting from both the pandemic and the affair may make it more difficult for couples to effectively regulate their emotions during this time, which may slow or even inhibit the healing process, as the couple may be more irritable and liable to strike out at the slightest provocation [106]. Additionally, while it is common for couples to take a break from each other (either by spending more time apart, or even moving to a different house for a period) after the discovery of an affair, the pandemic made such a break impossible due to strict rules related to social distancing. This may have seriously disturbed the healing time that such a separation provided [104].

Gordon and Mitchell observed that while communication is an important factor in healing, constantly discussing the affair and the details of the extradyadic relationship may be more harmful than helpful to healing, as partners may not yet be emotionally ready to discuss them [99]. Infidelity is a much-stigmatized phenomenon and responses such as shame, shock, anger, hurt and despair may result in constant friction at home. These intense emotions need space and time to be expressed and processed; being together 24/7 disallows this. Additionally, couples try to hide the affair from their children; this was especially true during the pandemic. Partners constantly being at home while dealing with infidelity and its aftermath means that these conflicts may have easily been overheard by the children, increasing their anxiety and familial stress.

An important component of the recovery process is rebuilding the trust that was lost as a result of the affair. This is, usually, a slow process which requires a concerted effort on the part of both partners, which is often not linear [104]. One of the first steps in rebuilding trust is for the "offending" partner to stop seeing the affair partner, which may require changing where one goes to the gym, shopping, etc. The pandemic has changed all of this. On the one hand, the strict social distancing rules may have decreased the chance that affair partners would continue to meet, but on the other hand, various forms of virtual contact may have continued [106].

Gordon and Mitchell concluded their study by observing that "infidelity is a wrenching and devastating event that is difficult for couples to navigate even under the best of circumstances [99]. Experiencing this relational trauma during a global pandemic that is also traumatic with far-reaching social and economic consequences is even more overwhelming. This context can intensify and exacerbate normal emotional reactions to affairs and complicates efforts toward recovery. Couples will need to dig deep and intentionally build emotional resources to meet these challenges. However, all is not lost in this context and there is hope for couples' recovery during this time. After many years of working with couples to deal with the discovery of an affair, we have found that couples can be astonishingly resilient ... Thus, COVID-19's vast and life-changing impacts can create added challenges and barriers in couples emotional and social lives, but as the cliche suggests, it also can create opportunities for immense growth for these couples and the clinicians who are trying to help them" [99].

6.3. Therapists Addressing Infidelity: Challenges and Attitudes

As infidelity remains one of the major causes of divorce, it is essential that therapists are trained to help couples deal with what can be a devastating personal and relational experience [107]. Irvine and Peluso explored therapists' subjective experiences with treating affairs [108]. Professional guidelines, such as those of the American Association of Marriage and Family Therapy or the American Psychological Association, state that therapists are expected to practice competently when treating individuals or couples [109,110]. Given the complex and morally laden nature of affairs, therapists may confront challenges that can significantly impact treatment outcomes. Among those challenges, the therapist may experience countertransference and then over-identify with one partner, which will hamper their neutral position as a counselor [111]. Garza conducted a study that revealed that therapists' attitudes toward infidelity can clearly influence their treatment decisions [112]. Specifically, therapists with more negative views towards infidelity guided the couple in reducing environmental risk factors (e.g., limiting Internet access) related to the affair, rather than addressing larger processes that impacted the couple's presenting issue. Other struggles that therapists face when dealing with clients facing infidelity may involve their need to strike a balance between addressing the needs of both partners while exploring the underlying causes of the affair. Additional challenges that emerge from this process include having to establish trust and forgiveness between the partners healing from the emotional injury, which could resemble symptoms of post-traumatic stress disorder such as hypervigilance and increased distress [113].

Irvine and Peluso were interested in exploring a myriad of therapist-related factors that impact counseling for couples faced with infidelity [108]. These included influences such as the personal and professional experiences and histories of therapists who treated infidelity, and the challenges they faced when treating couples in these circumstances. They found that the specific experiences of the counselor directly impact the competency of treatment for those recovering from a romantic affair. Therapists who had attended infidelity training, held their license for more than 16 years, held a doctoral degree and were licensed to practice marriage and family therapy showed the highest levels of comfort, preparedness, effectiveness and confidence in treating infidelity [113]. In turn, four factors in couples were identified by Irvine and Peluso that negatively affect recovery from romantic affairs [108]. This included things such as the betrayal continuing while the couple was in therapy, an unwillingness to commit to therapy, continual blame and resentment towards each other without forgiveness.

Ultimately, further training related to the issue of infidelity is suggested for clinicians working with couples [108]. Research has shown that the vast majority of therapists have never received any courses on infidelity, and that this had hampered their perceived competence when treating such individuals [114] Several factors which may impede effective treatment delivery have been identified by Irvine and Peluso [108]. These factors included learning how to manage one's countertransference reactions, knowing how to address trauma and manage emotional reactivity, possessing clinical experience and balancing needs that arise in the process of therapy.

7. Conclusions

Clearly, the consequential effects of infidelity vary widely according to the type of extradyadic behavior performed, in combination with the demographic and interpersonal factors of the people in question. Men and women react to emotional and sexual infidelity differently, as research suggests that women tend to judge more behaviors as unfaithful, while men hold more permissive attitudes towards extramarital sex [17]. This may be explained by evolutionary psychology as the genders' attempt to protect their union and offspring. Additionally, the literature on infidelity has also shown that younger people express greater negative attitudes toward infidelity and more often perceive sexual behaviors as infidelity than older people [115]. This is further supported by the work of Varga et al., who observed that age may have a moderating effect on the gender differences concerning sexual versus emotional jealousy [116]. Researchers further suggest that individuals who are most likely to commit infidelity are more educated, wealthier and less tied to a religious faith [74].

Infidelity may not only have a destructive impact on the relationship leading to separation or divorce; it can also negatively affect one's emotional wellbeing by enhancing depressive symptoms, highlighting low self-esteem and promoting remorse in the unfaithful party [3]. This type of attachment injury could impose psychological and emotional dysregulation for those facing these circumstances, which may emulate symptoms of conditions such as depression, anxiety and AD [28,30,38,41,51,53]. The impact of this life-altering event challenges the person's sense of self, safety and trust in another who is supposed to be their "secure base" for love and adoration [29,31]. Thus, infidelity leaves some at risk of turning towards unhealthy coping mechanisms such as excessive drinking, drug use, unprotected sex, and suicidal behavior in response to their emotional pain [63,64,70,117].

Overall, it is clear that the implications of a romantic affair have a substantial impact on one's life beyond their intimate relationships. Clinicians are encouraged to seek professional training when treating couples afflicted by infidelity and to be conscious about how their own moral and personal views related to the matter could impact their clients' recovery from these circumstances [108]. Scuka suggests clinicians normalize the experience of infidelity for their clients, as this can serve as the first step in identifying realistic expectations for the healing process [118]. However, communication regarding the details of an extradyadic affair should be guided between partners, as Gordon and Mitchell stress the importance of being emotionally ready for those conversations [99]. Therefore, it is recommended that therapists should be mindful of integrating high levels of sensitivity, care and honesty in these sessions to facilitate appropriate closure for those impacted by infidelity.

Author Contributions: Conceptualization, A.R. and S.H.C.; methodology, software, formal analysis, resources, data curation, investigation, writing—original draft preparation, writing—review and editing, visualization, A.R. and S.H.C.; supervision, project administration, A.R. All authors have read and agreed to the published version of the manuscript.

Funding: This research received no external funding.

Informed Consent Statement: Not applicable.

Conflicts of Interest: The authors declare no conflict of interest.

References

1. Grøntvedt, T.V.; Kennair, L.E.O.; Bendixen, M. Breakup Likelihood Following Hypothetical Sexual or Emotional Infidelity: Perceived Threat, Blame, and Forgiveness. *J. Relatsh. Res.* **2020**, *11*, 1–9.e7. [CrossRef]
2. Bendixen, M.; Kennair, L.E.O.; Grøntvedt, T.V. Forgiving the unforgivable: Couples' forgiveness and expected forgiveness of emotional and sexual infidelity from an error management theory perspective. *Evol. Behav. Sci.* **2018**, *12*, 322–335. [CrossRef]
3. Bozoyan, C.; Schmiedeberg, C. What is Infidelity? A Vignette Study on Norms and Attitudes toward Infidelity. *J. Sex Res.* **2022**, 272–275, *online ahead of print*. [CrossRef]
4. Drigotas, S.M.; Safstrom, C.A.; Gentilia, T. An investment model prediction of dating infidelity. *J. Pers. Soc. Psychol.* **1999**, *77*, 509–524. [CrossRef]
5. Blow, A.J.; Hartnett, K. Infidelity in committed relati0nships II: A substantive review. *J. Marital. Fam. Ther.* **2005**, *31*, 217–233. [CrossRef]
6. Urganci, B.; Sakman, E. Perceptions of infidelity. In *Encyclopedia of Evolutionary Psychological Science*; Shackelford, T.K., Weekes-Shackelford, V.A., Eds.; Springer International Publishing: Berlin/Heidelberg, Germany, 2019; pp. 1–3. Available online: https://doi.org/10.1007/978-3-319-16999-6_1805-1 (accessed on 22 January 2023). [CrossRef]
7. Weiser, D.A.; Lalasz, C.B.; Weigel, D.J.; Evans, W.P. A prototype analysis of infidelity. *Pers. Relatsh.* **2014**, *21*, 655–675. [CrossRef]
8. Bernard, J. Infidelity: Some moral and social issues. In *Beyond Monogamy: Recent Studies of Sexual Alternatives in Marriage*; Smith, J.R., Smith, L.G., Eds.; Johns Hopkins University Press: Baltimore, MD, USA, 1974; pp. 130–158.
9. Pittman, F.S.; Wagers, T.P. The relationship, if any, between marriage and infidelity. *J. Couple Relatsh. Ther.* **2005**, *4*, 135–148. [CrossRef]
10. Thompson, A.P. Extramarital sex: A review of the research literature. *J. Sex Res.* **1983**, *19*, 1–22. [CrossRef]
11. Leeker, O.; Carlozzi, A. Effects of Sex, Sexual Orientation, Infidelity Expectations, and Love on Distress related to Emotional and Sexual Infidelity. *J. Marital. Fam. Ther.* **2014**, *40*, 68–91. [CrossRef]
12. Edlund, J.E.; Heider, J.D.; Scherer, C.R.; Farc, M.-M.; Sagarin, B.J. Sex Differences in Jealousy in Response to Actual Infidelity. *Evol. Psychol.* **2006**, *4*, 462–470. [CrossRef]
13. Penke, L.; Asendorpf, J.B. Evidence for conditional sex differences in emotional but not in sexual jealousy at the automatic level of cognitive processing. *Eur. J. Pers.* **2008**, *22*, 3–30. [CrossRef]
14. Cramer, R.E.; Lipinski, R.E.; Meteer, J.D.; Houska, J.A. Sex Differences in Subjective Distress to Unfaithfulness: Testing Competing Evolutionary and Violation of Infidelity Expectations Hypotheses. *J. Soc. Psychol.* **2008**, *148*, 389–405. [CrossRef]
15. Luo, S.; Cartun, M.A.; Snider, A.G. Assessing extradyadic behavior: A review, a new measure, and two new models. *Pers. Individ. Differ.* **2010**, *49*, 155–163. [CrossRef]
16. Guitar, A.E.; Geher, G.; Kruger, D.J.; Garcia, J.R.; Fisher, M.L.; Fitzgerald, C.J. Defining and Distinguishing Sexual and Emotional Infidelity. *Curr. Psychol.* **2016**, *36*, 434–446. [CrossRef]
17. Labrecque, L.T.; Whisman, M.A. Extramarital Sex and Marital Dissolution: Does Identity of the Extramarital Partner Matter? *Fam. Process.* **2020**, *59*, 1308–1318. [CrossRef]
18. Fincham, F.D.; May, R.W. Infidelity in romantic relationships. *Curr. Opin. Psychol.* **2017**, *13*, 70–74. [CrossRef]
19. Whitty, M.T.; Quigley, L.-L. Emotional and Sexual Infidelity Offline and in Cyberspace. *J. Marital. Fam. Ther.* **2008**, *34*, 461–468. [CrossRef]
20. Harris, C.R.; Christenfeld, N. Gender, jealousy, and reason. *Psychol. Sci.* **1996**, *7*, 364–366. [CrossRef]
21. Buss, D.M.; Larsen, R.J.; Westen, D.; Semmelroth, J. Sex Differences in Jealousy: Evolution, Physiology, and Psychology. *Psychol. Sci.* **1992**, *3*, 251–256. [CrossRef]
22. Sabini, J.; Green, M.C. Emotional Responses to Sexual and Emotional Infidelity: Constants and Differences Across Genders, Samples, and Methods. *Pers. Soc. Psychol. Bull.* **2004**, *30*, 1375–1388. [CrossRef]
23. Symons, D.K.; Buss, D.M. The evolution of desire: Strategies of human mating. *J. Marriage Fam.* **1994**, *56*, 1052. [CrossRef]
24. Fisher, M.; Voracek, M.; Rekkas, P.V.; Cox, A. Sex Differences in Feelings of Guilt Arising from Infidelity. *Evol. Psychol.* **2008**, *6*, 147470490800600308. [CrossRef]
25. DeSteno, D.; Bartlett, M.Y.; Braverman, J.; Salovey, P. Sex differences in jealousy: Evolutionary mechanism or artifact of measurement? *J. Pers. Soc. Psychol.* **2002**, *83*, 1103–1116. [CrossRef]
26. Harris, C.R. A Review of Sex Differences in Sexual Jealousy, Including Self-Report Data, Psychophysiological Responses, Interpersonal Violence, and Morbid Jealousy. *Pers. Soc. Psychol. Rev.* **2003**, *7*, 102–128. [CrossRef] [PubMed]
27. Bowlby, J. Defensive processes in the light of attachment theory. In *Attachment and the Therapeutic Process Essays in Honor of Otto Allen Will, Jr., M.D.*; Schwartz, D.P., Sacksteder, J.L., Akabane, Y., Eds.; International Universities Press, Inc.: Madison, CT, USA, 1987; pp. 63–79.
28. Johnson, S.M.; Makinen, J.A.; Millikin, J.W. Attachment injuries in couple relationships: A new perspective on impasses in couples therapy. *J. Marital. Fam. Ther.* **2001**, *27*, 145–155. [CrossRef]
29. Hazan, C.; Shaver, P. Romantic love conceptualized as an attachment process. *J. Personal. Soc. Psychol.* **1987**, *52*, 511–524. [CrossRef]
30. Warach, B.; Josephs, L. The aftershocks of infidelity: A review of infidelity-based attachment trauma. *Sex. Relatsh. Ther.* **2021**, *36*, 68–90. [CrossRef]

31. Charny, I.W.; Parnass, S. The impact of extramarital relationships on the continuation of marriages. *J. Sex Marital. Ther.* **1995**, *21*, 100–115. [CrossRef]
32. Shrout, M.R.; Weigel, D.J. 'Should I stay or should I go?' Understanding the noninvolved partner's decision-making process following infidelity. *J. Soc. Pers. Relatsh.* **2019**, *36*, 400–442. [CrossRef]
33. Bird, M.H.; Butler, M.H.; Fife, S.T. The Process of Couple Healing Following Infidelity. *J. Couple Relatsh. Ther.* **2007**, *6*, 1–25. [CrossRef]
34. Cano, A.; O'Leary, K.D. Romantic jealousy and affairs: Research and implications for couple therapy. *J. Sex Marital. Ther.* **1997**, *23*, 249–275. [CrossRef]
35. Gordon, K.C.; Baucom, D.H. A multitheoretical intervention for promoting recovery from extramarital affairs. *Clin. Psychol. Sci. Pract.* **1999**, *6*, 382–399. [CrossRef]
36. Gossner, J.D.; Fife, S.T.; Butler, M.H. Couple healing from infidelity: A deductive qualitative analysis study. *Sex. Relatsh. Ther.* **2022**, 1–22, *in press*. [CrossRef]
37. Kaplánová, A.; Gregor, A. Guilt- and Shame-Proneness and Their Relation to Perceptions of Dating Infidelity. *Stud. Psychol.* **2019**, *61*, 145–158. [CrossRef]
38. Lonergan, M.; Brunet, A.; Rivest-Beauregard, M.; Groleau, D. Is romantic partner betrayal a form of traumatic experience? A qualitative study. *Stress Health* **2021**, *37*, 19–31. [CrossRef]
39. Moller, N.P.; Vossler, A. Defining infidelity in research and couple counseling: A qualitative study. *J. Sex Marital. Ther.* **2015**, *41*, 487–497. [CrossRef]
40. Shackelford, T.K.; Leblanc, G.J.; Drass, E. Emotional reactions to infidelity. *Cogn. Emot.* **2000**, *14*, 643–659. [CrossRef]
41. Laaser, D.; Putney, H.L.; Bundick, M.; Delmonico, D.L.; Griffin, E.J. Posttraumatic Growth in Relationally Betrayed Women. *J. Marital. Fam. Ther.* **2017**, *43*, 435–447. [CrossRef]
42. Cano, A.; O'Leary, K.D. Infidelity and separations precipitate major depressive episodes and symptoms of nonspecific depression and anxiety. *J. Consult. Clin. Psychol.* **2000**, *68*, 774–781. [CrossRef]
43. DeSteno, D.; Valdesolo, P.; Bartlett, M.Y. Jealousy and the threatened self: Getting to the heart of the green-eyed monster. *J. Pers. Soc. Psychol.* **2006**, *91*, 626–641. [CrossRef]
44. Ward, J.; Voracek, M. Evolutionary and social cognitive explanations of sex differences in romantic jealousy. *Aust. J. Psychol.* **2004**, *56*, 165–171. [CrossRef]
45. De Souza, A.A.L.; Verderane, M.P.; Taira, J.T.; Otta, E. Emotional and sexual jealousy as a function of sex and sexual orientation in a Brazilian sample. *Psychol. Rep.* **2006**, *98*, 529–535. [CrossRef]
46. Green, M.C.; Sabini, J. Gender, socioeconomic status, age, and jealousy: Emotional responses to infidelity in a national sample. *Emotion* **2006**, *6*, 330–334. [CrossRef]
47. Tagler, M.J.; Jeffers, H.M. Sex Differences in Attitudes toward Partner Infidelity. *Evol. Psychol.* **2013**, *11*, 821–832. [CrossRef]
48. American Psychiatric Association (Ed.) *Diagnostic and Statistical Manual of Mental Disorders: DSM-5*, 5th ed.; American Psychiatric Association: Washington, DC, USA, 2013.
49. Maercker, A.; Lorenz, L. Adjustment disorder diagnosis: Improving clinical utility. *World J. Biol. Psychiatry* **2018**, *19*, S3–S13. [CrossRef]
50. Lusterman, D.-D. Marital infidelity: The effects of delayed traumatic reaction. *J. Couple Relatsh. Ther.* **2005**, *4*, 71–81. [CrossRef]
51. Roos, L.G.; O'Connor, V.; Canevello, A.; Bennett, J.M. Post-traumatic stress and psychological health following infidelity in unmarried young adults. *Stress Health* **2019**, *35*, 468–479. [CrossRef]
52. Baucom, N.H.; Gordon, K.C.; Snyder, D.K.; Atkins, D.C.; Christensen, A. Treating Affair Couples: Clinical Considerations and Initial Findings. *J. Cogn. Psychother.* **2006**, *20*, 375–392. [CrossRef]
53. Steffens, B.A.; Rennie, R.L. The Traumatic Nature of Disclosure for Wives of Sexual Addicts. *Sex. Addict. Compulsivity* **2006**, *13*, 247–267. [CrossRef]
54. Gordon, K.C.; Baucom, D.H.; Snyder, D.K. An integrative intervention for promoting recovery from extramarital affairs. *J. Marital. Fam. Ther.* **2004**, *30*, 213–231. [CrossRef]
55. Dean, C.J. Psychoeducation: A First Step to Understanding Infidelity-Related Systemic Trauma and Grieving. *Fam. J.* **2011**, *19*, 15–21. [CrossRef]
56. Allen, E.S.; Atkins, D.C.; Baucom, D.H.; Snyder, D.K.; Gordon, K.C.; Glass, S.P. Intrapersonal, Interpersonal, and Contextual Factors in Engaging in and Responding to Extramarital Involvement. *Clin. Psychol. Sci. Pract.* **2005**, *12*, 101–130. [CrossRef]
57. Gordon, K.C.; Baucom, D.H.; Snyder, D.K. Optimal Strategies in Couple Therapy: Treating Couples Dealing with the Trauma of Infidelity. *J. Contemp. Psychother.* **2008**, *38*, 151–160. [CrossRef]
58. Bachem, R.; Casey, P. Adjustment disorder: A diagnosis whose time has come. *J. Affect. Disord.* **2018**, *227*, 243–253. [CrossRef]
59. Van Overmeire, R. Comment on Dutheil, Mondillon, and Navel (2020): The importance of adjustment disorders and resilience. *Psychol. Med.* **2020**, *52*, 3741–3742. [CrossRef]
60. Chia, B.-H.; Chia, A.; Tai, B.-C. Suicide Letters in Singapore. *Arch. Suicide Res.* **2008**, *12*, 74–81. [CrossRef]
61. Kazan, D.; Calear, A.L.; Batterham, P.J. The impact of intimate partner relationships on suicidal thoughts and behaviours: A systematic review. *J. Affect. Disord.* **2016**, *190*, 585–598. [CrossRef]

62. Snyder, D.K.; Baucom, D.H.; Gordon, K.C. An Integrative Approach to Treating Infidelity. *Fam. J.* **2008**, *16*, 300–307. [CrossRef]
63. Stephens, B.J. Suicidal Women and Their Relationships with Husbands, Boyfriends, and Lovers. *Suicide Life-Threat. Behav.* **1985**, *15*, 77–90. [CrossRef]
64. Martin, J.S.; Ghahramanlou-Holloway, M.; Englert, D.R.; Bakalar, J.L.; Olsen, C.; Nademin, E.M.; Jobes, D.A.; Branlund, S. Marital Status, Life Stressor Precipitants, and Communications of Distress and Suicide Intent in a Sample of United States Air Force Suicide Decedents. *Arch. Suicide Res.* **2013**, *17*, 148–160. [CrossRef]
65. Selterman, D.; Garcia, J.R.; Tsapelas, I. What Do People Do, Say, and Feel When They Have Affairs? Associations between Extradyadic Infidelity Motives with Behavioral, Emotional, and Sexual Outcomes. *J. Sex Marital. Ther.* **2021**, *47*, 238–252. [CrossRef]
66. Garcia, J.R.; Gesselman, A.N.; Massey, S.G.; Seibold-Simpson, S.M.; Merriwether, A.M. Intimacy Through Casual Sex: Relational Context of Sexual Activity and Affectionate Behaviours. *J. Relatsh. Res.* **2018**, *9*, 1–10. [CrossRef]
67. Mark, K.P.; Herbenick, D. The influence of attraction to partner on heterosexual women's sexual and relationship satisfaction in long-term relationships. *Arch. Sex. Behav.* **2014**, *43*, 563–570. [CrossRef] [PubMed]
68. Fife, S.T.; Weeks, G.R.; Stellberg-Filbert, J. Facilitating forgiveness in the treatment of infidelity: An interpersonal model. *J. Fam. Ther.* **2011**, *35*, 343–367. [CrossRef]
69. Allen, E.S.; Atkins, D.C. The Association of Divorce and Extramarital Sex in a Representative U.S. Sample. *J. Fam. Issues* **2012**, *33*, 1477–1493. [CrossRef]
70. Amato, P.R.; Previti, D. People's reasons for divorcing: Gender, social class, the life course, and adjustment. *J. Fam. Issues* **2003**, *24*, 602–626. [CrossRef]
71. Daly, M.; Wilson, M. *Homicide: Foundations of Human Behavior*; Routledge: New York, NY, USA, 1989.
72. Buunk, B.P.; Dijkstra, P. Men, women, and infidelity: Sex differences in extradyadic sex and jealousy. In *The State of Affairs: Explorations in Infidelity and Commitment*; Duncombe, J., Harrison, K., Allan, G., Marsden, D., Eds.; Lawrence Erlbaum: Mahwah, NJ, USA, 2004; pp. 103–120.
73. Burdette, A.M.; Ellison, C.G.; Sherkat, D.E.; Gore, K.A. Are there religious variations in marital infidelity? *J. Fam. Issues* **2007**, *28*, 1553–1581. [CrossRef]
74. Atkins, D.C.; Baucom, D.H.; Jacobson, N.S. Understanding infidelity: Correlates in a national random sample. *J. Fam. Psychol.* **2001**, *15*, 735–749. [CrossRef]
75. DeWall, C.N.; Lambert, N.M.; Slotter, E.B.; Pond, R.S.; Deckman, T.; Finkel, E.J.; Luchies, L.B.; Fincham, F.D. So far away from one's partner, yet so close to romantic alternatives: Avoidant attachment, interest in alternatives, and infidelity. *J. Pers. Soc. Psychol.* **2011**, *101*, 1302–1316. [CrossRef]
76. Whisman, M.A.; Gordon, K.C.; Chatav, Y. Predicting sexual infidelity in a population-based sample of married individuals. *J. Fam. Psychol.* **2007**, *21*, 320–324. [CrossRef]
77. Whisman, M.A.; Snyder, D.K. Sexual infidelity in a national survey of American women: Differences in prevalence and correlates as a function of method of assessment. *J. Fam. Psychol.* **2007**, *21*, 147–154. [CrossRef]
78. Treas, J.; Giesen, D. Sexual Infidelity Among Married and Cohabiting Americans. *J. Marriage Fam.* **2000**, *62*, 48–60. [CrossRef]
79. Barta, W.D.; Kiene, S. Motivations for infidelity in heterosexual dating couples: The roles of gender, personality differences, and sociosexual orientation. *J. Soc. Pers. Relatsh.* **2005**, *22*, 339–360. [CrossRef]
80. Janssen, E.; Bancroft, J. The dual-control model: The role of sexual inhibition & excitation in sexual arousal and behavior. In *The Psychophysiology of Sex*; Janssen, E., Ed.; Indiana University Press: Bloomington, IN, USA, 2007; pp. 197–222.
81. Bancroft, J.; Graham, C.A.; Janssen, E.; Sanders, S.A. The Dual Control Model: Current Status and Future Directions. *J. Sex Res.* **2009**, *46*, 121–142. [CrossRef]
82. Mark, K.P.; Janssen, E.; Milhausen, R.R. Infidelity in heterosexual couples: Demographic, interpersonal, and personality-related predictors of extradyadic sex. *Arch. Sex. Behav.* **2011**, *40*, 971–982. [CrossRef]
83. Previti, D.; Amato, P.R. Is infidelity a cause or a consequence of poor marital quality? *J. Soc. Pers. Relatsh.* **2004**, *21*, 217–230. [CrossRef]
84. Brooks, T.J.; Monaco, K. Your cheatin' heart: Joint production, joint consumption and the likelihood of extramarital sex. *Appl. Econ. Lett.* **2013**, *20*, 272–275. [CrossRef]
85. Abzug, R. Extramarital affairs as occupational hazard: A structural, ethical (cultural) model of opportunity. *Sexualities* **2016**, *19*, 25–45. [CrossRef]
86. Hertlein, K.M.; Webster, M. Technology, relationships, and problems: A research synthesis. *J. Marital. Fam. Ther.* **2008**, *34*, 445–460. [CrossRef]
87. Dew, J.P.; Saxey, M.T.; Mettmann, A. Money lies and extramarital ties: Predicting separate and joint occurrences of financial deception and extramarital infidelity. *Front. Psychol.* **2022**, *13*, 1038169. [CrossRef]
88. Thibault, J.; Kelley, H.H. *The Social Psychology of Groups*; Wiley: New York, NY, USA, 1959.
89. Nye, F.I. Choice, exchange, and the family. In *Contemporary Theories about the Family*; Burr, W.R., Hill, R., Nye, F.I., Reiss, I.L., Eds.; The Free Press: Hong Kong, 1979; Volume 2, pp. 1–41.

90. Wilcox, B.; Dew, J.P.; VanDenBerghe, B. State of Our Unions 2019: iFidelity: Interactive Technology and Relationship Faithfulness. 2019. Available online: http://nationalmarriageproject.org/wp-content/uploads/2019/07/SOU2019.pdf (accessed on 22 January 2023).
91. Johnson, M.P.; Caughlin, J.P.; Huston, T.L. The tripartite nature of marital commitment: Personal, moral, and structural reasons to stay married. *J. Marriage Fam.* **1999**, *61*, 160. [CrossRef]
92. Jeanfreau, M.M.; Mong, M. Barriers to Marital Infidelity. *Marriage Fam. Rev.* **2019**, *55*, 23–37. [CrossRef]
93. Rodrigues, D.; Lopes, D.; Pereira, M. Sociosexuality, Commitment, Sexual Infidelity, and Perceptions of Infidelity: Data from the Second Love Web Site. *J. Sex Res.* **2017**, *54*, 241–253. [CrossRef]
94. Rose, A.H.; Anderson, S.R.; Miller, R.B.; Marks, L.D.; Hatch, T.G.; Card, N.A. A Dyadic Exploration of Marital Satisfaction as a Mediator between Religiosity and Depressive Symptoms. *Marriage Fam. Rev.* **2020**, *57*, 243–266. [CrossRef]
95. Saxey, M.T.; LeBaron-Black, A.B.; Dew, J.P.; Curran, M.A. Less Than Fully Honest: Financial Deception in Emerging Adult Romantic Relationships. *Emerg. Adulthood* **2022**, *10*, 1529–1542. [CrossRef]
96. Obar, J.A.; Wildman, S. Social media definition and the governance challenge: An introduction to the special issue. *Telecommun. Policy* **2015**, *39*, 745–750. [CrossRef]
97. Facebook. Facebook Q3 2019 Earnings. 2019. Available online: https://investor.fb.com/investor-events/event-details/2019/Facebook-Q3-2019-Earnings/default.aspx (accessed on 22 January 2023).
98. Adam, A. Perceptions of infidelity: A comparison of sexual, emotional, cyber-, and parasocial behaviors. *Interpersona Int. J. Pers. Relatsh.* **2019**, *13*, 237–252. [CrossRef]
99. Gordon, K.C.; Mitchell, E.A. Infidelity in the Time of COVID-19. *Fam. Process.* **2020**, *59*, 956–966. [CrossRef]
100. Shaw, A.M.M.; Rhoades, G.; Allen, E.S.; Stanley, S.M.; Markman, H.J. Predictors of Extradyadic Sexual Involvement in Unmarried Opposite-Sex Relationships. *J. Sex Res.* **2013**, *50*, 598–610. [CrossRef]
101. Warren, T. Microsoft's Skype Struggles Have Created a Zoom Movement. The Verge. 31 March 2020. Available online: https://www.theverge.com/2020/3/31/21200844/microsoft-skype-zoom-houseparty-coronavirus-pandemicusage-growth-competition (accessed on 22 January 2023).
102. Takahashi, D. Ashley Madison: Affairs in the Time of Coronavirus. Venture Beat. 28 March 2020. Available online: https://venturebeat.com/2020/03/28/ashley-madison-affairs-in-the-time-of-coronavirus/ (accessed on 22 January 2023).
103. Crouch, E.; Dickies, L. Economic repercussions of marital infidelity. *Int. J. Sociol. Soc. Policy* **2016**, *36*, 53–65. [CrossRef]
104. Abrahamson, I.; Hussain, R.; Khan, A.; Schofield, M.J. What Helps Couples Rebuild Their Relationship After Infidelity? *J. Fam. Issues* **2012**, *33*, 1494–1519. [CrossRef]
105. Parker, K.; Menasce Horowitz, J.; Brown, A. About Half of Lower-Income American Report Household, Job, or Wage Loss due to COVID-19. Pew Research Center: Social & Demographic Trends. 21 April 2020. Available online: https://www.pewsocialtrends.org/2020/04/21/about-half-of-lower-income-americans-report-householdjob-or-wage-loss-due-to-cov (accessed on 22 January 2023).
106. Weiner-Davis, M. Incubated Infidelity: Is Sheltering in Place with Your Spouse after an Affair a Blessing or Curse? Psychology Today. 4 May 2020. Available online: https://www.psychologytoday.com/us/blog/divorce-busting/202005/incubated-infidelity (accessed on 22 January 2023).
107. Scott, S.B.; Rhoades, G.K.; Stanley, S.M.; Allen, E.S.; Markman, H.J. Reasons for divorce and recollections of premarital intervention: Implications for improving relationship education. *Couple Fam. Psychol. Res. Pract.* **2013**, *2*, 131–145. [CrossRef] [PubMed]
108. Irvine, T.J.; Peluso, P.R. An affair to remember: A mixed-methods survey examining therapists' experiences treating infidelity. *Fam. J.* **2022**, *30*, 324–333. [CrossRef]
109. American Association for Marriage and Family Therapy. AAMFT Code of Ethics. 2015. Available online: https://www.aamft.org/Legal_Ethics/Code_of_Ethics.aspx (accessed on 22 January 2023).
110. American Psychological Association. Ethical Principles of Psychologists and Code of Conduct (2002, Amended Effective 1 June 2010, and 1 January 2017). 2017. Available online: https://www.apa.org/ethics/code/ (accessed on 22 January 2023).
111. Peluso, P.R. *A Family Systems Guide to Infidelity: Helping Couples Understand, Recover from, and Avoid Future Affairs*; Routledge: London, UK, 2019.
112. Garza, L. The Role of Gender and Attitudes toward Infidelity in Therapists' Treatment Decisions for Couples Presenting with Physical Infidelity. Ph.D. Thesis, Fielding Graduate University, Santa Barbara, CA, USA, 2020. ProQuest Dissertations & Theses Global (Publication no. 2385373582).
113. Smithey, A.R. Counselors' Emotional Reactions when Treating Couples Facing Infidelity: A Generic Qualitative Inquiry. Ph.D. Thesis, Capella University, Minneapolis, MN, USA, 2015. ProQuest Dissertations & Theses Global (Publication no. 1671736541).
114. Softas-Nall, B.; Beadle, M.; Newell, J.; Helm, H.M. Spousal Disclosure of Extramarital Relationships: Attitudes of Marriage and Family Therapists. *Fam. J.* **2008**, *16*, 328–337. [CrossRef]
115. Moreno, N.; Kahumoku-Fessler, E.P. Understanding Infidelity: How Perceptions of Infidelity Behaviors Vary by Sex and One's Own Infidelity Experiences. *Am. J. Fam. Ther.* **2018**, *46*, 107–121. [CrossRef]
116. Varga, C.M.; Gee, C.B.; Munro, G. The Effects of Sample Characteristics and Experience with Infidelity on Romantic Jealousy. *Sex Roles* **2011**, *65*, 854–866. [CrossRef]

117. Klaar, C.M. Straight Wives of HIV-Positive Husbands Who Contracted the Virus Through Male-to-Male Sexual Contact. *J. GLBT Fam. Stud.* **2012**, *8*, 99–120. [CrossRef]
118. Scuka, R.F. A Clinician's Guide to Helping Couples Heal from the Trauma of Infidelity. *J. Couple Relatsh. Ther.* **2015**, *14*, 141–168. [CrossRef]

International Journal of
Environmental Research and Public Health

MDPI

Article

The Double Burden of Isolation and Unemployment: Suicide Risk in Structurally Vulnerable Populations in Japan—A Case Study of Akita Prefecture (2018–2022)

Roseline Yong

Department of Community-Based Psychosomatic Health Care, Graduate School of Medicine, Akita University, Akita 010-8543, Japan; roselineyong@med.akita-u.ac.jp

Abstract

Suicide in Japan remains elevated and uneven across regions. We hypothesized that (H1) unemployment and (H2) living alone each increase suicide mortality, and that (H3) their combination yields more-than-additive risk, especially among middle-aged men. Using specially tabulated mortality data (2018–2022) from the Japan Suicide Countermeasures Promotion Center, we cross-classified deaths and denominators into 24 strata by sex, age (20–39, 40–59, ≥60), employment (employed/unemployed), and cohabitation (with others/alone). Five-year average rates per 100,000 were computed; between-group differences were tested with chi-square (Holm-adjusted contrasts). Additive interaction between unemployment and living alone was quantified with the Interaction Contrast (ICR) and Synergy Index (SI), and Akita rates were benchmarked against national strata. Prefecture-level quantification and national benchmarking are rarely reported in Japan. Rates differed significantly across employment-by-cohabitation groups in every sex-by-age stratum ($p < 0.001$). Unemployment and living alone each elevated risk, with the highest rate reported among unemployed men aged 40–59 who were living alone (317.1; >14× employed, cohabiting peers at 22.1). Additive interaction was strongest in men aged 40–59 (ICR = 198.3; SI = 3.05) and present in men aged 20–39 and ≥60; among women, interaction was most evident at the ages of 40–59 and sub-additive at ≥60. Compounded effects among men were consistently larger in Akita than nationally, whereas the largest absolute burden fell on unemployed men aged ≥60 who were living with others (203 deaths). The novelty of this investigation lies in quantifying additive interaction with national benchmarking and contrasting per capita risk with absolute burden to guide dual-track prevention. The findings are ecological.

Keywords: suicide rates; social isolation; unemployment; living alone; Akita; Japan; rural aging and depopulation; middle-aged men; suicide prevention policy

1. Introduction

Suicide remains a critical global public health concern, responsible for over 700,000 deaths each year, with many more non-fatal attempts [1]. Risk is particularly heightened among individuals facing social isolation and unemployment—conditions which are increasingly prevalent in aging, economically unstable, and socially fragmented societies [2,3].

Japan exemplifies this paradox. Despite its economic prosperity and universal healthcare system, the country continues to report suicide rates higher than most other Organization for Economic Co-operation and Development (OECD) nations. Although national figures have declined since the early 2000s, suicide remains a leading cause of death—especially among working-age men and older adults [4]. Beneath these national averages lie deep regional disparities, most notably in rural, depopulating areas where demographic aging, economic stagnation, and social fragmentation converge [5].

Akita Prefecture illustrates these structural vulnerabilities. In 2022, its suicide mortality rate stood at 23.7 per 100,000—well above the national average of 16.3 [4]. The region is marked by rapid demographic aging (with over 38% of residents aged 65 or older), sustained youth outmigration, and limited economic diversification [6]. These conditions contribute to widespread solitary living, poor access to mental health services, and restricted employment opportunities—particularly outside of agriculture and small-scale industry. Vulnerability is especially acute among older adults and non-regular workers, who often lack job stability, social protection, and community support [7,8].

Theoretically, unemployment and isolation are established, independent risk factors for suicide—linked to depressive symptoms, suicidal ideation, and diminished social connectedness [9,10]. Among working-age adults—particularly men—these stressors can erode identity, purpose, and integration in settings where masculine identity is strongly tied to stable employment and family roles [11,12].

Joiner's Interpersonal Theory of Suicide [13] offers a useful framework here, highlighting "thwarted belongingness" and perceived burdensomeness as central psychological mechanisms that may be activated when social roles are lost or unattainable. In Japan's labor market, over 36% of jobs are non-regular [14], and men in precarious roles show an elevated suicide risk [15]. At the extreme end, consistent social isolation and withdrawal (hikikomori) underscore how chronic withdrawal compounds isolation and risk [16]. Notably, mere participation in work or school does not guarantee emotional connection; individuals with limited social integration may suffer more distress than those who are formally excluded [17]. This underscores the gap between physical inclusion and perceived belonging. Relatedly, higher odds of depressive symptoms among men living alone or in multigenerational households versus spouse-only households was found, with neighborhood social cohesion buffering this risk [18].

Despite extensive research on the individual effects of social isolation and unemployment, their combined impact remains underexplored—particularly among structurally vulnerable populations such as unemployed, middle-aged men living alone. This intersection warrants closer examination.

To address this gap, the present study investigates suicide mortality in Akita Prefecture from 2018 to 2022, analyzing variations by sex, age, employment status, and cohabitation and benchmarking against national data. Specifically, we hypothesize that

H1. *Unemployment is associated with higher suicide mortality.*

H2. *Living alone is associated with higher suicide mortality.*

H3. *The combination of unemployment and living alone produces compounded risk, particularly among middle-aged men.*

By focusing on a demographically and economically marginalized region, this study aims to illuminate how overlapping vulnerabilities interact to elevate suicide risk—and how broader structural forces shape the lived experience of isolation.

2. Methods

2.1. Data Source and Scope

This study utilizes specially tabulated suicide mortality data obtained from the Japan Suicide Countermeasures Promotion Center (JSCP), published annually as the Regional Suicide Profile. These profiles are compiled for every prefecture, designated city, and municipality in Japan, and have been distributed since 2017 under the national directive outlined in the 2017 Cabinet-approved General Principles of Suicide Prevention Policy. The aim of the Regional Suicide Profile is to support municipalities in designing and evaluating localized suicide prevention strategies by providing granular data on suicide cases and regional context.

Although the profiles are not publicly disclosed online, they are made available to all local governments upon request and are compiled using officially verified vital statistics (death certificates), municipal registry information, and other administrative records.

The dataset used in this study covers suicide deaths occurring between 2018 and 2022 (Heisei 30 to Reiwa 4) in Akita Prefecture, one of Japan's most demographically vulnerable regions. For comparative benchmarking, corresponding national data were used from the same JSCP sources.

Importantly, the JSCP aggregates suicide data by demographic attributes and contextual variables, including the following:

- Sex.
- Age group.
- Employment status.
- Living arrangement (cohabitation status).
- History of suicide attempts (in some profiles).
- Means of suicide.
- Stress, mental health status, and household structure (when available from municipal data).

In small population groups, even one additional suicide case can cause a significant fluctuation in the suicide rate. To minimize year-to-year volatility and better identify structural patterns among different segments of the population, we calculated a five-year average suicide mortality rate. This five-year average was computed based on the total number of suicide deaths and the estimated population in each demographic group, using annual statistics from the Ministry of Internal Affairs and Communications' Population Estimates.

2.2. Variables and Demographic Stratification

The data were stratified across four variables, yielding a total of 24 demographic subgroups:

- Sex: Male/Female.
- Age Group: 20–39, 40–59, $\geq$60.
- Employment Status: Employed/Unemployed.
- Cohabitation Status: Living with others/Living alone.

Each suicide case was assigned to 1 of these 24 strata based on the deceased's official records. Employment status and living arrangement were determined from municipal and welfare registries or, in some cases, inferred from available records at the time of death registration.

In the JSCP registry, the term "Unemployed" referred to individuals who were not formally registered in paid employment at the time of their death. This classification may include long-term unemployed persons, those engaged in irregular or informal work, and individuals who are outside the labor force for reasons such as retirement, disability, or caregiving. While useful for population-level comparisons, this category is heterogenous and should be interpreted with caution.

2.3. Outcome Measure: Suicide Mortality Risk

The main outcome variable was the suicide mortality risk per 100,000 population for each demographic stratum. This was calculated using the following formula:

$$\text{Suicide mortality risk} = \frac{\text{Number of suicides in subgroup}}{\text{Population of subgroup}} \times 100,000 \quad (1)$$

Population denominators were taken from Akita Prefecture's own regional data and national-level comparative groups. National risk rates for each demographic stratum were used as benchmarks, allowing for localized risk amplification to be observed in Akita. To protect confidentiality and minimize disclosure risk in small cells—and to reduce year-to-year volatility in strata with small denominators—we report five-year average rates and do not present annual, stratum-specific rates.

Population denominators and five-year averaging were implemented. The denominators for each sex–age-employment–cohabitation stratum were annual mean population estimates produced by the JSCP using the Ministry of Internal Affairs and Communications' 2020 Census "employment status" basic tabulations. JSCP apportioned individuals with "unknown" labor-force status across employed and unemployed categories (i.e., employed: "work in addition to housework/study"; unemployed: "unemployed"; plus non-labor-force groups) before deriving annual means. As the outcome is a five-year average (2018–2022), the denominator used for rate calculation is the JSCP one-year mean multiplied by five. Thus,

$$\text{Five-year average rate} = \frac{\text{Deaths over } 2018 - 2022}{(\text{JSCP annual mean population}) \times 5} \times 100,000 \quad (2)$$

2.4. Analytical Approach

The analysis was descriptive and comparative in nature. In addition to descriptive comparisons, we conducted simple statistical tests to confirm observed differences. Chi-square tests were applied to compare suicide counts across selected demographic subgroups, and z-tests for two proportions were used to assess differences in suicide mortality rates between Akita and national benchmarks. While the ecological design of the data limits the application of multivariate modeling, these tests provide statistical confirmation of key disparities.

Patterns were also interpreted with reference to the epidemiological concept of causal interaction, meaning that the joint effect of unemployment and solitary living on suicide mortality was greater than the sum of their independent effects. To examine this more explicitly, we calculated two measures of additive interaction [19]:

The Interaction Contrast (ICR),

$$\text{ICR} = \text{R}_{11} - \text{R}_{10} - \text{R}_{01} + \text{R}_{00} \quad (3)$$

where R_{00} = employed + living with others (reference), R_{10} = employed + living alone, R_{01} = unemployed + living with others, and R_{11} = unemployed + living alone. Interpretation, ICR > 0 → positive interaction (the joint effect is greater than the sum of the individual parts), ICR = 0 → no interaction on the additive scale, and ICR < 0 → antagonism (the joint effect is less than expected).

And the Synergy Index (SI),

$$SI = \frac{R_{11} - R_{00}}{(R_{10} - R_{00}) + (R_{01} - R_{00})} \quad (4)$$

Interpretation: SI = 1 → no interaction (joint effect = sum of individual effects), SI > 1 → positive interaction (joint effect greater than expected), and SI < 1 → antagonist interaction (joint effect smaller than expected).

Both metrics require the full 2 × 2 cross-classification of employment status (employed vs. unemployed) and cohabitation (living with others vs. living alone), and thus draw on all four corresponding subgroups. For readability, ICR and SI are reported in the table row corresponding to the joint-exposure group (unemployed, living alone), but they are derived from rates across all four exposure categories.

Special attention was paid to the following:

- Identifying the highest-risk subgroups.
- Comparing Akita's suicide rates for each stratum with national equivalents.
- Observing gendered and age-specific patterns of compounded vulnerability.

All between-group comparisons and interaction metrics (ICR, SI) used the five-year average rates defined above. The proportions shown in the descriptive tables/figures represent the the total share of deaths within Akita or Japan for 2018–2022; because persons aged <20 years and those in the age-unknown categories are excluded from our 24 strata, the within-table percentages do not sum to 100%.

2.5. Ethical Considerations

All data used in this study were aggregated, publicly available, and devoid of personally identifiable information. As the analysis did not involve human subjects or intervention, ethical approval was not required under institutional or national guidelines.

3. Results

Suicide mortality in Akita Prefecture from 2018 to 2022 revealed sharp disparities across demographic lines, shaped by age, sex, employment status, and cohabitation patterns. Table 1 (men) and Table 2 (women) report the counts, denominators, rates, and interaction metrics.

Table 1. Suicide mortality in men by age, employment, and cohabitation, Akita Prefecture (2018–2022).

Age Group	Employment	Cohabitation	Deaths	Population	Rate (100,000 Population)	Notes (ICR/SI)
20–39	Employed	With others	61	54,378	22.4	Ref group
20–39	Employed	Alone	6	9822	12.2	↓ vs. ref
20–39	Unemployed	With others	36	8884	81.0 (***)	↑ vs. ref
20–39	Unemployed	Alone	12	2060	116.5 (***)	ICR = 45.7; SI = 1.94
40–59	Employed	With others	107	96,845	22.1	Ref group
40–59	Employed	Alone	37	12,492	59.2 (***)	↑ vs. ref
40–59	Unemployed	With others	34	8325	81.7 (***)	↑ vs. ref
40–59	Unemployed	Alone	28	1766	317.1 (***)	ICR = 198.3; SI = 3.05
≥60	Employed	With others	71	69,102	20.5	Ref group
≥60	Employed	Alone	15	8168	36.7	↑ vs. ref
≥60	Unemployed	With others	203	83,619	48.6 (***)	↑ vs. ref
≥60	Unemployed	Alone	82	14,501	113.1 (***)	ICR = 48.3; SI = 2.09

Note: "Ref group" = employed, living with others within the same age stratum. ↑ vs. ref = rate higher than the reference; ↓ vs. ref = rate lower than the reference. Asterisks indicate Holm-adjusted pairwise significance (*** $p < 0.001$); no asterisk = not significant. ICR = Interaction Contrast (per 100,000); SI = Synergy Index—reported for the joint-exposure row (unemployed, alone) and calculated from all four exposure cells.

Table 2. Suicide mortality in women by age, employment, and cohabitation, Akita Prefecture (2018–2022).

Age Group	Employment	Cohabitation	Deaths	Population	Rate (100,000 Population)	Notes (ICR/SI)
20–39	Employed	With others	12	46,735	5.1	Ref group
20–39	Employed	Alone	7	6657	21.0 (*)	↑ vs. ref
20–39	Unemployed	With others	14	16,125	17.4 (*)	↑ vs. ref
20–39	Unemployed	Alone	3	1735	34.6 (*)	ICR = 1.3; SI = 1.05
40–59	Employed	With others	22	77,721	5.7	Ref group
40–59	Employed	Alone	2	6912	5.8	≈ref
40–59	Unemployed	With others	26	33,596	15.5 (**)	↑ vs. ref
40–59	Unemployed	Alone	6	2654	45.2 (***)	ICR = 29.6; SI = 3.99
≥60	Employed	With others	5	32,588	3.1	Ref group
≥60	Employed	Alone	5	5162	19.4 (*)	↑ vs. ref
≥60	Unemployed	With others	152	151,209	20.1 (**)	↑ vs. ref
≥60	Unemployed	Alone	37	36,582	20.2 (**)	ICR = −16.2; SI = 0.51

Note: "Ref group" = employed, living with others within the same age stratum. ↑ vs. ref = rate higher than the reference. Asterisks indicate Holm-adjusted pairwise significance (* $p < 0.05$; ** $p < 0.01$; *** $p < 0.001$); no asterisk = not significant. ICR = Interaction Contrast (per 100,000); SI = Synergy Index—reported for the joint-exposure row (unemployed, alone) and calculated from all four exposure cells.

3.1. Statistical Confirmation

Chi-square tests confirmed that suicide rates differed significantly across employment cohabitation groups within every sex-by-age stratum (men 20–39: $\chi^2(3) = 73.23$, $p < 0.001$; men 40–59; $\chi^2(3) = 264.42$, $p < 0.001$; men $\geq$ 60: $\chi^2(3) = 128.98$, $p < 0.001$; women 20-39, $\chi^2(3) = 19.00$, $p < 0.001$; women 40–59; $\chi^2(3) = 31.42$, $p < 0.001$; women $\geq$ 60: $\chi^2(3) = 22.97$, $p < 0.001$). Pairwise Holm-adjusted comparisons showed that the unemployed-alone group consistently had significantly higher rates than the employed-with-others reference group in men of all ages ($p < 0.001$) and in middle-aged women ($p = 0.038$); see the significance markers in Tables 1 and 2.

3.2. Independent Effects of Unemployment and Living Alone

Men (Table 1): Holding cohabitation constant, unemployment was associated with markedly higher suicide rates across all age groups. Among men aged 40–59 who were living alone, the rate was 317.1 vs. 59.2 per 100,000 when unemployed versus employed—about a 5-fold increase (+257.9). Elevations were also large in men ≥60 living alone (113.1 vs. 36.7; almost 3-fold, +76.4) and men 30–39 living alone (116.5 vs. 12.2; almost 10-fold, +104.3). Unemployment among cohabiting men likewise raised risk, e.g., 40–59 (81.7 vs. 22.1; almost f-fold, +59.6) and 20–39 (81.0 vs. 22.4; almost 4-fold, +58.6). Significance markers appear in Table 1.

Considering living arrangement within employment strata, living alone further amplified risk. The contrast was greatest for unemployed men 40–59 (317.1 vs. 81.7; almost 4-fold, +235.4) and unemployed men ≥60 (113.1 vs. 48.6; almost 2-fold, +64.5). Among employed men, living alone was associated with higher rates in 40–59 (59.2 vs. 22.1; almost 3-fold, +37.1) and ≥60 (36.7 vs. 20.5; almost 2-fold, +16.2), while 20–39 showed no elevation (12.2 vs. 22.4).

Women (Table 2): Within the same cohabitation status, unemployment generally conferred higher risk, with especially pronounced differences among women aged 40–59 living alone (45.2 vs. 5.8; almost 8-fold, +39.4) and women aged ≥60 living with others

(20.1 vs. 3.1; almost 6-fold, +17.0). Elevations were also evident for women aged 20–39 who were living with others (17.4 vs. 5.1; almost 3-fold, +12.3) and women aged 20–39 living alone (34.6 vs. 21.0; almost 1.7-fold, +13.6). By contrast, among women aged ≥60 living alone, unemployment had little effect (20.2 vs. 19.4).

Examining living arrangements alongside employment strata revealed that living alone was associated with higher rates among employed women aged 20–39 (21.0 vs. 5.1; almost 4-fold, +15.9) and employed women aged ≥60 (19.4 vs. 3.1; almost 6-fold, +16.3). Among unemployed women aged 40–59, living alone also raised the suicide risk (45.2 vs. 15.5; almost 3-fold, +29.7). Differences were minimal for employed women 40–59 (5.8 vs. 5.7) and unemployed women ≥ 60 (20.2 vs. 20.1).

3.3. *Joint Effects of Unemployment and Isolation*

When unemployment and living alone co-occurred, a more-than-additive joint effect emerged, consistent with the epidemiological concept of causal interaction. Table 1 shows that among men aged 20–39, the ICR was 45.7 per 100,000 and SI = 1.94. The most dramatic synergy occurred among middle-aged men (40–59), with rates rising from 81.7 (unemployed, cohabiting) to 317.1 (unemployed, alone), yielding an ICR of 198.3 and SI = 3.05, indicating that the joint effect was more than three times greater than the sum of individual risks. Men aged ≥60 also showed significant synergy (ICR = 48.3; SI = 2.09).

Table 2 shows that among women, synergy was most pronounced in the 40–59 age group (ICR = 29.6; SI = 3.99), despite overall lower absolute rates. In contrast, younger women showed little evidence of interaction (ICR = 1.3; SI = 1.05), while older women exhibited sub-additivity (ICR = −16.2; SI = 0.51), suggesting that solitary living added little incremental risk for this group.

3.4. *Akita Versus National Comparisons*

To examine whether these compounded effects were unique to Akita or reflected broader national trends, interaction metrics were benchmarked against national suicide rates (Table 3). Synergy among men was consistently stronger in Akita than nationally. For instance, among middle-aged men (aged 40–59), the Akita ICR was 198.3 compared to 117.8 nationally, and the SI was 3.05 versus 2.18. This indicates that the compounding disadvantage of unemployment and isolation was markedly more severe in Akita.

Table 3. Interaction metrics (ICR and SI) for suicide mortality in Akita Prefecture versus national benchmarks, 2018–2022.

Sex	Age Group	Akita ICR	Akita SI	National ICR	National SI	Difference (ICR)	Ratio (SI)
Men	20–39	45.7	1.94	26.9	1.57	+18.8	1.24
Men	40–59	198.3	3.05	117.8	2.18	+80.5	1.40
Men	≥60	48.3	2.09	36.7	2.07	+11.6	1.01
Women	20–39	1.3	1.05	13.7	1.86	−12.4	0.56
Women	40–59	29.6	3.99	20.4	2.21	+9.2	1.81
Women	≥60	−16.2	0.51	5.4	1.58	−21.6	0.32

Positive ICR values indicate more-than-additive joint effects of unemployment and solitary living; negative values indicate sub-additivity. Ratios > 1 for SI reflect stronger compounded effects in Akita than nationally.

Among women, patterns were more heterogeneous. In the 40–59 age group, synergy was stronger in Akita (ICR = 29.6; SI = 3.99) than nationally (ICR = 20.4; SI = 2.21). In contrast, older women (≥60) showed sub-additivity in Akita (ICR = −16.2; SI = 0.51), whereas nationally, the interaction remained modestly positive (ICR = 5.4; SI = 1.58).

3.5. Burden Versus Risk

Tables 1 and 2 and Figure 1 (counts) show that the largest burden of suicides was recorded for unemployed men aged ≥60 who were living with others (n = 203 deaths over 2018–2022). In contrast, Figure 2 (rates per 100,000) and Table 1 highlight a small but high-risk subgroup: unemployed men aged 40–59 living alone (317.1 per 100,000), who had over fourteen times the reference rate for employed, cohabiting men of the same age (22.1 per 100,000). For women, the burden was concentrated among those aged ≥60 who were unemployed and living with others (n = 152; Table 2), whereas the highest risk appeared among unemployed women aged 40–59 living alone (45.2 per 100,000; Table 2). Together, these complementary views justify dual policy targets: (i) reduce total deaths where numbers are highest, and (ii) mount high-intensity outreach for small, hyper-vulnerable groups.

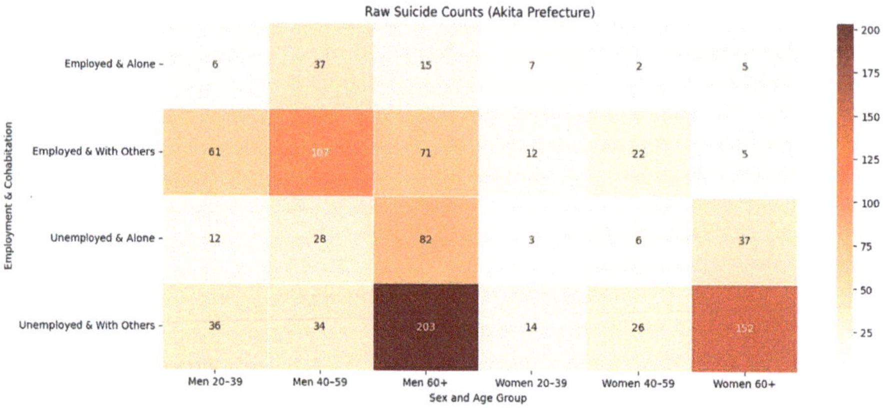

Figure 1. Heatmap of raw suicide counts by demographic group in Akita Prefecture, 2018–2022.

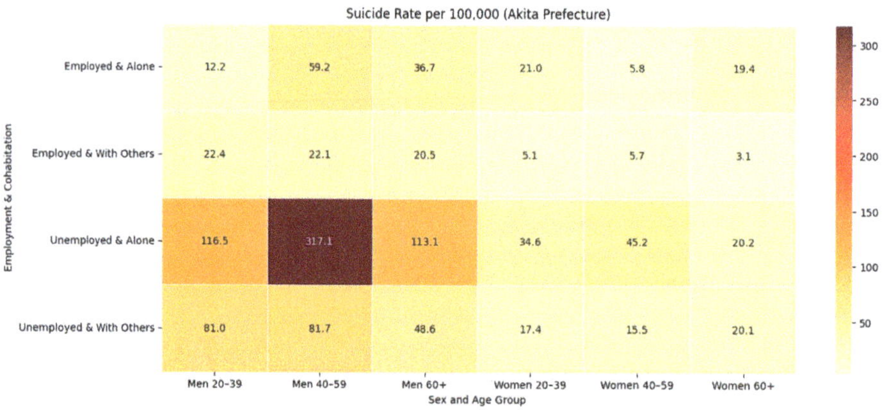

Figure 2. Heatmap of five-year suicide rate per 100,000 by demographic group in Akita Prefecture, 2018–2022.

4. Discussion

Taken together, these findings support H1, partially support H2 (with important sex- and age-specific exceptions), and strongly support H3, with the sharpest compounding among men. What is new here is that we (i) quantify how unemployment and solitary living combine on an additive scale (ICR, SI), (ii) show that this compounding is stronger in Akita than nationally, and (iii) separate high burden from high-risk groups to motivate a dual prevention strategy. These findings reveal stark social gradients in suicide mortality in Akita, shaped by structural precarity and social isolation. The highest relative risk was observed among unemployed, middle-aged men living alone, underscoring the compounding nature of economic exclusion and social living. This pattern reinforces earlier work in Japan linking unemployment to elevated suicide risk [15,16] and highlights how occupational instability continues to erode mental health in contexts where masculine identity is closely tied to employment and family roles.

Living alone also independently heightened risk, especially for men. This finding echoes broader evidence that solitary living can signify social detachment, diminished emotional integration, and limited access to informal care networks—particularly in aging rural communities [9,10]. For women, however, the association between cohabitation and suicide was less consistent. One plausible, but tentative, interpretation is that women may maintain stronger extra-household social ties or face different cultural expectations regarding disclosure and help-seeking [3]. Our ecological data cannot adjudicate mechanisms, and alternative explanations (e.g., reporting differences, cohort effects, health-selection process) should be considered.

Crucially, these structural risks did not operate additively, but interactively. The combination of unemployment and solitary living produced suicide rates far beyond either factor alone. This supports the epidemiological concept of causal interaction, quantified here with the ICR and SI [19]. Middle-aged men displayed especially strong synergy, with joint effects more than three times greater than expected from independent risks. Women aged 40–59 also showed evidence of compounded vulnerability, though older women exhibited sub-additivity, suggesting heterogeneous pathways across the life course.

These patterns align with Durkheim's typologies of anomic and egoistic suicide, where weakened social integration and disrupted norms elevate suicidality [20], and also with Joiner's Interpersonal Theory of Suicide, which emphasizes the role of thwarted belongingness, perceived burdensomeness, and acquired capability for suicide [13]. In the context of Akita, prolonged economic stagnation, demographic aging, and depopulation may collectively foster both social detachment and community-wide exposures to hardship, amplifying vulnerability through structural as well as psychological channels [5,7].

These patterns are also consistent with Japan's phenomenon of hikikomori—prolonged social withdrawal that can persist into midlife. Although our registry data cannot identify hikikomori directly, two features of the results align with this pathway: (i) extreme risk among unemployed, middle-aged men living alone and (ii) a weaker gradient by cohabitation in some strata. Many socially withdrawn adults do not live alone but remain secluded within the parental household; thus, "living with others" can still coincide with severe isolation. In Joiner's terms, long-term withdrawal may intensify thwarted belongingness and perceived burdensomeness, while unemployment erodes role identity; the elevated ICR and SI among middle-aged men in Akita are consistent with this mechanism [16].

The contrast between high-burden and high-risk groups is particularly instructive. Older, unemployed men living with others accounted for the largest number of suicide deaths, reflecting the cumulative burden of structural vulnerability. In contrast, middle-aged, unemployed men living alone faced the most extreme per capita risk, signaling acute concentration of vulnerability in a smaller subgroup. This duality indicates that prevention policy must simultaneously address the volume of suicide in large groups and the intensity of risk in smaller but hyper-vulnerable ones.

Compared with prior work that typically examines unemployment or living arrangement in isolation, this study quantifies their additive interaction at population level, benchmarks these interactions against national strata, and pairs rate-based risk with count-based burden to generate actionable, dual-track prevention guidance for structurally vulnerable regions.

When benchmarked nationally, Akita displayed consistently stronger interaction effects among men, particularly in midlife. This suggests that regional structural vulnerabilities—population aging, economic contraction, and outmigration—intensify the psychological costs of unemployment and isolation beyond national averages. Internationally, the compounded risks identified here echo patterns in other East Asian contexts, such as South Korea and Taiwan, where unemployment [21] and solitary living [22] have been linked to sharply elevated suicide rates. At the same time, evidence from European cohorts shows that strong neighborhood social capital can buffer the mental health harms of isolation [23], suggesting that community-level cohesion remains a critical protective factor across settings.

4.1. Strengths and Limitations

This study provides a rare ecological analysis quantifying the interaction effects of unemployment and solitary living on suicide mortality. The use of officially verified vital statistics across five years minimized random volatility and allowed for benchmarking against national data. However, several limitations must be acknowledged. First, its ecological design precludes individual-level causal inference, raising the risk of ecological fallacy. Second, the registry category of "unemployed" is heterogeneous, encompassing long-term unemployed, non-regular workers, and those outside the labor force for caregiving or health reasons. Third, cohabitation is an imperfect proxy for social isolation, which is fundamentally subjective and may persist even in multi-person households. This is particularly salient for people experiencing hikikomori, who may be classified as "living with others" despite marked isolation [16]. Fourth, unmeasured confounders such as mental health diagnoses, prior suicide attempts, or access to care were unavailable. Fifth, the exclusion of persons under 20 years limits generalizability to youth suicide patterns. Finally, the cross-sectional design treats 2018–2022 as a single snapshot, masking temporal dynamics—including the impact of the COVID-19 pandemic, which may have reshaped patterns of isolation and employment [4].

4.2. Policy and Prevention Implications

Our findings underscore the need for multilevel suicide prevention strategies that address both broad population burden and acute per capita risk, especially in structurally marginalized regions like Akita. The sharp contrast between groups with high suicide counts and those with extreme suicide rates reveals the necessity of dual-focus interventions: on the one hand, population-scale mental health infrastructure for high-burden groups, and on the other, precision-targeted support for acutely vulnerable subpopulations. Because the analysis is ecological, these patterns should guide place-based identification of communities and settings where individual-level screening and support are intensified, rather than stereotyping or universally targeting all persons within a demographic category.

Focused outreach should be targeted toward unemployed, middle-aged men living alone, who face suicide risks exceeding 300 per 100,000—indicating critical levels of structural and social disconnection. However, preventive action cannot stop at this group. Expanding community-based mental health services in rural and depopulating areas is essential, as in these areas, access to care is limited and stigma continues to deter help-seeking. At the same time, strengthening local social cohesion, such as neighborhood mutual aid, community centers, and intergenerational initiatives may buffer the risks of isolation—especially for solitary older adults.

Municipal outreach should include low-threshold, home-based psychosocial services for adults with hikikomori-like withdrawal, with family education, stepwise social re-engagement, and links to employment rehabilitation. These approaches directly address isolation that is not captured by living-alone status and align with the interaction patterns observed in Akita [11,15,16].

Economic interventions also remain critical. Employment reintegration programs that target non-regular and long-term unemployed workers—including skills retraining, job placement, and workplace-based social support—can help restore both material security and a sense of purpose. Complementary to these, early warning systems that draw on municipal and welfare registries could enable proactive engagement with individuals who have recently become unemployed, bereaved, or socially withdrawn, ensuring support reaches those at heightened risk before crises develop.

Finally, gender-sensitive approaches are necessary. Suicide pathways differ across men and women, shaped by varying social roles, caregiving responsibilities, and access to informal support networks. Interventions must therefore be flexible enough to recognize and respond to these gendered dynamics, rather than assuming uniform vulnerabilities.

To be effective, suicide prevention policy must move beyond the clinic and address the social, economic, and demographic structures that concentrate risk. Particularly in aging, economically declining prefectures, suicide cannot be separated from broader processes of disconnection, disenfranchisement, and demographic collapse. A structurally informed suicide prevention framework is therefore essential, and should align public health, labor policy, and community development to target both the volume and intensity of suicide risk.

4.3. Future Research

Further work should employ longitudinal and individual-level data to clarify causal pathways, including the sequencing of unemployment, isolation, and suicidality. Integrating measures of subjective isolation, social network quality, and neighborhood-level cohesion would allow more precise evaluation of protective and risk factors. Comparative research across regions and countries could also reveal how demographic, cultural, and policy contexts condition the interaction between structural precarity and suicide risk.

5. Conclusions

Consistent with our hypotheses, unemployment increased suicide mortality rate (H1), living alone increased mortality for many—but not for all—groups (H2), and a combination of the two produced the highest risks, particularly among middle-aged men (H3), in Akita Prefecture. In contrast, the largest absolute burden affected older unemployed men living with others, underscoring the need to distinguish per capita risk from case burden when prioritizing action. Effective prevention in aging, depopulating regions should be multi-sectoral—expanding timely access to care, strengthening social integration and employment stability, and coupling system-wide investments with intensive outreach to small, hyper-vulnerable groups at risk of being overlooked.

Funding: This research was funded by Akita University Research Support Program.

Institutional Review Board Statement: Not applicable. The study did not involve human participants or animal experiments. Field observations were non-invasive and conducted in compliance with all relevant local and national regulations; no capture, handling, or manipulation of organisms occurred.

Informed Consent Statement: Not applicable.

Data Availability Statement: The original data presented in the study are openly available in Zenodo at https://shorturl.at/9ekiT.

Acknowledgments: We gratefully acknowledge the Japan Suicide Countermeasures Promotion Center (JSCP) for providing the specially tabulated Regional Suicide Profile data (aggregated from the National Police Agency suicide statistics and related administrative records). We also thank the Akita Prefectural Government and municipal offices for their cooperation and assistance with contextual information. The interpretations and any errors are solely the authors' responsibility and do not necessarily reflect the views of JSCP or Akita Prefecture.

Conflicts of Interest: The author declares no conflicts of interest.

References

1. World Health Organization. Suicide Worldwide in 2021: Global Health Estimates. 2025. Available online: https://iris.who.int/bitstream/handle/10665/381495/9789240110069-eng.pdf?sequence=1 (accessed on 13 July 2025).
2. Näher, A.-F.; Rummel-Kluge, C.; Hegerl, U. Associations of suicide rates with socioeconomic status and social isolation: Findings from longitudinal register and census data. *Front. Psychiatry* **2020**, *10*, 898. [CrossRef] [PubMed]
3. Middleton, N.; Whitley, E.; Frankel, S.; Dorling, D.; Sterne, J.; Gunnell, D. Suicide risk in small areas in England and Wales, 1991–1993. *Soc. Psychiatry Psychiatr. Epidemiol.* **2004**, *39*, 45–52. [CrossRef] [PubMed]
4. Ministry of Health, Labour and Welfare. The 2024 White Paper on Suicide Countermeasures [Summary]. Available online: https://www.mhlw.go.jp/content/001464705.pdf (accessed on 11 September 2025).
5. Goto, H.; Kawachi, I.; Vandoros, S. The association between economic uncertainty and suicide in Japan by age, sex, employment status, and population density: An observational study. *Lancet Reg. Health West. Pac.* **2024**, *46*, 101069. [CrossRef] [PubMed]
6. Statistics Bureau of Japan. Current Population Estimates as of 1 October 2023. Available online: https://www.stat.go.jp/data/jinsui/2023np/index.html (accessed on 13 June 2025).
7. Inoue, Y.; Nakatani, H.; Ono, I.; Peng, X. Factors related to a sense of economic insecurity among older adults who participate in social activities. *PLoS ONE* **2024**, *19*, e0301280. [CrossRef]
8. Shimazaki, T.; Yamauchi, T.; Takenaka, K.; Suka, M. The link between involuntary non-regular employment and poor mental health: A cross-sectional study of Japanese workers. *Int. J. Psychol.* **2024**, *59*, 1–29. [CrossRef]
9. Luo, Z.; Wang, J.; Chen, X.; Cheng, D.; Zhou, Y. Assessment of the relationship between living alone and suicidal behaviors based on prospective studies: A systematic review and meta-analysis. *Front. Public Health* **2024**, *12*, 1444820. [CrossRef] [PubMed]
10. Niu, L.; Jia, C.; Ma, Z.; Wang, G.; Sun, B.; Zhang, D.; Zhou, L. Loneliness, hopelessness and suicide in later life: A case–control psychological autopsy study in rural China. *Epidemiol. Psychiatr. Sci.* **2020**, *29*, e119. [CrossRef] [PubMed]
11. Yong, R. Characteristics of and gender difference factors of hikikomori among the working-age population: A cross-sectional population study in rural Japan. *Nihon Koshu Eisei Zasshi* **2020**, *67*, 237–246. [PubMed]
12. Glei, D.A.; Lee, C.; Brown, C.L.; Weinstein, M. Are employment and social integration more strongly associated with deaths of despair than psychological or economic distress? *Soc. Sci. Med.* **2024**, *357*, 117197. [CrossRef] [PubMed]
13. Joiner, T. *Why People Die by Suicide*; Harvard University Press: Cambridge, MA, USA, 2005.
14. Statistics Bureau of Japan. Labour Force Survey (Basic Tabulation): 2024 Annual Average Results. Available online: https://www.stat.go.jp/data/roudou/sokuhou/nen/ft/index.html (accessed on 15 July 2025).
15. Kachi, Y.; Otsuka, T.; Kawada, T. Precarious employment and the risk of serious psychological distress: A population-based cohort study in Japan. *Scand. J. Work Environ. Health* **2014**, *40*, 465–472. [CrossRef] [PubMed]
16. Yong, R.; Nomura, K. Hikikomori is most associated with interpersonal relationships, followed by suicide risks: A secondary analysis of a national cross-sectional study. *Front. Psychiatry* **2019**, *10*, 247. [CrossRef] [PubMed]
17. Yong, R. Reevaluating hikikomori and challenging loneliness assumptions in Japan: A cross-sectional analysis of a nationwide internet sample. *Front. Psychiatry* **2024**, *15*, 1323846. [CrossRef] [PubMed]
18. Honjo, K.; Tani, Y.; Saito, M.; Sasaki, Y.; Kondo, K.; Kawachi, I.; Kondo, N. Living alone or with others and depressive symptoms, and effect modification by residential social cohesion among older adults in Japan: The JAGES longitudinal study. *J. Epidemiol.* **2018**, *28*, 315–322. [CrossRef] [PubMed]
19. Rothman, K.J. Causes. *Am. J. Epidemiol.* **1976**, *104*, 587–592. [CrossRef] [PubMed]

20. Durkheim, E. *Suicide: A Study in Sociology*, reprint ed.; Routledge: London, UK, 1897.
21. Chang, S.-S.; Gunnell, D.; Sterne, J.A.C.; Lu, T.-H.; Cheng, A.T.A. Was the economic crisis 1997–1998 responsible for rising suicide rates in East/Southeast Asia? A time-trend analysis for Japan, Hong Kong, South Korea, Taiwan, Singapore and Thailand. *Soc. Sci. Med.* **2009**, *68*, 1322–1331. [CrossRef] [PubMed]
22. Kim, J.; Lee, Y.S.; Lee, J. Living arrangements and suicidal ideation among Korean older adults. *Aging Ment. Health* **2016**, *20*, 1305–1313. [CrossRef] [PubMed]
23. Baranyi, G.; Sieber, S.; Cullati, S.; Pearce, J.R.; Dibben, C.J.L.; Courvoisier, D.S. The longitudinal associations of perceived neighborhood disorder and lack of social cohesion with depression among adults aged 50 years or older: An individual-participant-data meta-analysis from 16 high-income countries. *Am. J. Epidemiol.* **2020**, *189*, 343–353. [CrossRef] [PubMed]

International Journal of
Environmental Research and Public Health

MDPI

Article

Reducing Loneliness through the Power of Practicing Together: A Randomized Controlled Trial of Online Dyadic Socio-Emotional vs. Mindfulness-Based Training

Hannah Matthaeus [1,2], Malvika Godara [1,3], Sarita Silveira [1], Martin Hecht [4], Manuel Voelkle [2] and Tania Singer [1,*]

1 Social Neuroscience Lab, Max Planck Society, 10557 Berlin, Germany; hannah.matthaeus@social.mpg.de (H.M.); malvika.godara@social.mpg.de (M.G.)
2 Department of Psychology, Humboldt-Universität zu Berlin, 12489 Berlin, Germany; manuel.voelkle@hu-berlin.de
3 Institute of Medical Psychology, Charité—Universitätsmedizin Berlin, 10117 Berlin, Germany
4 Faculty of Humanities and Social Sciences, Helmut Schmidt University, 22043 Hamburg, Germany; martin.hecht@hsu-hh.de
* Correspondence: singer@social.mpg.de

Abstract: Loneliness has become a pressing topic, especially among young adults and during the COVID-19 pandemic. In a randomized controlled trial with 253 healthy adults, we evaluated the differential efficacy of two 10-week app-delivered mental training programs: one based on classic mindfulness and one on an innovative partner-based socio-emotional practice (Affect Dyad). We show that the partner-based training resulted in greater reductions in loneliness than the mindfulness-based training. This effect was shown on three measures of loneliness: general loneliness assessed with the 20-item UCLA Loneliness Scale, state loneliness queried over an 8-day ecological momentary assessment in participants' daily lives, and loneliness ratings required before and after daily practice. Our study provides evidence for the higher efficacy of a mental training approach based on a 12 min practice conducted with a partner in reducing loneliness and provides a novel, scalable online approach to reduce the increasing problem of loneliness in society.

Keywords: mental training; social connectedness; app-delivered intervention; randomized controlled trial; mental health

1. Introduction

Loneliness has been defined as the feeling of deficiencies in the frequency and quality of social contact [1]. Research has shown that subjectively experienced loneliness is relevant for predicting objective outcomes, such as increased mortality [2], cardiovascular diseases [3], and cognitive functioning [4]. Higher loneliness has also been linked to an increased risk of depression, anxiety, and suicidal ideation [5]. While research findings have been mixed regarding the relationship between age and loneliness [6–8], recent studies have consistently noted a trend toward increased loneliness among young adults [9,10], with younger individuals often reporting the highest levels of loneliness [11,12]. This rising trend in loneliness, also referred to as a loneliness epidemic [13], has been amplified in recent years by the COVID-19 pandemic [14]. In Germany, loneliness increased during the first lockdown, particularly affecting young adults [15,16]. These alarming developments call for effective measures and intervention programs to mitigate loneliness on a large scale, with a focus on digital approaches that are scalable and easily accessible, even in times and under conditions that require staying at home.

Several approaches for the reduction of loneliness have been developed to address the growing issue of loneliness, with meditation, mindfulness, and social cognitive training rated as particularly promising solutions [17]. The field of contemplative science has gained prominence in recent years for improving mental health and well-being [18,19] as well as social connectedness [20]. Previous research has shown that classic 8-week mindfulness programs such as mindfulness-based stress reduction (MBSR) [21] and more compassion-based approaches can reduce loneliness [22]. While a review from Veronese et al. (2021) [17] reports successful loneliness reduction through mindfulness, a closer look at the studies referenced reveals that most interventions were conducted in person. These in-person trainings typically involved weekly sessions led by a teacher [23]. However, research on training based on online applications is limited. One study, which utilized a two-week smartphone-based training program focusing on daily attention and acceptance practices, reported reductions in state loneliness as assessed with ecological momentary assessment (EMA) but not in trait measures of loneliness [24]. There remains a lack of research on the efficacy of low-dose mindfulness or compassion-based mental training delivered online and via mobile apps, despite evidence suggesting that digital interventions can be beneficial for combating loneliness, specifically among non-elderly adults [25].

In addition to the specific content and skills a practice focuses on, mental training programs also differ in the modality in which they are practiced. Although most contemplative practices are performed alone due to their origin in classic meditation, there is a growing interest in intersubjective, dyadic approaches such as inquiry methods [26] or other intersubjective practice formats [27]. In the ReSource project [28], new contemplative partner-based practices called Contemplative Dyads were introduced. They involve a structured dialogue where two randomly assigned partners take turns answering and exploring specific questions while the other partner is empathically listening without interrupting. These interactions were found to increase social connectedness and social disclosure over a 3-month period of practice [20]. Research has shown that social connectedness can act as a buffer against loneliness [29] and can be increased through both intrapersonal interventions based on compassion [30] and socio-emotional partner-based dyadic training [20]. This suggests that the novel types of daily Dyads, which emphasize social connections with a partner, may serve as an auspicious approach to reducing subjective loneliness. However, in the ReSource project, which was an extensive in-person large-scale study that included 3-day in-person retreats and weekly in-person sessions with teachers, both types of Dyads (Affect Dyad and Perspective Dyad), introduced as core practices, were always combined with more classic meditation practices [28]. Studies have yet to explore the isolated effects of socio-emotional dyadic practice (Affect Dyad) on reducing loneliness and enhancing social connectedness, especially its differential efficacy in comparison to classic mindfulness practices and in app-delivered formats.

To address these gaps, we compared the efficacy of a purely online partner-based socio-emotional training (Affect Dyad) with classic mindfulness training performed over 10 weeks with weekly online sessions with teachers and daily 12 min practice in reducing loneliness using a multi-method approach. To assess different aspects of loneliness, we employed (1) a validated trait scale, the UCLA Loneliness Scale [31], (2) an 8-day EMA of loneliness dynamics assessed in participants' daily lives, and (3) a daily state measure of perceived loneliness assessed directly before and after each daily practice session over the 10 weeks of training.

Given the social nature of the novel partner-based practice, we expected the dyadic training to be more effective in increasing social connectedness and reducing loneliness than a comparable mindfulness practice performed alone. This expectation stems from the fact that the dyadic practice involves more self-disclosure, which is known to be associated with decreasing loneliness [32]. Additionally, we aimed to explore potential factors that could drive changes in loneliness in the two different interventions. Previous studies have identified common humanity [33], social contacts [24], social support [34], a sense of belonging [35], and a low fear of compassion [36] as mediators of loneliness. However, these factors have not been directly compared in the context of different contemplative practices and were therefore assessed in this study.

2. Materials and Methods

The data reported in this study were gathered as part of the CovSocial project, a longitudinal mental-health study initiated during the early weeks of the first lockdown in Germany due to the COVID-19 pandemic (for the study protocol, see [37]). The main objectives of the project were to investigate changes in psychological vulnerability, resilience, and social cohesion resulting from a crisis such as the COVID-19 pandemic (phase 1) and to examine the differential effects of online mental training programs in a randomized controlled trial (RCT; phase 2; Trial Registration: ClinicalTrials.gov NCT04889508 on 17 May 2020).

2.1. Sample

The CovSocial project's phase 2 recruited participants from a community sample in Berlin, initially selected from phase 1 participants (Figure 1). Various recruitment methods, including registration office sampling and social media advertising, led to 7214 registrations, with 3522 completing the phase 1 questionnaires. These 3522 individuals were invited to a pre-screening for phase 2, in which eligibility based on specific criteria was assessed. Phase 1 inclusion criteria comprised age (18–65), Berlin residency, and German proficiency. Participants were excluded from phase 2 if they lacked internet access or necessary technical equipment, had a background in psychology, engaged in regular spiritual practices, took specific medications, participated in stress reduction programs, suffered from chronic illness or pain, had a psychiatric history, or exceeded cutoff scores on questionnaires assessing alexithymia [38], depression [39], and anxiety [40], including an item for suicidality. Eligible participants were randomly assigned to three groups, initially oversampling for ideal group sizes. Detailed information about the recruitment process, study design, and interventions can be found in Supplementary Material S1 and the study protocol [37].

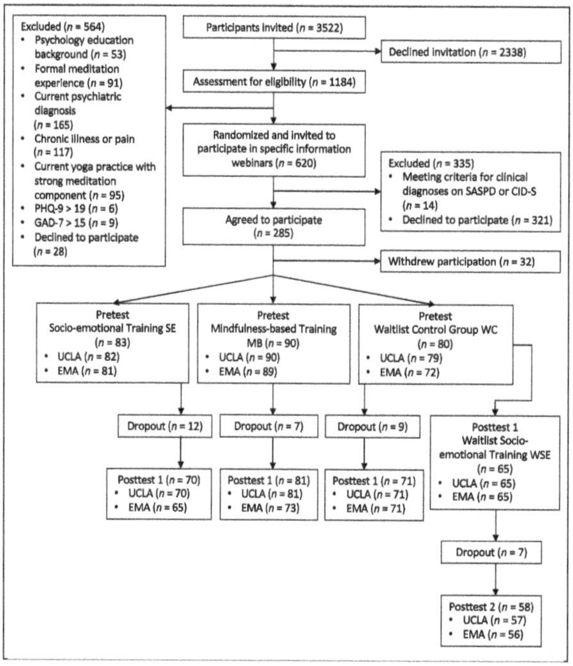

Figure 1. CONSORT flow diagram. EMA = ecological momentary assessment; UCLA = University of California Loneliness Scale; SASPD = standardized assessment of severity of personality disorder; CID-S = composite international diagnostic screener; GAD-7 = Generalized Anxiety Disorder-7; PHQ-9 = Patient Health Questionnaire-9.

A total of 253 participants (age: M = 44.36, SD = 11.48; 75.5% female) participated in the pretest of phase 2. After 10 weeks of treatment in the two intervention groups, we assessed measures in posttest 1 from 70 participants of the socio-emotional training (SE), 81 of the mindfulness-based training (MB), and 71 of the Waitlist Control Group (WC). In addition, 65 participants in WC continued after posttest 1, undergoing socio-emotional training in a second intervention phase as well as assessments at posttest 2 (WSE). Figure 2 depicts the study design, including the measurements relevant to the reported analyses.

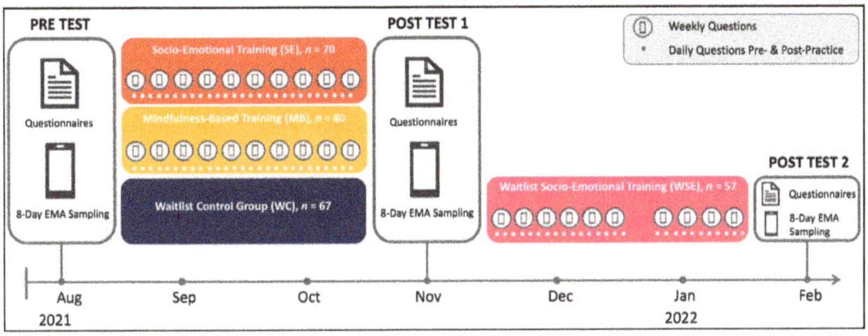

Figure 2. Study design of the CovSocial project phase 2, including study measures for loneliness assessment.

This study was preregistered at the Open Science Framework (https://osf.io/3nsjc, accessed on 23 April 2024; see Supplementary Material S3) and is in accordance with the Declaration of Helsinki. Ethical approval was received by the institutional review board of Charité—Universitätsmedizin Berlin (#EA4/081/21). All participants provided written informed consent and were reimbursed for their time spent on testing at the rate of EUR 10 per hour. Table 1 displays sample descriptives for this study.

Table 1. Characteristics of Participants at Pretest Split by Intervention Group (n = 253).

	Socio-Emotional Training (n = 83)	Mindfulness-Based Training (n = 90)	Waitlist Control Training (n = 80)
Age in years, mean ± SD	43.14 ± 11.80	44.14 ± 11.44	45.86 ± 11.15
Females, n (%)	65 (78.3%)	64 (71.1%)	62 (77.5%)
Married or cohabiting, n (%)	27 (32.5%)	32 (35.6%)	32 (40%)
Background of migration to current country of residence, n (%)	4 (4.8%)	10 (11.1%)	3 (3.8%)
Years of education, mean ± SD	18.49 ± 3.97	17.06 ± 3.52	18.41 ± 3.20
Employed full-time, n (%)	42 (50.6%)	57 (63.3%)	46 (57.5%)
Income > Berlin average monthly net (EUR 2175) [a], n (%)	52 (62.7%)	61 (67.8%)	56 (70.0%)
Lifetime prevalence of mental disorder, n (%)	17 (20.5%)	16 (17.8%)	18 (22.5%)

Note: [a] Amt für Statistik, Berlin-Brandenburg, 2019; https://www.statistik-berlin-brandenburg.de/publikationen (accessed on 23 April 2024).

2.2. Procedure

All participants in SE, MB, and WSE underwent a 10-week training program with a 12 min daily app-based practice six times per week and a weekly 2 h online coaching session in smaller groups of 15 to 20 participants, supported by four expert mindfulness and Dyad teachers randomly assigned to these subgroups. The training differed between MB and SE/WSE.

In MB, the CovSocial app provided guided meditation recordings on breathing, listening, and open awareness (see presence module [28]).

In SE and WSE, the participants engaged in mental training through contemplative Dyads, which are structured meditations performed with a partner [20]. During this training, they were paired with a randomly assigned partner from their group, with the partners changing after each weekly coaching session. During each practice, one partner began the session by talking for 2.5 min about a situation from the last 24 h in which they experienced a difficult emotion and how they felt this emotion in their body, followed by talking for 2.5 min about a gratitude-eliciting situation and related bodily experiences. The listener was instructed to remain silent and listen empathically without judgment, both externally and internally, while resonating with the feelings of the other person. After those 5 minutes, the roles of speaker and listener switched, and the partner that was listening in the first half of the practice got to share their respective difficult and grateful situations with the related bodily sensations. Before and after each practice, participants of all groups answered questions about their subjective state at that moment. A detailed description of the intervention protocol, including the onboarding procedure and training, can be found in Supplementary Material S1.

2.3. Measures

This study presents data on loneliness and social connectedness, as well as compliance and motivation for the two types of mental training programs offered in the CovSocial phase 2 study. The number of completed practices measured compliance during the intervention period and during the voluntary continuation of practice for 10 weeks after each posttest. Motivation was assessed before each practice using a rating scale from 0 ("not at all") to 4 ("very much").

The primary outcome of loneliness was evaluated at pretest, posttest 1, and posttest 2 using two different methods. The first was a validated psychometric questionnaire, the 20-item UCLA Loneliness Scale (UCLA-20; score range, 1–5; [31,41]), with a higher score indicating greater loneliness. The second method was an 8-day ecological momentary assessment (EMA), in which participants were asked to rate their level of loneliness on a scale of 0–8 when receiving push notifications on their mobile devices every three hours from the time of awakening until 9 pm. Additionally, loneliness was assessed daily with a self-generated item (rating scale 0–8; "How lonely do you feel right now?"), immediately before and after each daily practice during the 10-week intervention program. Social closeness with the respective Dyad partner was measured only in Dyad groups (SE, WSE) using the Inclusion of Other Scale (IOS; [42]). Further, the extent of personal self-disclosure during each Dyad was assessed on a rating scale from 0 ("not at all") to 4 ("very personal").

In addition, variables that might be considered mediating factors of change in loneliness were assessed once a week during the two intervention periods in a pseudorandomized design. Using one item each, these measures included common humanity (State Self-Compassion Scale (SSCS) [43]; "I reminded myself that there are many other people in the world who feel as I do"), frequency and valence of social contacts (self-generated, "How often did you have social contact during the past week?" and "On average, how pleasant were these social contacts?"), social support (Brief-COPE [44]; "I have sought help and support from others"), belonging to friends and the world (Inclusion of Other in the Self Scale [42]; "Draw the circles to best represent your affiliation with the following group: Me and Friends, Me and World Population"), and fear of compassion (FoC [45]; "I do not want to be compassionate with myself because it might make me soft and easy to take advantage of", "I do not want to be compassionate with myself because I do not want to become dependent on it").

2.4. Statistical Analyses

Descriptive statistics for UCLA and EMA ratings and the internal consistency of UCLA are reported in Supplementary Tables S1 and S2. Power analyses were conducted using G*Power [46] for analysis of variance with repeated measurements and interactions between group and within-group variables using elements: $\alpha = 0.05$, power $(1 - \beta) = 0.80$, 3 groups, 2 measurement occasions, $f = 0.10$, and $r = 0.39$ for repeated measurements (see Supplementary Material S2 for further details). All outcome variables were standardized by their overall standard deviation (pooled across time points and groups) to ensure comparability across the different measurement time points and groups. Participants' sex and age were included as covariates in all models. Analyses of change in primary outcomes used linear mixed-effects models with fixed effects for the intervention group and time (pretest, posttest 1, posttest 2), an interaction between group and time, and individual-level random intercepts. The WC group was used as the reference group, with backward difference coding for the time factor. Planned contrasts considered the effect of treatment in SE, MB, and WSE as contrasted against the WC group. We report standardized estimates and *p*-values. Model estimates of planned contrasts reflect effect size estimates classified as small ($\geq$0.20), medium ($\geq$0.50), or large ($\geq$0.80). Data are analyzed using the intention-to-treat approach, ensuring that all participants who provided data for at least the pretest timepoint are included in the analysis for each outcome.

Changes in daily measured variables before and after daily practice in SE and MB were analyzed using linear mixed-effects models with fixed effects for group, day, and measurement occasion (dummy coded variable for whether the measurement occasion was before or after the practice; reference group: pre-practice scores) as well as their two- and three-way interactions, individual-level random intercepts, and correlated random slopes for time and measurement occasion with SE as the reference group. A second model included WSE with fixed effects for time, measurement occasion, and their interaction, as well as individual-level random intercepts and correlated random slopes. For variables assessed either before (i.e., motivation) or after (i.e., self-disclosure) daily practice, models included fixed effects for group, day, their interaction, and individual-level random intercepts and slopes.

Planned contrasts included change over time (day and measurement occasion) for each group separately (SE, MB, and WSE) and for differential effects between SE and MB. Preregistered hypotheses were tested one-sidedly. Outcome analyses were conducted using the lme4 [47] and multcomp packages [48] in R (version 4.0.2; [49]). Change slopes of weekly assessed mediator variables were extracted in the form of estimated fixed effects of time from linear mixed-effects models that included random intercepts and slopes. Mediation models were conducted using the lavaan package [50], with the pre-to-posttest change in each outcome variable defined as the dependent variable, group as an independent variable, and extracted slopes as mediators of change. Since mediator variables were not assessed in WC, the mediation models used a dummy-coded group variable with MB defined as the reference group. An effect was deemed significant if zero was not included in the 95% confidence interval. Bootstrap confidence intervals will be reported using 5000 bootstrap iterations in each model.

3. Results

3.1. Engagement

Compliance to practice (Figure 3) showed no significant change over time in SE ($\beta_{SE} = -0.02, p = 1$) but decreased significantly in MB ($\beta_{MB} = -0.10, p < 0.001$), with a significant difference in change over time between the groups ($\beta_{diff} = -0.08, p = 0.001$). Baseline levels at week 1 showed no significant difference between SE and MB ($\beta_{diff} = 0.15$, $p = 1$). In WSE, compliance showed no significant change over time ($\beta_{WSE} = -0.01, p = 0.435$).

Voluntary continuation of practice (Figure 3) for a further 10 weeks after the posttest showed no significant change over time in SE ($\beta_{SE} = -0.02$, $p = 0.889$). In MB, the decrease was significant ($\beta_{MB} = -0.08$, $p < 0.001$), with a significant difference between groups ($\beta_{diff} = -0.06, p = 0.027$). A significant difference in baseline levels at week 1 reflected a significantly higher continuation attendance in SE compared to MB ($\beta_{diff} = -0.82$, $p < 0.001$). In WSE, continuation compliance significantly decreased over time ($\beta_{WSE} = -0.11, p < 0.001$).

No significant change in motivation (Figure 3) was found over time in SE ($\beta_{SE} = -0.01$, $p = 1$), MB ($\beta_{MB} = -0.05$, $p = 0.055$), or WSE over time ($\beta_{WSE} = 0.00$,

p = 0.985), and motivation did not differ between SE and MB in week 1 (β_{diff} = −0.13, p = 0.747).

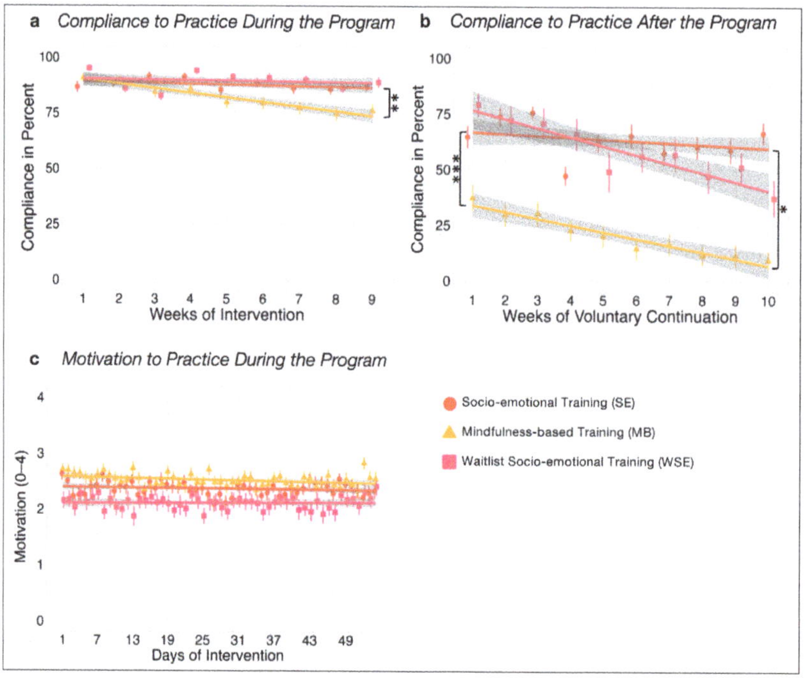

Figure 3. Time courses with group mean and standard errors of (**a**) compliance of training during the intervention period, (**b**) compliance of voluntary continuation for another 10 weeks of training after the posttest with the study app, and (**c**) self-rated motivation of training during the intervention period. Bonferroni corrected significance level of * α = 0.05, ** α = 0.01, and *** α = 0.001.

3.2. Primary Outcome

A significant decrease in UCLA-20 scores (Figure 4) was observed for SE compared to WC (β_{SE} = −0.23, p = 0.035) but not to MB (β_{diff} = −0.13, p = 0.343), indicating a small effect size for the reduction in loneliness within the SE group. MB vs. WC (β_{MB} = −0.10, p = 0.551), as well as WSE vs. WC (β_{WSE} = −0.12, p = 0.619), showed no significant change.

Loneliness ratings measured with an EMA design (Figure 4) showed a significant training-related reduction for SE compared to WC (β_{SE} = −0.19, p < 0.001) and MB (β_{diff} = −0.13, p < 0.001), with small effect sizes observed for both comparisons. No significant change was found for MB compared to WC (β_{MB} = −0.07, p = 0.123) and WSE compared to WC (β_{WSE} = −0.10, p = 0.055).

A significantly greater decrease in change in loneliness from before to after each daily practice (Figure 4), i.e., a direct practice effect, was observed for SE (β_{SE} = −0.15, p < 0.001) and MB (β_{MB} = −0.08, p < 0.001), indicating small effect sizes for both groups. Differences between groups were not significant (β_{diff} = 0.07, p = 0.055), with a trend indicating a possibly greater direct decrease in loneliness for SE. No change over time was found for daily pre-practice loneliness in SE (β_{SE} = −0.00, p = 1) or MB (β_{MB} = −0.03, p = 0.414). WSE showed a significant decrease over time (β_{WSE} = −0.05, p = 0.035) and a significant direct practice effect (β_{WSE} = −0.15, p < 0.001), with small effect sizes observed for both findings.

Social closeness ratings showed a significant increase after each practice compared to before in both socio-emotional training groups, SE (β_{SE} = 0.48, p < 0.001) and WSE (β_{WSE} = 0.47, p < 0.001; Figure 5). No significant change over time (Figure 5) was observed in SE (β_{SE} = −0.01, p = 0.651) or WSE (β_{WSE} = −0.00, p = 0.854). Ratings of self-disclosure after each practice showed no change over time in either socio-emotional training groups (Figure 5), SE ($\beta_{SE} = -0.01$, $p = 0.603$), or WSE ($\beta_{WSE} = -0.02$, $p = 0.695$).

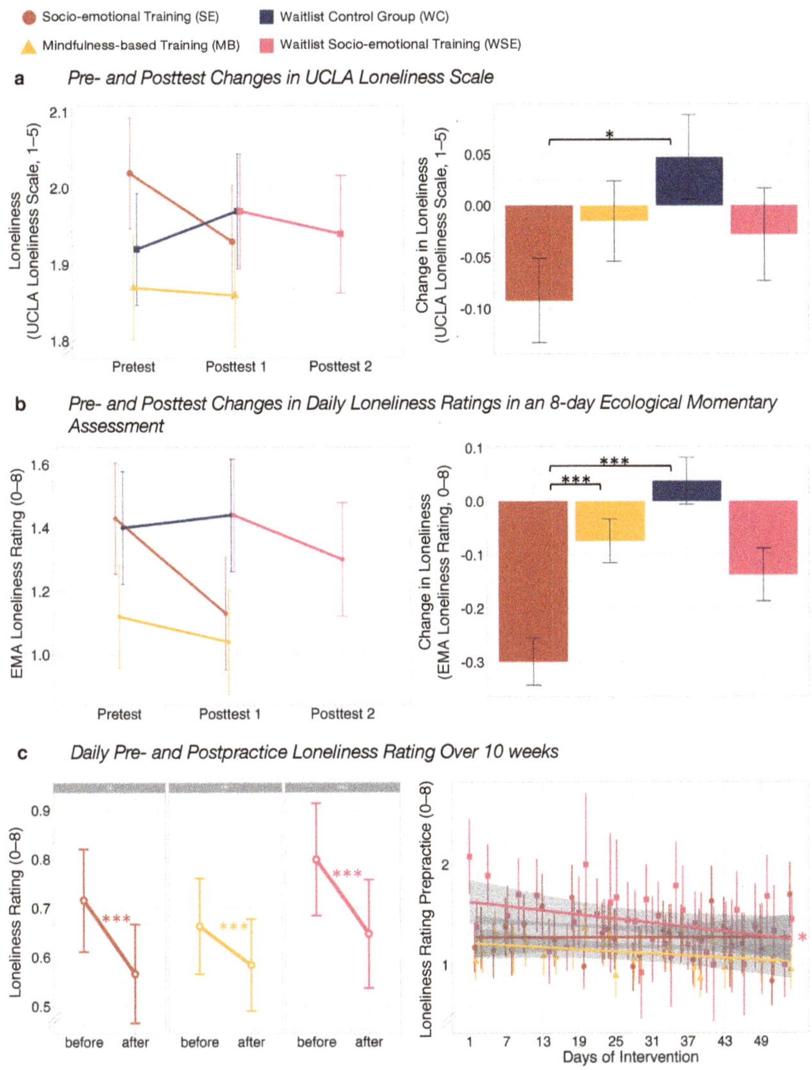

Figure 4. Group differences at pretest, posttest 1 and posttest 2, and of pre- to posttest changes using unstandardized estimates of the linear mixed model of (**a**) UCLA-20 and (**b**) ecological momentary assessment (EMA). Group differences in (**c**) mean daily pre- to post-practice changes in loneliness ratings and trajectories over 10 weeks of training in daily pre-practice loneliness ratings. Difference Scores are extracted from linear mixed models with sex and age as covariates. Data are presented as means and standard errors. Bonferroni corrected significance level of * $\alpha = 0.05$ and *** $\alpha = 0.001$.

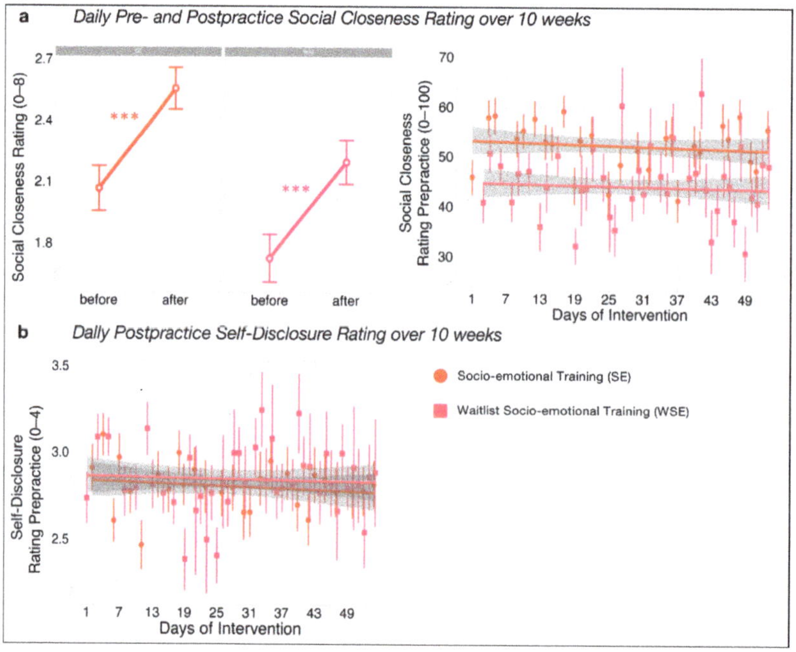

Figure 5. Group differences in (**a**) mean daily pre- to post-practice changes in social closeness ratings and trajectories over 10 weeks of training in daily pre-practice social closeness ratings. Group differences in trajectories over 10 weeks of training in daily post-practice self-disclosure ratings (**b**). Difference Scores are extracted from linear mixed models with sex and age as covariates. Data are presented as means and standard errors. Bonferroni corrected significance level of *** $\alpha = 0.001$.

3.3. Potential Mediator Factors of Change

Potential mediators of change in loneliness were assessed by change over the intervention in weekly measured variables of common humanity, frequency and valence of social contacts, social support, sense of belonging to friends and the world, and fear of compassion. Fear of compassion ($\beta = -0.07$, $p < 0.001$) and sense of belonging to friends ($\beta = -0.92$, $p = 0.008$) decreased significantly over time in all groups (SE, MB, and WSE). No significant change was found for common humanity ($\beta = 0.00$, $p = 0.919$), frequency of social contacts ($\beta = -0.03$, $p = 0.177$), valence of social contacts ($\beta = 0.03$, $p = 0.340$), social support ($\beta = -0.01$, $p = 0.682$), and sense of belonging to the world ($\beta = -0.50$, $p = 0.190$).

Mediation analyses did not reveal any indirect significant effects of the intervention group on changes in primary outcomes via changes in common humanity, frequency and valence of social contacts, social support, sense of belonging to friends and the world, and fear of compassion (see Tables S3 and S4 in the Supplementary Materials). No mediation effects were found for changes in UCLA-20 and loneliness ratings of EMA from pretest to posttest 1 in SE and MB and from posttest 1 to posttest 2 for WSE.

4. Discussion

The present RCT aimed at investigating the differential efficacy of two 10-week app-delivered mental training—a classic mindfulness-based intervention and a novel partner-based socio-emotional training (Affect Dyad), both involving 12 min daily practice—on different outcomes of loneliness and social connectedness.

First, we compared motivation, compliance, and voluntary continuation between the two types of mental training. Participants in the dyadic socio-emotional training groups (SE and WSE) showed higher compliance and voluntary continuation after the official training program compared to the mindfulness-based intervention (MB), despite both intervention groups reporting similar levels of motivation to perform the daily practice. The higher compliance levels observed in the socio-emotional training, requiring daily scheduled joint sessions throughout both the 10-week main program and the 10-week voluntary continuation period, may be due to the inherent accountability fostered by their shared commitments. In contrast to solitary practices, where skipping a session is easier, the social expectation inherent in dyadic training fosters a sense of obligation, hence translating individual motivation into tangible behavioral outcomes. This adherence to social norms likely contributes to increased attendance and engagement sustainability with daily mental training sessions, speaking for the sustainability of this novel dyadic format.

Second, we aimed to investigate the differential efficacy of the two online interventions on different markers of subjective loneliness. We found evidence that both groups of socio-emotional dyadic training (SE and WSE) led to greater reductions in dynamic state loneliness (EMA) compared to the mindfulness training group and waitlist control group. Similarly, we also observed greater reductions in general trait-level loneliness (UCLA) for the Affect Dyad training group as compared to the control group. However, this effect could only be observed in the SE group and not in the WSE group. Concerning daily ratings of loneliness immediately before and after practice, we found, on average, a decrease in loneliness in all three intervention groups. However, we could clearly observe a trend towards higher loneliness reduction in both Dyad groups as compared to the mindfulness group. Loneliness ratings before daily practice did not change over the 10-week intervention period for SE and MB but significantly decreased in WSE.

The reduction of loneliness after daily practice in both groups is in line with previous studies showing mindfulness- or compassion-based practices, typically performed alone, to be effective in reducing loneliness [17]. Thus, for example, a previous study on daily online meditation practice focusing on mentalizing and attention has demonstrated effectiveness in reducing state loneliness. Importantly, however, we extend these findings by showing, as predicted, that a novel partner-based practice, the Affect Dyad, outperforms mindfulness-based practice on all primary outcome measures in significantly decreasing loneliness in participants' daily lives (EMA), as well as on the UCLA trait measure. In contrast, findings suggest that mindfulness practice, when applied as low-dose online training only, was not able to significantly reduce loneliness on both of these primary outcome measures.

Overall, we observed slightly stronger effects for the first Dyad cohort as compared to participants of the waitlist control group, who were administered active mental training in late winter. Multiple reasons could explain this finding. Firstly, the waitlist control group had a drop-out for the continuation of the training program and, therefore, had a lower sample size ($n = 65$) and, thus, less statistical power to detect an effect [51]. Additionally, seasonal effects might have influenced the efficacy of Affect Dyad training in WSE conducted in late winter 2021 during increasing numbers of COVID-19 infections, while SE received their training in early autumn.

The third aim of the present work was to assess improvements in social connectedness resulting from dyadic practice. Indeed, in line with previous findings [20], we observed an immediate increase in perceived social closeness after each daily Dyad. In contrast to previous findings, however, neither aspect of social connectedness showed improvement over the 10-week training period. It is possible that the smaller range of the scale utilized in the current study may have been insufficient to capture the subtle shifts in self-disclosure levels. Additionally, the absence of in-person meetings among participants may have contributed to a higher baseline level of self-disclosure due to anonymity [52]. On the contrary, the lack of replicable increase in social closeness over the course of the intervention might be due to the anonymity. These results suggest that while in-person meetings might facilitate the generalization of feelings of social connectedness during training, they could potentially lead to lower baseline levels of self-disclosure. Future research on Affect Dyad training will have to investigate these effects further.

Finally, we explored potential factors that may mediate intervention-related changes in loneliness observed before and after the 10-week training. No significant mediation effects could be observed. This may be due to the explorative nature of assessing potential mediators through one-item scales, which might lack sufficient reliability over time. Future studies will have to investigate possible mechanisms of change in loneliness using task-based measures and a more comprehensive assessment of the potential mediator variables.

5. Conclusions

Given the global rise of subjective loneliness in recent years, particularly amplified by the COVID-19 pandemic, many people, especially among younger demographics, experience loneliness and deficits in social connectedness. We found that purely online low-dose partner-based socio-emotional training was more effective than a comparable classic mindfulness-based program in reducing different aspects of state and trait-related loneliness. Furthermore, the dyadic practice seemed to result in higher compliance during and after the training, suggesting its potential for sustainable practice with enduring effects. Thus, we conclude that these daily dyadic intersubjective mental pieces of training provide a potentially scalable, low-cost digital approach to counter the threat of rising loneliness and its associated burdens, including severe mental health problems. Further, such socio-emotional partner-based pieces of training are even more promising as they come with additional benefits in reducing other aspects of mental health like depression and anxiety while at the same time boosting social skills such as empathy and (self-)compassion as well as resilience.

Supplementary Materials: The following supporting information can be downloaded at: https://www.mdpi.com/article/10.3390/ijerph21050570/s1, Supplementary Material S1: Mental Training Intervention Protocol CovSocial Phase 2: Summary; Supplementary Material S2: Power Analysis; Supplementary Material S3: Deviations from preregistration; Table S1: Descriptive statistics for loneliness (UCLA Loneliness Scale) and loneliness ratings measured with EMA, split by measurement occasion and group; Table S2: Cronbach's alpha values for UCLA Loneliness Scale; Table S3: Mediation effects of slopes on change in outcome variables in the (waitlist) socio-emotional (SE and WSE) mental training compared to mindfulness-based mental training (MB); Table S4: Mediation effects of slopes on change in outcome variables in the socio-emotional (SE) mental training compared to waitlist socio-emotional (WSE) mental training.

Author Contributions: Conceptualization: H.M., M.G., S.S., M.V., and T.S.; methodology: H.M., M.G., S.S., M.H., M.V., and T.S.; development of intervention program and teacher training: T.S.; formal analysis: H.M., M.G., S.S., M.H., and M.V.; investigation: H.M., M.G., S.S., and T.S.; writing—original draft preparation: H.M.; writing—review and editing: H.M., M.G., S.S., M.H., M.V., and T.S.; supervision: M.V. and T.S.; PI of CovSocial and project administration: T.S. All authors have read and agreed to the published version of the manuscript.

Funding: This study forms part of the CovSocial project, headed by Tania Singer (principal investigator) and funded in the majority by funds from the Social Neuroscience Lab of the Max Planck Society. Tania Singer and five other cooperation partners received a kick-off grant for the CovSocial Project in 2020, funded through the Berlin University Alliance (BUA) as part of the Excellence Strategy of the German federal and state governments (grant agreement number 114_GC_Pandemie_23).

Institutional Review Board Statement: This study was preregistered at the Open Science Framework (https://osf.io/3nsjc; see Supplementary Material S3) and is in accordance with the Declaration of Helsinki. Ethical approval was received by the institutional review board of Charité—Universitätsmedizin Berlin (#EA4/081/21). All participants provided written, informed consent.

Informed Consent Statement: All participants provided written, informed consent.

Data Availability Statement: Data and R code are available from the corresponding author to other researchers on reasonable request.

Acknowledgments: We thank Juliane Domke, Carmen Martinez-Moura, Birgit Severin, Karen Joachim, and all researchers and student assistants at the Social Neuroscience Lab for their help in organizing, preparing, and collecting the data for this project, and Cäcilia Krämer, Martin Büchele, Katharina Schacht, and Oliver Kirchhof for teaching the intervention program.

Conflicts of Interest: T.S. was honorary co-founder, scientific and curriculum advisor for Humanize from 2021 to summer 2023. Humanize is a start-up that is inspired by T.S.'s mental intervention research as well as her ReConnect Masterclasses and courses focusing on dyadic interventions, including the Affect Dyad, and is releasing modified and extended versions of these dyad intervention programs on a commercial digital platform and app. These additional offices of T.S. have all been formally approved by the Max Planck Society. At the present moment, T.S. no longer has any active role nor any shares in Humanize.

References

1. Perlman, D.; Peplau, L. Toward a social psychology of loneliness. *Pers. Relatsh. Disord.* **1981**, *3*, 31–43.
2. Holt-Lunstad, J.; Smith, T.B.; Baker, M.; Harris, T.; Stephenson, D. Loneliness and Social Isolation as Risk Factors for Mortality: A Meta-Analytic Review. *Perspect. Psychol. Sci.* **2015**, *10*, 227–237. [CrossRef] [PubMed]
3. Valtorta, N.K.; Kanaan, M.; Gilbody, S.; Ronzi, S.; Hanratty, B. Loneliness and social isolation as risk factors for coronary heart disease and stroke: Systematic review and meta-analysis of longitudinal observational studies. *Heart* **2016**, *102*, 1009–1016. [CrossRef]
4. Lara, E.; Martín-María, N.; De la Torre-Luque, A.; Koyanagi, A.; Vancampfort, D.; Izquierdo, A.; Miret, M. Does loneliness contribute to mild cognitive impairment and dementia? A systematic review and meta-analysis of longitudinal studies. *Ageing Res. Rev.* **2019**, *52*, 7–16. [CrossRef] [PubMed]
5. Beutel, M.E.; Klein, E.M.; Brähler, E.; Reiner, I.; Jünger, C.; Michal, M.; Wiltink, J.; Wild, P.S.; Münzel, T.; Lackner, K.J.; et al. Loneliness in the general population: Prevalence, determinants and relations to mental health. *BMC Psychiatry* **2017**, *17*, 97. [CrossRef]
6. Clark, D.M.T.; Loxton, N.J.; Tobin, S.J. Declining loneliness over time: Evidence from American colleges and high schools. *Personal. Soc. Psychol. Bull.* **2015**, *41*, 78–89. [CrossRef]
7. Mund, M.; Freuding, M.M.; Möbius, K.; Horn, N.; Neyer, F.J. The stability and change of loneliness across the life span: A meta-analysis of longitudinal studies. *Personal. Soc. Psychol. Rev.* **2020**, *24*, 24–52. [CrossRef]
8. Xin, S.; Xin, Z. Birth cohort changes in Chinese college students' loneliness and social support: One up, as another down. *Int. J. Behav. Dev.* **2016**, *40*, 398–407. [CrossRef]
9. Buecker, S.; Mund, M.; Chwastek, S.; Sostmann, M.; Luhmann, M. Is loneliness in emerging adults increasing over time? A preregistered cross-temporal meta-analysis and systematic review. *Psychol. Bull.* **2021**, *147*, 787. [CrossRef]
10. Twenge, J.M.; Spitzberg, B.H.; Campbell, W.K. Less in-person social interaction with peers among U.S. adolescents in the 21st century and links to loneliness. *J. Soc. Pers. Relatsh.* **2019**, *36*, 1892–1913. [CrossRef]
11. Barreto, M.; Victor, C.; Hammond, C.; Eccles, A.; Richins, M.T.; Qualter, P. Loneliness around the world: Age, gender, and cultural differences in loneliness. *Personal. Individ. Differ.* **2021**, *169*, 110066. [CrossRef] [PubMed]
12. Hawkley, L.C.; Buecker, S.; Kaiser, T.; Luhmann, M. Loneliness from young adulthood to old age: Explaining age differences in loneliness. *Int. J. Behav. Dev.* **2022**, *46*, 39–49. [CrossRef] [PubMed]
13. Jeste, D.V.; Lee, E.E.; Cacioppo, S. Battling the Modern Behavioral Epidemic of Loneliness: Suggestions for Research and Interventions. *JAMA Psychiatry* **2020**, *77*, 553–554. [CrossRef] [PubMed]
14. Ernst, M.; Niederer, D.; Werner, A.M.; Czaja, S.J.; Mikton, C.; Ong, A.D.; Rosen, T.; Brähler, E.; Beutel, M.E. Loneliness before and during the COVID-19 pandemic: A systematic review with meta-analysis. *Am. Psychol.* **2022**, *77*, 660. [CrossRef] [PubMed]
15. Berger, K.; Riedel-Heller, S.; Pabst, A.; Rietschel, M.; Richter, D. Einsamkeit während der ersten Welle der SARS-CoV-2-pandemie–Ergebnisse der NAKO-Gesundheitsstudie. *Bundesgesundheitsblatt-Gesundheitsforschung-Gesundheitsschutz* **2021**, *64*, 1157–1164. [CrossRef]
16. Buecker, S.; Horstmann, K.T. Loneliness and social isolation during the COVID-19 pandemic. *Eur. Psychol.* **2022**, *26*, 272–284. [CrossRef]
17. Veronese, N.; Galvano, D.; D'Antiga, F.; Vecchiato, C.; Furegon, E.; Allocco, R.; Smith, L.; Gelmini, G.; Gareri, P.; Solmi, M.; et al. Interventions for reducing loneliness: An umbrella review of intervention studies. *Health Soc. Care Community* **2021**, *29*, e89–e96. [CrossRef] [PubMed]
18. Gu, J.; Strauss, C.; Bond, R.; Cavanagh, K. How do mindfulness-based cognitive therapy and mindfulness-based stress reduction improve mental health and wellbeing? A systematic review and meta-analysis of mediation studies. *Clin. Psychol. Rev.* **2015**, *37*, 1–12. [CrossRef]
19. Singer, T.; Engert, V. It matters what you practice: Differential training effects on subjective experience, behavior, brain and body in the ReSource Project. *Curr. Opin. Psychol.* **2019**, *28*, 151–158. [CrossRef]
20. Kok, B.E.; Singer, T. Effects of Contemplative Dyads on Engagement and Perceived Social Connectedness Over 9 Months of Mental Training: A Randomized Clinical Trial. *JAMA Psychiatry* **2017**, *74*, 126–134. [CrossRef]

21. Kabat-Zinn, J. Mindfulness-based interventions in context: Past, present, and future. *Clin. Psychol. Sci. Pract.* **2003**, *10*, 144. [CrossRef]
22. Teoh, S.L.; Letchumanan, V.; Lee, L.-H. Can Mindfulness Help to Alleviate Loneliness? A Systematic Review and Meta-Analysis. *Front. Psychol.* **2021**, *12*, 633319. Available online: https://www.frontiersin.org/article/10.3389/fpsyg.2021.633319 (accessed on 23 April 2024). [CrossRef] [PubMed]
23. Hickin, N.; Käll, A.; Shafran, R.; Sutcliffe, S.; Manzotti, G.; Langan, D. The effectiveness of psychological interventions for loneliness: A systematic review and meta-analysis. *Clin. Psychol. Rev.* **2021**, *88*, 102066. [CrossRef] [PubMed]
24. Lindsay, E.K.; Young, S.; Brown, K.W.; Smyth, J.M.; Creswell, J.D. Mindfulness training reduces loneliness and increases social contact in a randomized controlled trial. *Proc. Natl. Acad. Sci. USA* **2019**, *116*, 3488–3493. [CrossRef] [PubMed]
25. Bessaha, M.L.; Sabbath, E.L.; Morris, Z.; Malik, S.; Scheinfeld, L.; Saragossi, J. A Systematic Review of Loneliness Interventions Among Non-elderly Adults. *Clin. Soc. Work. J.* **2020**, *48*, 110–125. [CrossRef]
26. Richardson, L.; St Pierre, E. A method of inquiry. *Handb. Qual. Res.* **2000**, *48*, 923–948.
27. Kramer, G.P. Insight Dialogue and Insight Dialogic Inquiry. PhD Thesis, California Institute of Integral Studies, San Francisco, CA, USA, 1997.
28. Singer, T.; Kok, B.E.; Bornemann, B.; Bolz, M.; Bochow, C. *The ReSource Project: Background, Design, Samples, and Measurements*, 2nd ed.; Max Planck Institute for Human Cognitive and Brain Sciences: Leipzig, Germany, 2016. Available online: http://hdl.handle.net/21.11116/0000-0003-FEC8-E (accessed on 23 April 2024).
29. Cacioppo, J.T.; Patrick, W. *Loneliness: Human Nature and the Need for Social Connection*; WW Norton & Company: New York, NY, USA, 2008.
30. Hutcherson, C.A.; Seppala, E.M.; Gross, J.J. Loving-kindness meditation increases social connectedness. *Emotion* **2008**, *8*, 720. [CrossRef]
31. Russell, D.; Peplau, L.A.; Cutrona, C.E. The revised UCLA Loneliness Scale: Concurrent and discriminant validity evidence. *J. Personal. Soc. Psychol.* **1980**, *39*, 472–480. [CrossRef]
32. Wei, M.; Russell, D.W.; Zakalik, R.A. Adult attachment, social self-efficacy, self-disclosure, loneliness, and subsequent depression for freshman college students: A longitudinal study. *J. Couns. Psychol.* **2005**, *52*, 602. [CrossRef]
33. Akin, A. Self-compassion and Loneliness. *Int. Online J. Educ. Sci.* **2010**, *2*, 702–718.
34. Zhang, N.; Fan, F.; Huang, S.; Rodriguez, M.A. Mindfulness training for loneliness among Chinese college students: A pilot randomized controlled trial. *Int. J. Psychol.* **2018**, *53*, 373–378. [CrossRef] [PubMed]
35. Gierveld, J.d.J. A review of loneliness: Concept and definitions, determinants and consequences. *Rev. Clin. Gerontol.* **1998**, *8*, 73–80. [CrossRef]
36. Jazaieri, H.; Jinpa, G.T.; McGonigal, K.; Rosenberg, E.L.; Finkelstein, J.; Simon-Thomas, E.; Cullen, M.; Doty, J.R.; Gross, J.J.; Goldin, P.R. Enhancing Compassion: A Randomized Controlled Trial of a Compassion Cultivation Training Program. *J. Happiness Stud.* **2013**, *14*, 1113–1126. [CrossRef]
37. Godara, M.; Silveira, S.; Matthäus, H.; Heim, C.; Voelkle, M.; Hecht, M.; Binder, E.B.; Singer, T. Investigating differential effects of socio-emotional and mindfulness-based online interventions on mental health, resilience and social capacities during the COVID-19 pandemic: The study protocol. *PLoS ONE* **2021**, *16*, e0256323. [CrossRef]
38. Bagby, R.M.; Parker, J.D.A.; Taylor, G.J. The twenty-item Toronto Alexithymia scale—I. Item selection and cross-validation of the factor structure. *Journal of Psychosomatic Research* **1994**, *38*, 23–32. [CrossRef] [PubMed]
39. Kroenke, K.; Spitzer, R.L.; Williams, J.B.W. The PHQ-9: Validity of a brief depression severity measure. *Journal of General Internal Medicine* **2001**, *16*, 606–613. [CrossRef]
40. Spitzer, R.L.; Kroenke, K.; Williams, J.B.W.; Löwe, B. A Brief Measure for Assessing Generalized Anxiety Disorder: The GAD-7. *Arch. Intern. Med.* **2006**, *166*, 1092. [CrossRef]
41. Döring, N.; Bortz, J. Psychometrische Einsamkeitsforschung: Deutsche Neukonstruktion der UCLA Loneliness Scale. *Diagnostica* **1993**, *39*, 224–239.
42. Aron, A.; Aron, E.N.; Smollan, D. Inclusion of other in the self scale and the structure of interpersonal closeness. *J. Personal. Soc. Psychol.* **1992**, *63*, 596. [CrossRef]
43. Neff, K.D.; Tóth-Király, I.; Knox, M.C.; Kuchar, A.; Davidson, O. The development and validation of the state self-compassion scale (long-and short form). *Mindfulness* **2021**, *12*, 121–140. [CrossRef]
44. Carver, C.S. You want to measure coping but your protocol'too long: Consider the brief cope. *Int. J. Behav. Med.* **1997**, *4*, 92–100. [CrossRef] [PubMed]
45. Gilbert, P.; McEwan, K.; Gibbons, L.; Chotai, S.; Duarte, J.; Matos, M. Fears of compassion and happiness in relation to alexithymia, mindfulness, and self-criticism. *Psychol. Psychother. Theory Res. Pract.* **2012**, *85*, 374–390. [CrossRef] [PubMed]
46. Faul, F.; Erdfelder, E.; Lang, A.-G.; Buchner, A. G* Power 3: A flexible statistical power analysis program for the social, behavioral, and biomedical sciences. *Behav. Res. Methods* **2007**, *39*, 175–191. [CrossRef] [PubMed]
47. Bates, D.; Mächler, M.; Bolker, B.; Walker, S. Fitting Linear Mixed-Effects Models Using lme4. *J. Stat. Softw.* **2015**, *67*, 1–48. [CrossRef]
48. Hothorn, T.; Bretz, F.; Westfall, P. Simultaneous inference in general parametric models. *Biom. J. J. Math. Methods Biosci.* **2008**, *50*, 346–363. [CrossRef] [PubMed]

49. R Core Team. *R: A Language and Environment for Statistical Computing;* R Foundation for Statistical Computing: Vienna, Austria, 2022. Available online: https://www.R-project.org/ (accessed on 23 April 2024).
50. Rosseel, Y. lavaan: An R package for structural equation modeling. *J. Stat. Softw.* **2012**, *48*, 1–36. [CrossRef]
51. Cohen, J. A power primer. *Psychol. Bull.* **1992**, *112*, 155–159. [CrossRef]
52. Clark-Gordon, C.V.; Bowman, N.D.; Goodboy, A.K.; Wright, A. Anonymity and online self-disclosure: A meta-analysis. *Commun. Rep.* **2019**, *32*, 98–111. [CrossRef]

International Journal of
Environmental Research and Public Health

MDPI

Article

Preventing Loneliness and Reducing Dropout: Results from the COMPLETE Intervention Study in Upper Secondary Schools in Norway

Helga Bjørnøy Urke *, Torill Bogsnes Larsen and Sara Madeleine Eriksen Kristensen

Department of Health Promotion and Development, University of Bergen, 5009 Bergen, Norway; torill.larsen@uib.no (T.B.L.); madeleine.kristensen@uib.no (S.M.E.K.)
* Correspondence: helga.urke@uib.no

Abstract: This study examines the impact of interventions aimed at improving psychosocial health on students' perception of a caring school climate, their feelings of loneliness, and school completion in Norwegian upper secondary education. Two intervention conditions were tested: a universal single-tier intervention focused on improving the psychosocial school climate: the Dream School Program, and a multi-tier intervention combining the Dream School Program with a targeted measure, the Mental Health Support Team. The direct and indirect effects of these interventions on school completion were analyzed using structural equation models (SEM), with data from 1508 students (mean age at Time 1: 17.02 (SD = 0.92); 60.7% girls; 72.1% Norwegian-born). The results indicated that loneliness levels did not differ significantly between the intervention conditions. However, students in the multi-tier intervention group reported a significantly higher perception of a caring school climate compared to those in the single-tier intervention group. The multi-tier intervention group had a lower rate of school completion compared to the control group and the single-tier intervention group. The SEM analysis revealed that the multi-tier intervention reduced loneliness in the second year of upper secondary school by promoting a caring school climate in the first school year. In contrast, the single-tier intervention was associated with increased loneliness due to a decrease in the perception of a caring school climate. The implications of these findings are discussed.

Keywords: loneliness; school climate; dropout; completion; intervention; adolescence

1. Introduction

Given the strong link between education, health, and accomplishments in life, schools are one of the most important settings for stimulating positive adolescent development [1]. Moreover, school dropout is shown to be a significant determinant for future social and economic adversity [2], and in Norway, preventing school dropout is an explicit national goal [3]. The reasons why young people leave school before completing upper secondary education are many, varied and complex, and its reduction requires efforts at many levels. At the school level, research has found relational factors, such as teacher support and loneliness, to be significant predictors of intentions to drop out [4]. Further, an inclusive environment, the quality of peer relations, and teacher support are predictors for reduced loneliness [5].

The importance of teacher–student and peer relationships for youth well-being has long been acknowledged [6]. The only activity that youth spend more time engaged in than school is sleeping [7], and close to half of their waking time is spent in school. Hence, their emotional well-being is likely influenced by the quality of their school-related relationships, such as those with their teachers and peers [6]. As such, when the school safeguards socially nurturing environments, it represents an important arena for academic development, as well as positive adjustment and socioemotional functioning [8,9]. This aspect of school is the psychosocial school environment, and it can be defined as "the social situations at school in relation to pupils' work situation (such as teacher support, work demands, and influence over school work) as well as in relation to pupils' peer relations at school..." [10], p. 169.

Creating a school environment where everyone feels included and where everyone wants to be is therefore an important prevention effort, both from a socio-economic and a human perspective [1]. Such an environment is possible to target through interventions intended to reduce loneliness, prevent dropout, and stimulate completion. School interventions to prevent or reduce complex phenomena such as loneliness and dropout are recommended to address the wider social school climate [3,11]. Further, previous research regarding evidence-based interventions in school mental health work indicates that effective interventions are characterized by (among others) combining universal and targeted measures and taking a whole-school approach that involves a range of relevant stakeholders [12]. While there are indications of what type of intervention efforts can be effective in the landscape of loneliness and school completion, there is still a call for more rigorous testing of such interventions, taking local context into consideration [11], and determining the right balance between universal and targeted interventions [12]. Acknowledging that universal interventions are easier, less burdensome for schools, and often less expensive to implement than more targeted measures or combinations of universal and targeted interventions, it is prudent to assess how various combinations of interventions contribute to mitigating the challenges of loneliness and dropout [13].

The aim of the present study was to investigate whether systematic work within the classroom and school environment through a universal (single-tier) and a combination of a universal and a targeted (multi-tier) intervention affected students' experiences in the psychosocial environment (i.e., perceptions of a caring school climate and feelings of loneliness) and the completion of upper secondary education in Norway.

1.1. The Need to Belong and Loneliness

The need to belong is considered a fundamental human need [14], and during adolescence, peer relationships become increasingly important [15,16], while the vulnerability to feelings of loneliness can become more salient [17]. The prevalence of loneliness peaks during adolescence, and this is assumed to be related to changes in the youths' personal identities and their needs and expectations in relation to the importance of social relationships [18–20]. In Norway, nationally representative surveys found that 10% of youth experience loneliness, and that girls report twice the level of loneliness than do boys. Further, a trend of increasing loneliness prevalence has been observed over the past decade [21]. According to the evolutionary theory of loneliness [22], there are three core aspects of loneliness: (1) it is a subjective experience not synonymous with objective isolation, (2) it is due to deficient social relations or a discrepancy between desired and actual social relations, and (3) it is experienced as distressful [23]. Loneliness can therefore be seen as an unpleasant subjective experience of a deficiency in one's social relations. The adverse impact that loneliness can have on adolescents' well-being has been widely documented in the literature. For instance, studies have linked loneliness during adolescence and early adulthood with poorer general health [18,20], reduced sleep quality [24], and higher mortality rates [25].

1.2. Loneliness and Dropout

In addition to health consequences, loneliness is a risk factor for dropout [4,26,27], while completing and passing upper secondary education is an important basis for further education and entry into work life. Studies show that those who do not complete upper secondary education have a weaker connection to the labor market and a more extensive use of public social security and benefit programs than those who complete this education [2]. Young people who do not complete or are left out of education run a great risk of permanent exclusion in relation to work life [2,28]. In addition to burdens for the individual, research suggests that dropping out of upper secondary education can contribute to significant socio-economic costs at the societal level [2].

Studies have found that being liked and accepted by fellow students is important for young people's positive development [29–31]. In contrast, students reporting low social integration or not experiencing a connection to others are also more likely to have lower life satisfaction and experience mental health difficulties [30]. Inevitably, adolescence involves socially challenging periods, including the transition from lower to upper secondary education, which for many, can encompass losing important social relationships that have been built up over the years. For some, establishing new relationships can be a daunting task, and as such, the school transition represents a risk factor for loneliness. To ensure a good transition between lower and upper secondary school, it is therefore important to work to establish a good psychosocial environment to counteract loneliness through the development of good relationships from the very beginning of the school year. Research has suggested that one of the most important factors for success in school is making at least one friend during the first few weeks of starting a new school [32]. An inclusive and caring environment can contribute to the experience of connection or belonging, thus decreasing the feeling of loneliness [33], and in turn promote school well-being and completion.

1.3. School Psychosocial Environment (Caring Climate) and Loneliness

Researchers have emphasized the vital role of teachers in contributing to reducing student loneliness [34,35]. Empirical data on this association is limited, but the existing studies support the proposition that the quality of teacher–student relationships can influence student loneliness, e.g., with more emotional support from the teacher being associated with less student loneliness [4,36,37]. Although the teacher–student relationship and its association with loneliness is less explored, research on the overall psychosocial school environment has also been conducted in relation to loneliness, with one study finding that the perception of an unsupportive social classroom environment was the strongest predictor of school loneliness [5]. This implies that a positive social classroom environment is an important safeguard against student loneliness, and that teachers play a key role in ensuring such an environment.

1.4. The Aim of the Study

Against the backdrop of increasing loneliness reporting by young people [21], the suggested association between loneliness and intentions to drop out of school [4,26], and the overwhelming evidence for the benefits of education [2], the need for effective efforts to tackle this complex issue is clear. Focusing on a caring psychosocial school environment and improving the contact between teachers and students, as well as strengthening the relationships among students in the classroom and in the school, might be effective in preventing dropout [3]. However, the school environment is a complex, living organization, and each school is different when it comes to staff, student population, and academic tracks, not to mention socioeconomic, cultural, and geographic contexts. To gain a more nuanced understanding of specific viable efforts in the Norwegian context, more rigorous evaluations are needed. In this study, we introduce the Dream School Program and the Mental Health Support Team (MHST) (detailed descriptions below in Section 2.2), which are measures that have been implemented in Norwegian upper secondary schools to systematically promote these aspects of the psychosocial environment [38]. The main purpose of the present study was to investigate whether systematic work within the classroom and school environment by means of a single-tier (Dream School Program) and a multi-tier (Dream School Program and MHST) intervention affected the students' experiences with the psychosocial environment (measured as a caring climate) and their connection to their peers (measured as feelings of loneliness) and its relation to completion of upper secondary education. Considering the comparably larger efforts in the multi-tier intervention through the combination of a universal and a targeted approach, we anticipated that the multi-tier intervention would have the strongest effect on the outcomes of interest.

2. Materials and Methods

This study is a part of the COMPLETE study [38], trial number NCT03382080, a school-based, three-armed cluster RCT with the aim of improving the psychosocial school environment and increasing completion rates in Norwegian upper secondary schools. Sixteen schools across four counties participated in the study, of which five schools received a single-tier intervention, six schools received a multi-tier intervention, and five schools made up the control group. The trial started in August 2016 and ended in June 2019, following students from when they started upper secondary school until they graduated. The study was non-blinded. Data were collected through individual surveys (psychosocial aspects) and school registries (school grades, absences, and completion (T3/grade 12)).

2.1. Participants

This paper utilized data collected from 1508 students in the general education track from the 16 schools in March 2017 (T1/grade 1) and 2018 (T2/grade 2). At T1, there were 1184 participants, and 949 responded at T2. School completion information was available from registry data for 1138 students. Concerning the intervention and control groups, 40.5% (n = 610) were in the single-tier intervention group, 40.6% (n = 613) were in the multi-tier intervention group, and 18.9% (n = 285) were in the control group. There were 60.7% girls (n = 916) and 39.3% boys (n = 592) in the sample. Regarding immigration background, 72.1% (n = 1088) were Norwegian-born and 6% (n = 89) were immigrants. The participants' ages ranged from 16 to 26 years old, wherein the majority (93.5%) were under 18 and 19 at T1 and T2, respectively. Concerning the participants' perceived family wealth, 0.7% (n = 10) responded that their family was 'not well off at all', 3.4% (n = 52) reported that their family was 'not well off', 18.4% (n = 278) said their family was 'moderately well off', 36.3% (n = 548) said their family was 'well off', and 16.5% (n = 249) perceived their family to be 'very well off' economically.

2.2. The Intervention Measures

The Dream School is a universal school program aimed at improving the psychosocial environment by applying a whole-school approach. The program is developed by the Norwegian NGO Adults for Children [39]. The goals of the Dream School, as stated by Adults for Children, are: (a) to establish a framework and tools for holistic work within the psychosocial learning environment in the school, (b) to increase the competence of employees regarding working to promote a good psychosocial environment, (c) to strengthen the relationship between students, as well as between students and staff, (d) to strengthen students' belonging, participation, mastery, and motivation, (e) to increase students' motivation to complete and pass school, and (f) to use students as resources in a systematic manner to promote a good psychosocial environment. The core elements of the program are Dream Classes 1 and 2, which are three-hour gatherings with a focus on classroom climate for students in grade 1, carried out the first or second week after school starts and at the beginning of the spring semester, respectively. The Dream Classes are organized and implemented by student mentors, which are older students at the school, in collaboration with contact teachers. Prior to the implementation of the program, the student mentors and contact teachers are specifically trained in the Dream School Program and the Dream Classes by workers from Adults for Children. Contact teachers are also responsible for following up on the action plan that the class creates and are important partners for the student mentors in their work with the class. At each school, a resource group is appointed consisting of members from school management, teachers, students, and possibly other employees who are responsible for following up the Dream School Program in their respective schools.

The MHST, on the other hand, is an indicated and selective measure to give special attention to students at risk of dropping out of school. More specifically, it is aimed at the psychosocial follow-up and the academic guidance of young people who, for various reasons, are struggling with regular attendance and academic progress. The aim is that the

MHST works systematically with vulnerable students from the transition from lower to upper secondary school and throughout the upper secondary school period. The MHST is a structural effort to strengthen the system for follow-up of individual students who need it. It is organized as a multidisciplinary and co-located team and can have somewhat different compositions across schools, but the school health nurse, follow-up services (from the school owner), and social counsellors or social workers within the schools are key players on the teams. The teams should be co-located, have an "open door" policy, work towards keeping students present at school, and help with transition work between the lower and upper secondary school, or assist if students switch schools during upper secondary education. The follow-up should be collaborative with the student, and in many cases, with their guardians to develop plans for academic progress. Such plans could, among other efforts, include closer academic or social support, alternative school schedules, or reducing the number of subjects that a student completes within a given academic year to increase the chances of passing, prolonging the study period. In the COMPLETE project, at the start of the first school year of upper secondary school, the school health nurse implemented Kidscreen [40] as a mapping tool for all students to gain an indication of students in special need of follow-up. All teachers were instructed to be in immediate and close contact with the team, in case of concern for specific students, as well as to collaborate on how to adjust for or facilitate students in need of special care. Beyond this, the teams did not have a set schedule with specific elements to implement during the project period, but rather the focus was on building a more robust and collaborative system within each school to quickly identify and support students at risk.

2.3. Instruments

2.3.1. Intervention Conditions

The intervention conditions were divided into three groups: the control group, the single-tier intervention group, and the multi-tier intervention group. We created a dummy variable for each intervention group so that individuals were either in that specific intervention group (coded as 1) or not (coded as 0).

2.3.2. Loneliness

We measured the participant's loneliness with an adapted short version of the UCLA loneliness scale developed for use in a Norwegian setting [41,42]. The participants assessed six questions on a scale ranging from 1 (not at all) to 5 (extremely). An example indicator is, "I feel as if nobody really understands me." The scale has achieved acceptable reliability in previous studies ($\alpha > 0.77$) [42].

2.3.3. Caring School Climate

To what extent students perceived their school climate to be caring was measured using an adapted, short version of the caring climate scale [43]. The scale consists of eight indicators which were assessed on a 5-point Likert scale, ranging from 1 (completely disagree) to 5 (completely agree). A sample indicator is as follows: "students feel that they are treated fairly".

2.3.4. Completion

The completion data were based on data obtained from county or school registries. In this study, completion is defined as graduation after three years of upper secondary school, which reflects normal progress for the general study track in Norwegian upper secondary schools [44]. It should be noted that the formal definition of not completing upper secondary education on which Norwegian dropout statistics are based is the completion of three years of upper secondary school within five years following enrollment [44].

2.3.5. Control Variables

We used several control variables in the hypothesized model. Gender was coded as 0 (boys) and 1 (girls). Socioeconomic position was measured by a single indicator, assessing how wealthy the participants perceived their families to be [45], ranging from 1 (not well off) to 5 (very well off). Symptoms of anxiety and depression were included as a control variable due to the substantial association of mental health with the study variables [46,47]. Anxiety and depressive symptoms were measured by a Norwegian short version of the Symptom Check List-90-R (SCL-5; [48–50]. The participants assessed the extent to which they had experienced distress during the last 14 days on a 4-point scale ranging from 1 (not at all) to 4 (very much). A sample indicator is: "feeling hopelessness about the future."

2.4. Missing Data Considerations

We examined the missing data patterns of the study variables using Little's Missing Completely at Random (MCAR) test and partial correlations. The MCAR test indicated that the missingness mechanism was not completely at random ($X^2 = 512.155$, $df = 297$, $p < 0.001$). We performed several correlation and partial correlation analyses to investigate the association between missingness in one variable and the subsequent level of another variable [51]. Missingness in caring school climate was not significantly related to the level of loneliness participants reported at the subsequent time point ($p > 0.05$). However, the relationship between missingness in loneliness and degree of completion was significantly associated when we controlled for the previous level of loneliness ($p < 0.05$). Thus, we assume that the missingness mechanism is approaching missing at random (MAR), and we used the full information maximum likelihood (FIML) estimation to handle potential missingness.

2.5. Analytical Plan

To investigate the effect of the interventions regarding a caring school climate, loneliness, degree of completion, and the longitudinal associations between these, we (1) performed a one-way analysis of variance (ANOVA), with a post hoc Tukey test and (2) used intervention condition as a predictor in the hypothesized model and compared the direct and indirect regression coefficients across groups. We used SPSS version 28 to perform the ANOVA analysis. For the structural equation modeling (SEM), we used robust maximum likelihood (MLR) estimation in M*plus* version 8 [52]. The following fit criteria were examined to assess the model fit of the SEM models: CFI > 0.90, RMSEA < 0.08, SRMR < 0.08 [48,49]. The Chi-square test was administered, but was not decisive in model fit evaluation due to sample size sensitivity [48].

3. Results

3.1. Descriptive Statistics

Details of the descriptive statistics are presented in Table 1. The reliability test of the caring school climate and loneliness constructs indicated good omega values ($\omega > 0.82$).

Table 1. Descriptive statistics of the study variables.

				Intervention Group		
				Control	Single-Tier	Multi-Tier
	n	*Ω*	Min-Max	*M (SD)*	*M (SD)*	*M (SD)*
T1 Caring school climate	1132	0.93	1–5	3.85 (0.66)	3.74 (0.73)	3.94 (0.73)
T2 Loneliness	915	0.82	1–5	2.31 (0.79)	2.27 (0.77)	2.33 (0.78)
Degree of completion	1138	–	1–6	5.79 (0.75)	5.71 (0.87)	5.48 (1.23)

3.2. Analysis of Variance

The one-way ANOVA with post-hoc Tukey test indicated that caring school climate and degree of completion significantly varied across intervention conditions, but the level of loneliness did not. Specifically, the participants in the multi-tier intervention group reported a significantly higher level of caring school climate ($M = 3.94$, $SD = 0.73$) compared to the single-tier intervention group ($M = 3.74$, $SD = 0.73$, $F(2, 1129) = 8.956$, $p < 0.001$). Regarding the degree of completion, the opposite was found. The multi-tier intervention group had a significantly lower degree of completion ($M = 5.48$, $SD = 1.23$) compared to the control group ($M = 5.79$, $SD = 0.75$) and the single-tier intervention group ($M = 5.71$, $SD = 0.87$), $F(2, 1135) = 8.947$, $p < 0.001$).

3.3. Hypothesized Model

We investigated three separate models, using the different intervention groups as a predictor in the hypothesized model. All models included gender and baseline socioeconomic position, with symptoms of anxiety and depression as control variables. Each model produced acceptable model fit (RMSEA < 0.04, CFI > 0.97, SRMR < 0.05), and the results are presented in Figure 1. There were several regression coefficients that were different across the intervention groups. First, the single-tier predictor variable had a significantly stronger effect on caring school climate compared to that of the control group ($\beta_{diff} = -0.10$, $p < 0.05$). Second, the multi-tier predictor variable had a significantly stronger effect on caring school climate compared to that of the control group ($\beta_{diff} = 0.11$, $p < 0.05$). Third, the multi-tier predictor variable had a significantly different effect on loneliness compared to that of the single-tier predictor variable ($\beta_{diff} = 0.12$, $p < 0.05$). Lastly, the multi-tier predictor variable had a significantly different effect on the degree of completion compared to that of the single-tier predictor variable ($\beta_{diff} = -0.14$, $p < 0.001$) and the control group variable ($\beta_{diff} = -0.18$, $p < 0.001$).

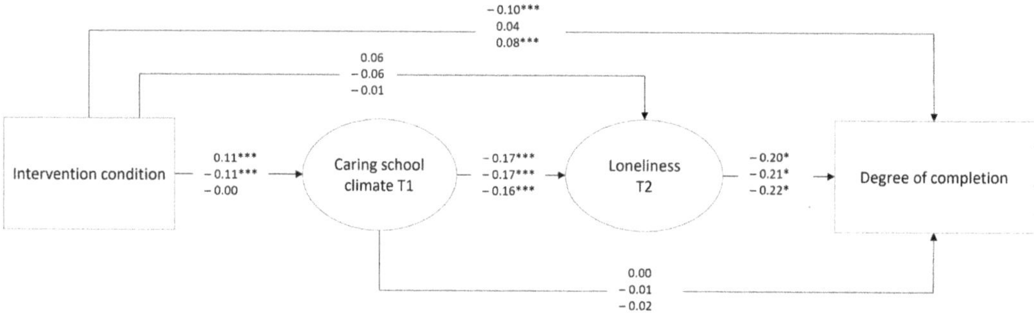

Figure 1. Hypothesized model of caring school climate, loneliness, and degree of completion. Note. The standardized results from all three models are presented in the figure, with the control group model on the bottom line, the single-tier model on the middle line, and the multi-tier model on the top line. * $p < 0.05$, *** $p < 0.001$.

Concerning the indirect effects in the model, only two effects were significant. The multi-tier predictor variable had a significant negative indirect effect on loneliness through the caring school climate variable ($\beta = -0.02$, $p < 0.01$). This implies that the multi-tier intervention reduced loneliness in the second year of upper secondary school through an increase in a caring school climate in the first school year. The opposite effect was found in the single-tier model, wherein the single-tier predictor had a significant positive effect on loneliness through a caring school climate ($\beta = 0.02$, $p < 0.01$). Thus, the single-tier intervention was related to an increase in loneliness through a reduction in the caring school climate.

4. Discussion

The main purpose of this study was to assess whether a single-tier (Dream School Program) and a multi-tier (Dream School Program and MHST) intervention improved the psychosocial school environment and increased completion of upper secondary school within three years when compared to the results of the control group schools. As indicators of the psychosocial environment, we used students' perceptions of a caring school climate and loneliness. The results were somewhat mixed and showed that perceptions of a caring school climate and degree of completion, but not the level of loneliness, significantly varied across intervention conditions. Specifically, the participants in the multi-tier intervention group reported a significantly higher level of a caring school climate compared to the single-tier intervention group. Regarding the degree of completion, the opposite was found: the multi-tier intervention group had a significantly lower degree of completion within three years compared to the control group and the single-tier intervention group. Further, when examining the indirect effects of the intervention, the results were that the multi-tier intervention reduced loneliness in the second year of upper secondary school through an increase in a caring school climate in the first school year. The opposite effect was found in the single-tier group, where the single-tier intervention was related to an increase in loneliness through a reduction in a caring school climate.

4.1. Completion of Upper Secondary School in Context of Vulnerability and Follow-Up

Research has indicated that good psychosocial school environments can promote positive social development and prevent students from dropping out of school [53]. Contrary to the initial prediction that a multi-tier intervention (consisting of the universal Dream School Program and the MHST) would lead to an increase in completion rate, the present study suggests that fewer students in the multi-tier group completed within the standard time of three years compared to the control group and the single-tier group. On the one hand, this is somewhat surprising, considering the comprehensive efforts on several levels (universal, selected, and indicated) that could be expected to help students with their progression. We can only speculate on possible explanations, but it could be that the range of measures within the multi-tier intervention was too comprehensive to implement within the project period to be effective in reaching its aims for school completion [13]. Previous research shows that interventions must be implemented according to their intentions to be effective [12]. In previous descriptive analyses of our material, we found that within the multi-tier group, the schools with higher implementation fidelity and integration showed higher completion rates compared to schools with lower implementation fidelity and integration [13]. As such, it could be that the very comprehensiveness of the intervention prevented sufficient implementation to reach the potential for higher completion rates.

However, an alternative explanation for our findings of a lower completion rate after three years in the multi-tier compared to the single-tier group could be that the follow-up of the students that struggled at school was more comprehensive in the multi-tier group, with a stronger focus on how to manage school life. In line with the principles of the MHSTs for exploring the most viable ways for coping with school for each adolescent who needs this assistance, the guidance may, in many cases, have included an adjusted educational plan that might lead to completion in the long run, but not within the three years of the standard completion time. Many of the measures used by the MHST, e.g., reducing the number of academic subjects each year or a combination of subjects and practical tasks outside of school, often lead to a prolonged track within upper secondary education. Acknowledging this aspect is also a reason to view completion within five years (or even longer) of enrollment, but this was not possible in our study. As such, although at first glance, our results on completion seem undesirable, they could reflect closer and more individually adjusted follow-up. To further understand the role of teams such as MHSTs, future intervention studies should make efforts to collect systematic information on what type of guidance and follow-up students receive, e.g., prolonging study period, more academic support, etc. Positively, previous research show that keeping students within the school system, even if it means that they do not pass all subjects within the three year norm, has a positive effect in a life course perspective [28], although statically, these students are classified as not completing school. Consequently, adjusting the educational plan towards a prolonged time to fulfill upper secondary education can have a positive effect in the long run. There is a need for additional research that differentiates more specifically between classifications of completion and dropout through following up with the students over a longer period.

4.2. Reducing Loneliness through a Whole School Approach to a Caring Psychosocial Environment

Regarding the perception of the psychosocial environment within the schools, our findings show that it was only in the multi-tier group that loneliness decreased through an increase in a perceived caring school climate. As shown by previous research [5], a positive social classroom environment can be an important safeguard against student loneliness, with teachers as important facilitators. Our results support this, to some degree, as we found that in the multi-tier group, perception of a caring school climate increased, and subsequently, loneliness decreased. Interestingly, the same results were not observed in the single-tier group. These results suggest that a combination of a universal program together with a selective and indicated measure, had a stronger effect on reducing loneliness compared to no intervention and a single-tier intervention only. For example, making the MHST available may have provided an additional focus on the school's efforts to improve its psychosocial environment in general, e.g., through better support to teachers in their work with the universal program, in turn increasing their efficacy in building a caring climate for the students [54,55]. Further, the MHST is intended to support particularly vulnerable students [38]. Although we do not have information regarding the prevalence of students that received follow-up from the MHST team, nor what specific efforts resulted from the follow-up, our results may reflect that students who are vulnerable, including with regards to social aspects, may have benefited from the team, and perhaps also due to a synergy effect of the two interventions efforts.

Moreover, it is interesting that despite lower completion rates in the multi-tier intervention, SEM analyses showed that students in this group were less lonely in the second year due to the perception of a caring climate in the first year. This finding suggests that even if the multi-tier intervention did not lead to increased completion rates, it may have led to an overall improvement in their social thriving, further supporting the multi-tier approach for these outcomes. Although the results of decreased loneliness, but not increased completion, within the same intervention group may seem puzzling or contradicting, it could be due to the fact that loneliness and school completion are affected by differential factors, as well as factors and mechanisms not considered in this study. For example, whereas increased socioemotional support and individual guidance on school functioning could speak to the emotional, social, and perhaps also academic thriving of an adolescent, it may not be enough to tackle the complexity of school completion in the same adolescent. Autonomous motivation and the positive outcomes associated with it, such as deep learning, engagement, improved performance, and interest, is important for positive development, flourishing, and wellbeing in an educational setting [56]. However, several factors are important for the development of autonomous motivation, including teacher autonomy support (i.e., supporting the students' volition and self-determination) [57]; a supportive home environment, with engaged parents or guardians [58]; and academic success [59]. In further studies on school completion, a more comprehensive assessment of the adolescents' socio-ecological system could be beneficial to understand where and how intervention efforts should be implemented.

The results from the analyses of the single-tier model showed an increase in loneliness in the second year through a reduction in a perceived caring school climate in the first year. This is somewhat surprising, as universal measures are generally considered important for ensuring good psychosocial conditions for all [12]. However, it could be that efforts through a universal program do not sufficiently reach the most vulnerable students, or that they can even reinforce feelings of exclusion and loneliness through, e.g., feelings of poor mastery in relation to social activities that are implemented. Previous studies on school-based mental health interventions have found indications of increased internalization of symptoms, in some students [60], indicating the need to take the possibility of such effects into account in school-based interventions in general. However, we cannot conclude this, based on our results.

4.3. Limitations

The study has limitations that should be considered. First, although perceptions of a caring school climate and loneliness reflect important characteristics, these are not exhaustive measures of the psychosocial school environment. Hence, it could be the case that the interventions have influenced other significant aspects of the students' social lives that we have not captured in this study, e.g., more directly, the teacher–student relationship, previously shown to be of importance for dropout [3,53]. Second, although for many, if not most, the adolescents' social life in general will be greatly reflected in their school social life, our loneliness measure is not school-specific. For example, if an adolescent is lonely in all arenas of life (e.g., leisure time, etc.), it may not be "enough" to mitigate loneliness through psychosocial interventions at the school level. That having been said, there is often overlap in the social connections between school and leisure time activities, and as such, the loneliness measure still has relevance in relation to the question which is the focus of our study. Third, it should also be noted that the proportion and number of students not completing in the single-tier, multi-tier, and control groups was relatively low, and therefore, statistical differences between the groups related to completion should be interpreted with caution.

5. Conclusions

Multi-tier interventions are more demanding to implement than single-tier interventions [13], but our results suggest that they may be more effective in catering deeper change regarding how a larger proportion of students experience social life in and outside of school. Further, the completion and dropout of upper secondary education is a complex field that is not merely a matter of counting students who pass subjects. Today, as most Norwegian adolescents enroll in upper secondary education, the need to recognize the diversity in the student body is crucial, and a range of options must be available to guide and facilitate individual adolescents' needs. Although completion (either within three or five years) is desired, it will not be the solution for every adolescent. Within this context, both universal and targeted measures may constitute a positive contribution in supporting adolescents in their transition to adult life. Meanwhile, for good reason, the national goal to increase completion remains. Efforts to achieve this goal must also reflect a recognition that school interventions alone will likely not suffice but need to be complemented by coordinated action across key adolescent developmental arenas.

Author Contributions: Conceptualization, H.B.U., T.B.L. and S.M.E.K.; methodology, H.B.U., T.B.L. and S.M.E.K.; formal analysis, S.M.E.K.; writing—original draft preparation, H.B.U., T.B.L. and S.M.E.K.; writing—review and editing, H.B.U., T.B.L. and S.M.E.K.; visualization, S.M.E.K.; funding acquisition, T.B.L. All authors have read and agreed to the published version of the manuscript.

Funding: This research was funded by the Norwegian Research Council, grant number 20161789.

Institutional Review Board Statement: The study was conducted in accordance with the Declaration of Helsinki and approved by the Institutional Review Board of the Norwegian Center for Research Data (NSD) (protocol code 48551, 24.06.2016).

Informed Consent Statement: Informed consent was obtained from all subjects involved in the study.

Data Availability Statement: The data presented in this study are available on request from the corresponding author. The data are not publicly available due to ethical restrictions.

Acknowledgments: We gratefully acknowledge all collaborating partners in the project. A special thanks to all students and staff at our participating schools.

Conflicts of Interest: The authors declare no conflict of interest.

References

1. Larsen, T. Shifting towards positive youth development in schools in Norway–challenges and opportunities. *Int. J. Ment. Health Promot.* **2016**, *18*, 8–20. [CrossRef]
2. Falch, T.; Johannesen, A.B.; Strøm, B. *The Social Costs of Dropouts in Upper Secondary Education in Norway*; Centre for Economic Research, NTNU: Trondheim, Norway, 2010.
3. Lillejord, S.; Halvorsrud, K.; Ruud, E.; Morgan, K.; Freyr, T.; Fischer-Griffiths, P.; Eikeland, O.J.; Hauge, T.E.; Homme, A.D.; Manger, T. *Frafall i Videregående Opplæring: En Systematisk Kunnskapsoversikt [Student Dropout in Upper Secondary Education–A Systematic Review]*; Kunnskapssenter for Utdanning: Oslo, Norway, 2015.
4. Frostad, P.; Pijl, S.J.; Mjaavatn, P.E. Losing All Interest in School: Social Participation as a Predictor of the Intention to Leave Upper Secondary School Early. *Scand. J. Educ. Res.* **2015**, *59*, 110–122. [CrossRef]
5. Morin, A.H. Teacher support and the social classroom environment as predictors of student loneliness. *Soc. Psychol. Educ.* **2020**, *23*, 1687–1707. [CrossRef]
6. Rutter, M. *Fifteen Thousand Hours: Secondary Schools and Their Effects on Children*; Harvard University Press: Cambridge, MA, USA, 1979.
7. Eccles, J.S.; Roeser, R.W. Schools as Developmental Contexts During Adolescence. *J. Res. Adolesc.* **2011**, *21*, 225–241. [CrossRef]
8. Aldridge, J.M.; McChesney, K. The relationships between school climate and adolescent mental health and wellbeing: A systematic literature review. *Int. J. Educ. Res.* **2018**, *88*, 121–145. [CrossRef]
9. Baker, J.A.; Dilly, L.J.; Aupperlee, J.L.; Patil, S.A. The developmental context of school satisfaction: Schools as psychologically healthy environments. *Sch. Psychol. Q.* **2003**, *18*, 206. [CrossRef]
10. Gillander Gadin, K.; Hammarström, A. Do changes in the psychosocial school environment influence pupils' health development? Results from a three-year follow-up study. *Scand. J. Public Health* **2003**, *31*, 169–177. [CrossRef]
11. Jefferson, R.; Barreto, M.; Verity, L.; Qualter, P. Loneliness During the School Years: How It Affects Learning and How Schools Can Help*. *J. Sch. Health* **2023**, *93*, 428–435. [CrossRef]
12. Weare, K.; Nind, M. Mental health promotion and problem prevention in schools: What does the evidence say? *Health Promot. Int.* **2011**, *26*, i29–i69. [CrossRef]
13. Larsen, T.; Holsen, I.; Urke, H.B.; Anvik, C.H.; Waldahl, R.H. Doing Collaborative Health Promotion Research in a Complex Setting: Lessons Learned from the COMPLETE Project in Norway. In *Global Handbook of Health Promotion Research*; Potvin, L., Jourdan, D., Eds.; Springer International Publishing: Cham, Switzerland, 2022; Volume 1, pp. 247–260. [CrossRef]
14. Baumeister, R.F.; Leary, M.R. The need to belong: Desire for interpersonal attachments as a fundamental human motivation. *Psychol. Bull.* **1995**, *117*, 497. [CrossRef]
15. Buhrmester, D. Intimacy of Friendship, Interpersonal Competence, and Adjustment during Preadolescence and Adolescence. *Child Dev.* **1990**, *61*, 1101–1111. [CrossRef]
16. Steinberg, L.; Morris, A.S. Adolescent Development. *J. Cogn. Educ. Psychol.* **2001**, *2*, 55–87. [CrossRef]
17. Laursen, B.; Hartl, A.C. Understanding loneliness during adolescence: Developmental changes that increase the risk of perceived social isolation. *J. Adolesc.* **2013**, *36*, 1261–1268. [CrossRef]
18. Harris, R.A.; Qualter, P.; Robinson, S.J. Loneliness trajectories from middle childhood to pre-adolescence: Impact on perceived health and sleep disturbance. *J. Adolesc.* **2013**, *36*, 1295–1304. [CrossRef]
19. Heinrich, L.M.; Gullone, E. The clinical significance of loneliness: A literature review. *Clin. Psychol. Rev.* **2006**, *26*, 695–718. [CrossRef]
20. Mahon, N.E.; Yarcheski, A.; Yarcheski, T.J. Health consequences of loneliness in adolescents. *Res. Nurs. Health* **1993**, *16*, 23–31. [CrossRef]
21. Bakken, A. *Ungdata 2022. Nasjonale Resultater*; NOVA, OsloMet: Oslo, Norway, 2022.
22. Cacioppo, J.T.; Cacioppo, S. Chapter Three-Loneliness in the Modern Age: An Evolutionary Theory of Loneliness (ETL). In *Advances in Experimental Social Psychology*; Olson, J.M., Ed.; Academic Press: Cambridge, MA, USA, 2018; Volume 58, pp. 127–197. [CrossRef]
23. Perlman, D.; Peplau, L.A. Toward a social psychology of loneliness. *Pers. Relatsh.* **1981**, *3*, 31–56.
24. Cacioppo, J.T.; Hawkley, L.C.; Crawford, L.E.; Ernst, J.M.; Burleson, M.H.; Kowalewski, R.B.; Malarkey, W.B.; Van Cauter, E.; Berntson, G.G. Loneliness and Health: Potential Mechanisms. *Psychosom. Med.* **2002**, *64*, 407–417. [CrossRef]
25. Holt-Lunstad, J.; Smith, T.B.; Baker, M.; Harris, T.; Stephenson, D. Loneliness and Social Isolation as Risk Factors for Mortality: A Meta-Analytic Review. *Perspect. Psychol. Sci.* **2015**, *10*, 227–237. [CrossRef]
26. Haugan, J.A.; Frostad, P.; Mjaavatn, P.-E. A longitudinal study of factors predicting students' intentions to leave upper secondary school in Norway. *Soc. Psychol. Educ.* **2019**, *22*, 1259–1279. [CrossRef]
27. Ramsdal, G.; Gjærum, R.G.; Wynn, R. Dropout and early unemployment. *Int. J. Educ. Res.* **2013**, *62*, 75–86. [CrossRef]

28. Markussen, E. Education pays off! On transition to work for 25 year olds in Norway with upper secondary education or lower as their highest educational level. *Educ. Res. Policy Pract.* **2017**, *16*, 27–42. [CrossRef]
29. Birkeland, M.S.; Breivik, K.; Wold, B. Peer Acceptance Protects Global Self-esteem from Negative Effects of Low Closeness to Parents During Adolescence and Early Adulthood. *J. Youth Adolesc.* **2014**, *43*, 70–80. [CrossRef] [PubMed]
30. Park, N. The Role of Subjective Well-Being in Positive Youth Development. *Ann. Am. Acad. Pol. Soc. Sci.* **2004**, *591*, 25–39. [CrossRef]
31. Currie, C.; Roberts, C.; Morgan, A.; Smith, R.; Settertobulte, W.; Samadal, O.; Rasmussen, V.B. (Eds.) *Young People's Health in Context: International Report from the HBSC 2001/02 Survey, (Health Policy for Children and Adolescents, No.4)*; WHO Regional Office for Europe: Copenhagen, Denmark, 2004.
32. Hattie, J.; Yates, G.C.R. *Visible Learning and the Science of How We Learn*; Routledge: London, UK, 2013. [CrossRef]
33. Eccles, A.M.; Qualter, P. Review: Alleviating loneliness in young people—A meta-analysis of interventions. *Child Adolesc. Ment. Health* **2021**, *26*, 17–33. [CrossRef]
34. Galanaki, E.P.; Vassilopoulou, H.D. Teachers and children's loneliness: A review of the literature and educational implications. *Eur. J. Psychol. Educ.* **2007**, *22*, 455. [CrossRef]
35. Rokach, A. *The Correlates of Loneliness*; Bentham Science Publishers: Sharjah, United Arab Emirates, 2016.
36. Dobson, J.E.; Campbell, N.J.; Dobson, R. Relationships Among Loneliness, Perceptions of School, and Grade Point Averages of High School Juniors. *Sch. Couns.* **1987**, *35*, 143–148.
37. Zhang, B.; Gao, Q.; Fokkema, M.; Alterman, V.; Liu, Q. Adolescent interpersonal relationships, social support and loneliness in high schools: Mediation effect and gender differences. *Soc. Sci. Res.* **2015**, *53*, 104–117. [CrossRef]
38. Larsen, T.; Urke, H.B.; Holsen, I.; Anvik, C.H.; Olsen, T.; Waldahl, R.H.; Antonsen, K.M.; Johnson, R.; Tobro, M.; Brastad, B.; et al. COMPLETE—A school-based intervention project to increase completion of upper secondary school in Norway: Study protocol for a cluster randomized controlled trial. *BMC Public Health* **2018**, *18*, 340. [CrossRef]
39. Voksne for Barn. Om Drømmeskolen. Voksne Barn. 2023. Available online: https://vfb.no/produkter-og-tjenester/skoleprogrammer/drommeskolen-2/om-drommeskolen/ (accessed on 24 April 2023).
40. KIDSCREEN. Welcome to Our KIDSCREEN Website. kidscreen.org. 2023. Available online: http://www.kidscreen.org/english/ (accessed on 24 April 2023).
41. Kraft, P.; Loeb, M. *Sogn og Fjordane Prosjektet*; National Institute of Public Health: Oslo, Norway, 1997.
42. Mittelmark, M.B.; Aarø, L.E.; Henriksen, S.G.; Siqveland, J.; Torsheim, T. Chronic Social Stress in the Community and Associations with Psychological Distress: A Social Psychological Perspective. *Int. J. Ment. Health Promot.* **2004**, *6*, 5–17. [CrossRef]
43. Newton, M.; Fry, M.; Watson, D.; Gano-Overway, L.; Kim, M.S.; Magyar, M.; Guivernau, M. Psychometric properties of the Caring Climate Scale in a physical activity setting. *Rev. Psicol. Deporte* **2007**, *16*, 67–84.
44. Statistics Norway. Gjennomføring i Videregående Opplæring. SSB. 2022. Available online: https://www.ssb.no/utdanning/videregaende-utdanning/statistikk/gjennomforing-i-videregaende-opplaering (accessed on 6 May 2023).
45. Iversen, A.C.; Holsen, I. Inequality in Health, Psychosocial Resources and Health Behavior in Early Adolescence: The Influence of Different Indicators of Socioeconomic Position. *Child Indic. Res.* **2008**, *1*, 291–302. [CrossRef]
46. Kristensen, S.M.; Urke, H.B.; Larsen, T.B.; Danielsen, A.G. Hello Darkness, My Old Friend: Moderating a Random Intercept Cross-lagged Panel Model of Loneliness and Symptoms of Anxiety and Depression. *Res. Child Adolesc. Psychopathol.* **2023**, *51*, 383–397. [CrossRef]
47. Urke, H.B.; Kristensen, S.M.; Bøe, T.; Gaspar de Matos, M.; Wiium, N.; Årdal, E.; Larsen, T. Perceptions of a caring school climate and mental well-being: A one-way street? Results from a Random Intercept Cross-Lagged Panel Model. Under review in Applied Developmental Science n.d. *(in press)*
48. Chen, F.F. Sensitivity of Goodness of Fit Indexes to Lack of Measurement Invariance. *Struct. Equ. Model. Multidiscip. J.* **2007**, *14*, 464–504. [CrossRef]
49. Hu, L.; Bentler, P.M. Cutoff criteria for fit indexes in covariance structure analysis: Conventional criteria versus new alternatives. *Struct. Equ. Model. Multidiscip. J.* **1999**, *6*, 1–55. [CrossRef]
50. Tambs, K.; Moum, T. How well can a few questionnaire items indicate anxiety and depression? *Acta Psychiatr. Scand.* **1993**, *87*, 364–367. [CrossRef]
51. Newman, D.A. Missing Data: Five Practical Guidelines. *Organ. Res. Methods* **2014**, *17*, 372–411. [CrossRef]
52. Muthén, L.K.; Muthén, B.O. *Mplus User's Guide*, 8th ed.; Muthén & Muthén: Los Angeles, CA, USA, 1998.
53. Krane, V.; Karlsson, B.; Ness, O.; Kim, H.S. Teacher–student relationship, student mental health, and dropout from upper secondary school: A literature review. *Scand. Psychol.* **2016**, *3*, e11. [CrossRef]
54. Zee, M.; Koomen, H.M.Y. Teacher Self-Efficacy and Its Effects on Classroom Processes, Student Academic Adjustment, and Teacher Well-Being: A Synthesis of 40 Years of Research. *Rev. Educ. Res.* **2016**, *86*, 981–1015. [CrossRef]
55. Warner, L.M.; French, D.P. Self-Efficacy Interventions. In *The Handbook of Behavior Change*; Hagger, M.S., Cameron, L.D., Hamilton, K., Hankonen, N., Lintunen, T., Eds.; Cambridge University Press: Cambridge, MA, USA, 2020; p. 461.
56. Ryan, R.M.; Deci, E.L. *Self-Determination Theory. Basic Psychological Needs in Motivation, Development and Wellness*; Guilford Press: New York, NY, USA, 2017.
57. Núñez, J.L.; León, J. Autonomy Support in the Classroom: A Review From Self-Determination Theory. *Eur. Psychol.* **2015**, *20*, 275–283. [CrossRef]

58. Katz, I.; Kaplan, A.; Buzukashvily, T. The role of parents' motivation in students' autonomous motivation for doing homework. *Learn. Individ. Differ.* **2011**, *21*, 376–386. [CrossRef]
59. Taylor, G.; Jungert, T.; Mageau, G.A.; Schattke, K.; Dedic, H.; Rosenfield, S.; Koestner, R. A self-determination theory approach to predicting school achievement over time: The unique role of intrinsic motivation. *Contemp. Educ. Psychol.* **2014**, *39*, 342–358. [CrossRef]
60. Foulkes, L.; Stringaris, A. Do no harm: Can school mental health interventions cause iatrogenic harm? *BJPsych Bull.* **2023**, 1–3. [CrossRef] [PubMed]

International Journal of
Environmental Research and Public Health

MDPI

Article

The Impact of Urban Allotment Gardens on Physical and Mental Health in Norway

Mari Johnsrud [1], Ursula Småland Goth [2] and Hilde Skjerve [1,*]

[1] Department of Health and Exercise, School of Health Sciences, Kristiania University College, 0107 Oslo, Norway; marijohnsrud@hotmail.com
[2] NLA University College, Campus Oslo, 0103 Oslo, Norway; ursula.goth@nla.no
* Correspondence: hilde.skjerve@kristiania.no; Tel.: +47-92211819

Abstract: In Norway, many communities offer low-rent plots of land on which city dwellers can build summer cottages and grow crops. These allotment gardens serve as recreational escapes from urban life. However, little is known about the impact these gardens have on their members. This study attempts to shed light on today's impact of allotment gardens in a public health setting in Norway. The study was based on 17 semi-structured interviews and 2 in-depth interviews with allotment house owners. Informants were mainly recruited by "snowball sampling". Our data show that maintaining an allotment promotes exercise and provides a positive impact on self-perceived well-being and physical health through outdoor activities. Spending time in the garden contributes to new knowledge and experiences. Owning an allotment garden has provided new knowledge, new skills, new hobbies, and thereby an improvement in lifestyle. The allotment garden has a strong impact on perceived health, well-being, and sense of coherence (SOC) for the individuals. It promotes outdoor activities along with social interaction and can prevent feelings of loneliness and isolation.

Keywords: allotment house; allotment garden; quality of life; physical health; mental health; perceived health

1. Introduction

Allotment gardens often include simple cabins, usually built out of recycled materials on a small plot of land. The garden plots are given to local community members to serve as getaways from city life with opportunities to grow one's own vegetables and live closer to nature. The first allotment gardens were established in Norway in 1907. At the time, many Norwegians, especially those living in big cities like Oslo, faced difficult social conditions. Allotment gardens were therefore established to improve the lives of city dwellers. Today in Oslo alone, there are nine separate allotment gardens with 1097 houses, and as of 31 May 2022, there were 7672 people on a waiting list to obtain one [1,2]. The gardens are open for use between 1 April and 1 October. During the fall and winter, the water supply and sewage are cut off to avoid freezing.

There is a growing consensus that the places where people live and the various social processes, relationships, and psychosocial concepts are associated with healthy communities, and that neighborhoods contribute to health [3]. Only recently have studies begun to shed light on the allotment gardens' positive impact on experienced health, lifestyle, and activity levels [4] due to the higher intake of fruits and vegetables [5–7] and the reduction in lifestyle diseases [4,5,8,9].

In recent years, the number of people with mental health challenges has increased [10]. In the Coyle and Dugan study, there was an observed connection between loneliness and a higher risk of having some form of mental illness [11]. In one survey, 62% of those persons who were experiencing loneliness answered that they were dissatisfied with their lives ([12] p. 49). Elderly people (65+) are more likely to be affected by loneliness [13,14].

Fortunately, several studies have found that activities such as gardening helped to reduce the incidence of social isolation and exclusion [5,6,15]. Findings from Martens et al. showed that the allotment garden had a positive impact on the quality of life for older gardeners [16]. Gardening has been shown to prevent the development of poor self-rated health [15,17] and improve feelings of mental well-being [5,6]. People with cognitive disorders can benefit from gardening activities [5,6] as they can have a therapeutic impact on health both mentally and physically [18]. One study found that gardening had a positive effect on mental health regardless of the person's state of health [17]. Martens indicated that allotment gardens should be used as part of a low-threshold preventive health measure [16]. Being part of a social environment can have a positive impact on stress management and, under the right circumstances, lead to increased internal motivation and better self-regulation ([19] p. 16).

This study aims to shed light on the impact of allotment gardens today in a public health setting in Norway. By doing so, the study aims to identify factors that improve self-perceived health, well-being, and the impacts on inhabitants' everyday life.

2. Materials and Methods

This study was conducted in 2022 and is based on 17 semi-structured interviews and 2 in-depth interviews with allotment house dwellers. Four of the informants were between 31 and 55 years of age and the remaining fifteen informants were in the 56–85 age group.

2.1. Interview Guide and Recruitment

A semi-structured interview based on mapping, lifestyle in the allotment garden, and the perceived importance of the allotment garden (Supplementary File S1) was developed in collaboration with allotment house owners. All informants were over 18 years of age and had owned an allotment for at least six months. Informants were recruited via "snowball sampling", whereby study subjects are invited to recruit new subjects in an ever-growing, self-enlarging sample ([20] pp. 21, 77) and via an advertisement in one garden's Facebook group. The inclusion of 17 interviews during the COVID-19 restrictions showed data saturation. During the process of writing the article after the restrictions were lifted, we wanted to ensure data saturation and included two more interviews in the study. ([20] pp. 78–79). The in-depth interviews with allotment owners took place at their compound and lasted between 65 and 90 min.

2.2. Interview Method and Analysis of the Data

The initial study took place during the COVID-19 restrictions. As a consequence, only 13 interviews could be performed in person. Three interviews were conducted over the telephone, and one took place through a Zoom video meeting. The telephone interviews lasted from 25 to 40 min while the physical semi-structured interviews lasted a duration of 30–90 min. The telephone informants answered the questions more comprehensively and directly than the physical interviewees did.

After the COVID-19 restrictions were lifted and the first analysis was performed, data from two additional in-depth interviews were collected at the allotment compound. Those interviews lasted between 60 and 90 min.

Before an interview took place, the informants were told about the purpose of the study, the study design, and our intention to publish the results ([20] Ch. 5). The interviews were performed by M.J. and U.S.G. After each interview, the researcher showed the informant their notes and quotes, which the informant verified [21]. Only verified notes and quotes were included in the data. Immediately after the interview, the interviewers reflected on what was said This allowed us to register more reflections. The reflection took place immediately after the interview and reduced any recall bias ([20] p. 118).

The analysis was performed in collaboration with the authors. During the analyses, a template for deduction was used [22]. This stepwise analysis was an aid to coding and dividing the data into thematic groups [23]. The analysis divided our data into three thematic groups: (1) well-being and physical activity; (2) social activity/sense of coherence (SOC) and routine; and (3) place for the family. To reduce potential bias and assess the data's consistency, the authors validated the results, which were then summarized to give an overview. The analysis was seen as a process of examining and interpreting data to elicit meaning, gain understanding, and develop empirical knowledge. Empirical data were collected inductively and after that coded and grouped. Pre-existing theories found within the previous analysis were compared with data from the following interview.

2.3. Weaknesses of the Study That May Have Affected the Result

By using "Snowball recruiting" instead of collecting a random sample, representativeness could not be guaranteed. Therefore, a sampling bias might have occurred.

Snowball recruiting also had an impact on gender distribution. Even though we encouraged equal participation of both genders, only five men participated in the study.

We used no recording devices during the interviews to get the informants to speak freely, implicating no independent means to check the accuracy of the notes.

2.4. Ethics

The study followed the ethical guidelines of Norwegian Centre for Research Data that state that participation in research should be based on information, consent, anonymity and confidentiality. An informed consent form was given to each informant prior to starting the interview. Data were collected anonymously so no identifying information was collected and interviewers' responses were recorded through handwritten notes. This way, the study did not require ethical approval [24].

3. Results

3.1. Well-Being and Physical Activity

> *"Since I struggle with musculoskeletal disorders, I have days where I must pay extra attention and listen to the body when it needs rest. But gardening helps me to maintain normal function."* (Informant 1)

> *"I used to look at weeding as a chore, whereas now it's a bit like meditation."* (Informant 10)

> *"Being at my allotment house makes me feel young and active. I have a place to be with my family, socialize with my friends, and at the same time be physically active."* (Informant 18)

Our findings show that keeping an allotment is a great form of exercise. Most free time goes to gardening. Younger members had less time because of childcare and job requirements. Informants older than 56 spent more time growing plants, weeding, and carrying out maintenance work. Weather and time of year were the two factors affecting the amount of activity in the garden. During the winter, only short visits were made to the garden.

3.2. Life-Style: Experience and Knowledge

> *"My partner and I have learned a lot about cultivation and got green thumb after acquiring an allotment garden. We have become better at utilizing the raw materials we have in the garden."* (Informant 3)

> *"Through active gardening, I have experienced both physical and mental mastery because I get to do new things."* (Informant 1)

> *"I have learned to be more outdoors and become more aware of nature."* (Informant 4)

Spending time in an allotment garden contributes to new knowledge and experiences, and this contribution had an impact on lifestyle. As Table 1 indicates, all informants stated that they had gained new knowledge after acquiring an allotment garden. Fruit and vegetable cultivation, beekeeping, and tree pruning were some of the activities the informants mentioned. They affirmed that they gained knowledge through their own experience, through friends, family, or other gardeners, and that they experienced mastery through various activities.

Table 1. Usage of the allotment house and social interaction.

	31–55 Years (Percentages)	56–85 Years (Percentages)
Stay during season		
Full time	1 (25%)	11 (73%)
Part time	3 (75%)	4 (27%)
Garden (social) events and voluntary work		
Participated	1 (25%)	8 (54%)
Participated if required	3 (75%)	5 (33%)
Did not participate	0	2 (13%)
Importance of SOC/social interaction		
Participated in various activity groups and events	4 (100%)	13 (87%)
Did not participate in activity groups or events	0	2 (13%)
Was social with family, friends	4 (100%)	15 (100%)
Was not social with family, friends	0	0
Gained interest and knowledge (maintenance and gardening)		
Learned something new	4	15

Table 1, which is based on the interviews, illustrates that informants over 55 took more time to participate in social activities or voluntary work. Social interaction was more important for allotment owners between 56 and 85 years, and all participants expressed the importance of socializing with family and friends. Finally, all our informants gained interest and knowledge in growing vegetables and fruits and by maintaining the allotment house.

3.3. Social Activity and Sense of Coherence

> *"I think that having access to an allotment garden is the biggest factor that protects against loneliness, depression, isolation, and diseases. And you get a sense of belonging. It also helps to even out socio-cultural differences."* (Informant 4)

> *"The social life in the allotment garden has meant a lot for my health and well-being, especially during COVID-19. Had it not been for the allotment garden, I probably would have climbed the walls."* (Informant 5)

As the quotes reveal, social interactions with family, friends, and other gardeners were and are an important part of life in the allotment community. For most of our informants the garden can counter loneliness. Particularly, vulnerable people and those over 55 will find SOC through social interaction with others (Table 1). Our data also showed that the social environment was especially important among those who spent every day in the garden during the growing season. This was not the case for allotment owners under 55. For them, work, childcare, and household activities took up most of their time; therefore, they could not spend every day in the garden.

Social events are a central part of the allotment garden. Most informants were positive about attending events. Only 2 of the 19 informants stated that they never or rarely participated in social events.

The feeling of belonging and social interaction is central to one's well-being. During the outbreak of COVID-19 in 2020, two of the informants mentioned that the garden was a life saver for their mental, physical, and social health.

3.4. Daily Routine and Physical Activity

> *"I feel a responsibility to manage the existing natural basis that is in the garden in the most sustainable way possible."* (Informant 6)

> *"I feel a responsibility that my daughter should have a nice and green place to grow up."* (Informant 4)

As our data show, many of the informants' lives centered around he allotment garden. Many informants also mentioned the garden's positive impact on both physical and mental health. For instance, informants that recently experienced disruptive situations like retirement or divorce found allotment activities to be a stabilizing factor in their lives.

Our data also indicate that, by keeping an allotment garden, which requires a lot of hard work and advanced planning, our informants had the feeling of SOC and mastery when seeing a project through from start to finish.

3.5. Place for the Family

> *"I cannot afford a garden and a house. It would have been a completely different upbringing for my daughter if we had not had an allotment garden. There's the freedom, the belonging, and things she has learned from being here. She would have had a much poorer upbringing without the allotment garden. This also applies to many of her friends from school and the neighborhood."* (Informant 4)

> *"The allotment house gives me the opportunity to interact with my family and see several members at the same time. It looks like the garden has been a place where we meet and have time for each other."* (Informant 17)

> *"The allotment garden is a great place for all of us. Here, we can also teach our children where the food comes from."* (Informant 2)

4. Discussion

Communities like those we find at urban allotment gardens are more likely to experience better self-reported health and well-being [3]. Allotment gardens have been in existence since 1907, yet we still have little knowledge about their benefits for the people who tend them [3,25].

4.1. Well-Being and Physical Activity

Salutogenesis predicts that organized physical activity can be a health resource [13,14]. Previous studies have confirmed that an allotment garden lowers the threshold for being outdoors and socializing with other people [6,8,18]. We found similar results in our study, indicating that allotment gardens have a significant impact on well-being and physical health and thereby on the individual's mental health.

4.2. Knowledge

Living in an allotment garden has provided new knowledge, new skills, new hobbies, and therefore a change in lifestyle. The experience of learning and mastering has a beneficial effect on self-development and self-esteem in humans [19]. Genter et al. found that allotment gardens could facilitate self-development and a sense of mastery [18]. In our study, several informants described their involvement with activities such as beekeeping, gardening, organizing social events, or coffee meetings. As other studies [8] show, the feeling of belonging and SOC is essential for one's well-being, and we saw how an allotment garden fulfilled at least some of those needs.

4.3. Mental Health

Green spaces can play an important role in health promotion ([26] Ch. 18). During the COVID-19 pandemic, there was considerable research about the role of private gardens and digital nature, which demonstrated that natural environments have the potential to buffer the impact of stressful events [27]. Lachowycz and Jones suggest that there are psychological benefits that can be derived from contact with nature such as stress reduction and positive emotions [28]. Seen from a salutogenic perspective, physical activity in an allotment garden has been shown to be a meaningful, comprehensible, and manageable way for older people to maintain their health [26] and that gardening might help reduce stress [6,18,29]. In addition, our findings show that gardening can be recommended for elderly people, ethnical minorities, and people with long-term health challenges by preventing social exclusion. Our finding was also seen in a study by Hajek and Köning [15,30].

4.4. Social Interactions, Room for Family and Friends, and the Perceived Significance of the Allotment Garden

SOC is a construct that refers to the extent to which one sees one's world as comprehensive, manageable, and meaningful [27]. In our study, we saw that the nature of the links between coherence and adaption reinforced each other.

Social interaction is an essential part of everyday life in an allotment garden, and especially important for vulnerable groups such as, the elderly, migrants, and single families, for example [30]. Gardeners contribute to and benefit the local environment [4], which increases social interaction [25]. Several informants pointed out their participation in various groups and events, and our study results show that carrying out gardening was important for their well-being.

The allotment garden's role in residents' well-being must not be underestimated [31]. It is therefore natural to understand that the loss of an allotment garden will affect a person's health.

5. Conclusions

Clearly, living in a garden house boosts one's health and social life and could be an important facility for vulnerable groups in the population. As our data show, allotment gardens are experienced as an arena for the inclusion of vulnerable groups such as the elderly, migrants, or single parents for various reasons. Therefore, our study concludes that the impact of public allotment gardens is characterized by a social and physically active lifestyle. Age, life situation, and interests determine how the residents utilize their garden. A garden has a significant impact on the lives of the owners, family members, friends, and the public visiting the compound. A garden has a strong impact on perceived health, well-being, and SOC for the individual, leading to increased outdoor activities and social interaction. While the findings suggest potential benefits, more comprehensive research is needed to confirm these outcomes.

Further Research

Further research is needed. Until recently, there have been few scientific studies on allotment gardens. This study used a qualitative approach and covered only one of Norway's allotment gardens. Follow-up studies could include other gardens within Norway, Denmark, or Austria where allotment gardens are common, and include a balance of genders, ages, and educational levels.

Supplementary Materials: The following supporting information can be downloaded at: https://www.mdpi.com/article/10.3390/ijerph21060720/s1, File S1: Questionnaire (translated from Norwegian).

Author Contributions: Conceptualization, M.J.; methodology, M.J. and H.S.; formal analysis, M.J., H.S. and U.S.G.; investigation/interviews, M.J. and U.S.G.; writing/original draft preparation, M.J.; writing/review and editing, U.S.G. and H.S.; visualization, M.J.; supervision, H.S. All authors have read and agreed to the published version of the manuscript.

Funding: This research received no external funding.

Institutional Review Board Statement: Ethical review and approval were waived for this study due to the fact that the research project did not collect personal data.

Informed Consent Statement: Informed consent was obtained from all subjects involved in the study and to publish this paper.

Data Availability Statement: The original contributions presented in the study are included in the article, further inquiries can be directed to the corresponding author.

Acknowledgments: The authors want to acknowledge their appreciation to Sogn kolonihage (Sogn Allotment Association) in Oslo, Norway.

Conflicts of Interest: The authors declare no conflicts of interest.

References

1. FAQ—Ventelisten. Oslo Krets av NKHF. Available online: https://oslokolonihager.com/ventelisten/ (accessed on 20 October 2021).
2. Kolonihagene i Oslo. Oslo Krets av NKHF. Available online: https://oslokolonihager.com/ (accessed on 20 October 2021).
3. Vaandrager, L.; Kennedy, L. The Application of Salutogenesis in Communities and Neighborhoods. In *The Handbook of Salutogenesis*; Mittelmark, M.B., Sagy, S., Eriksson, M., Bauer, G.F., Pelikan, J.M., Lindström, B., Espnes, G.A., Eds.; Springer: Cham, Switzerland, 2017; ISBN 978-3-319-04599-3.
4. Alaimo, K.; Beavers, A.W.; Crawford, C.; Snyder, E.H.; Litt, J.S. Amplifying Health Through Community Gardens: A Framework for Advancing Multicomponent, Behaviorally Based Neighborhood Interventions. *Curr. Environ. Health Rep.* **2016**, *3*, 302–312. [CrossRef]
5. Howarth, M.; Brettle, A.; Hardman, M.; Maden, M. What Is the Evidence for the Impact of Gardens and Gardening on Health and Well-Being: A Scoping Review and Evidence-Based Logic Model to Guide Healthcare Strategy Decision Making on the Use of Gardening Approaches as a Social Prescription. *BMJ Open* **2020**, *10*, e036923. [CrossRef]
6. Wood, C.J.; Pretty, J.; Griffin, M. A Case–Control Study of the Health and Well-Being Benefits of Allotment Gardening. *J. Public Health* **2016**, *38*, e336–e344. [CrossRef]
7. Machida, D. Relationship between Community or Home Gardening and Health of the Elderly: A Web-Based Cross-Sectional Survey in Japan. *Int. J. Environ. Res. Public Health* **2019**, *16*, 1389. [CrossRef]
8. Soga, M.; Cox, D.T.C.; Yamaura, Y.; Gaston, K.J.; Kurisu, K.; Hanaki, K. Health Benefits of Urban Allotment Gardening: Improved Physical and Psychological Well-Being and Social Integration. *Int. J. Environ. Res. Public Health* **2017**, *14*, 71. [CrossRef]
9. Blair, C.K.; Adsul, P.; Guest, D.D.; Sussman, A.L.; Cook, L.S.; Harding, E.M.; Rodman, J.; Duff, D.; Burgess, E.; Quezada, K.; et al. Southwest Harvest for Health: An Adapted Mentored Vegetable Gardening Intervention for Cancer Survivors. *Nutrients* **2021**, *13*, 2319. [CrossRef]
10. *Voluntary National Review 2021 Norway. Report on the Implementation of the 2030 Agenda for Sustainable Development*; Norwegian Ministry of Local Government and Modernisation: Oslo, Norway, 2021; p. 123.
11. Coyle, C.E.; Dugan, E. Social Isolation, Loneliness and Health Among Older Adults. *J. Aging Health* **2012**, *24*, 1346–1363. [CrossRef]
12. Støren, K.S.; Rønning, E.; Gram, K.H. *Livskvalitet i Norge 2020*; Rapporter; Statistisk Sentralbyrå: Oslo-Kongsvinger, Norway, 2020; p. 76.
13. Omsorgsdepartementet, H. Meld. St. 19 (2018–2019); regjeringen.no, 2019. Available online: https://www.regjeringen.no/contentassets/84138eb559e94660bb84158f2e62a77d/nn-no/pdfs/stm201820190019000dddpdfs.pdf (accessed on 20 October 2021).
14. Omsorgsdepartementet, H. Meld. St. 15 (2017–2018); regjeringen.no, 2018. Available online: https://www.regjeringen.no/contentassets/196f99e63aa14f849c4e4b9b9906a3f8/no/pdfs/stm201720180015000dddpdfs.pdf (accessed on 20 October 2021).
15. Hajek, A.; König, H.-H. Self-Rated Health and Social Exclusion: Does Gardening Moderate This Relation? Evidence from the German Ageing Survey. *Int. J. Environ. Res. Public Health* **2019**, *16*, 1834. [CrossRef]
16. Martens, N.E.; Nordh, H.; Gonzalez, M.T. Visiting the Allotment Garden—A Complete Experience. *J. Hous. Elder.* **2018**, *32*, 121–134. [CrossRef]
17. Shiue, I. Gardening Is Beneficial for Adult Mental Health: Scottish Health Survey, 2012–2013. *Scand. J. Occup. Ther.* **2016**, *23*, 320–325. [CrossRef]
18. Genter, C.; Roberts, A.; Richardson, J.; Sheaff, M. The Contribution of Allotment Gardening to Health and Wellbeing: A Systematic Review of the Literature. *Br. J. Occup. Ther.* **2015**, *78*, 593–605. [CrossRef]
19. Samdal, O.; Wold, B.; Harris, A.; Torsheim, T. *Stress og Mestring*; Helsedirektoratet: Oslo, Norway, 2017.
20. Green, J.; Thorogood, N. *Qualitative Methods for Health Research*, 4th ed.; SAGE Publication Ltd.: London, UK, 2018; ISBN 978-1-4739-9710-3.
21. Naderifar, M.; Goli, H.; Ghaljaei, F. Snowball Sampling: A Purposeful Method of Sampling in Qualitative Research. *Strides Dev. Med. Educ.* **2017**, *in press*. [CrossRef]
22. Hansen, E.C. *Successful Qualitative Health Research: A Practical Introduction*; Routledge: London, UK, 2020; ISBN 978-1-00-024654-4.
23. Kvalitative Forskningsmetoder i Praksis by Tjora, Aksel. 9788205546530. Heftet—2021. Akademika.No. Available online: https://www.akademika.no/realfag/naturvitenskap-filosofi-teori-og-metode/kvalitative-forskningsmetoder-i-praksis/9788205546530?gclid=Cj0KCQjwtamlBhD3ARIsAARoaEw9KOLa-LYZv0WFDCpMa71qlLk54GK4nU_dVjgJib_REb9lee2tBecaAqFxEALw_wcB (accessed on 10 July 2023).

24. Publisert: 6 September 2022, T.K.F. Kvalitativ Metode. Available online: https://www.forskningsetikk.no/ressurser/fbib/metoder/kvalitativ-metode/ (accessed on 10 July 2023).
25. Litt, J.S.; Soobader, M.-J.; Turbin, M.S.; Hale, J.W.; Buchenau, M.; Marshall, J.A. The Influence of Social Involvement, Neighborhood Aesthetics, and Community Garden Participation on Fruit and Vegetable Consumption. *Am. J. Public Health* **2011**, *101*, 1466–1473. [CrossRef]
26. Ericson, H.; Quennerstedt, M.; Geidne, S. Physical Activity as a Health Resource: A Cross-Sectional Survey Applying a Salutogenic Approach to What Older Adults Consider Meaningful in Organised Physical Activity Initiatives. *Health Psychol. Behav. Med.* **2021**, *9*, 858–874. [CrossRef]
27. Nigg, C.; Petersen, E.; MacIntyre, T. Natural Environments, Psychosocial Health, and Health Behaviors in a Crisis—A Scoping Review of the Literature in the COVID-19 Context. *J. Environ. Psychol.* **2023**, *88*, 102009. [CrossRef]
28. Lachowycz, K.; Jones, A.P. Towards a Better Understanding of the Relationship between Greenspace and Health: Development of a Theoretical Framework. *Landsc. Urban Plan.* **2013**, *118*, 62–69. [CrossRef]
29. Antonovsky, A. *Unraveling the Mystery of Health: How People Manage Stress and Stay Well*; Jossey-Bass: San Francisco, CA, USA, 1987; p. 218, ISBN 978-1-55542-028-4.
30. Goth, U.; Lyshol, H.; Tellnes, G.; Berg, J.; Ihle, R.; Sudmann, T.; Bonsaksen, T.; Fevang, M.; Moser, T.; Misvaer, N.; et al. Goth, US (Red). In *2014. Folkehelse i et Norsk Perspektiv. Gyldendal Akademisk*; Gyldendal Akademiske: Oslo, Norway, 2014; ISBN 978-82-05-46395-0.
31. Young, C.; Bauer, N. Eviction from Paradise: Lived Experience, Psycho-Social and Health Effects of Allotment Garden Loss. *Urban For. Urban Green.* **2022**, *75*, 127708. [CrossRef]

International Journal of
Environmental Research and Public Health

MDPI

Article

Conceptualising a Community-Based Response to Loneliness: The Representational Anchoring of Nature-Based Social Prescription by Professionals in Marseille, Insights from the RECETAS Project

Lucie Cattaneo [1], Alexandre Daguzan [1], Gabriela García Vélez [2] and Stéphanie Gentile [1,3,*]

[1] Service d'Evaluation Médicale, Hôpital sainte Marguerite, Assistance Publique des Hôpitaux de Marseille, 13009 Marseille, France; lucie.cattaneo@ap-hm.fr (L.C.); alexandre.daguzan@ap-hm.fr (A.D.)
[2] City Preservation Management Research Group, Faculty of Architecture and Urbanism, University of Cuenca, Cuenca 010150, Ecuador; gabriela.garcia@ucuenca.edu.ec
[3] School of Medicine, Aix Marseille Université, SSA, RITME, 13005 Marseille, France
* Correspondence: stephaniemarie.gentile@ap-hm.fr

Abstract

Background: Urban loneliness is rising worldwide and is a recognised public-health threat. Nature-Based Social Prescriptions (NBSPs), guided group activities in natural settings, are being piloted in six cities through the EU project RECETAS. However, in new contexts such as Marseille, its implementation is constrained by professionals' limited knowledge of the concept. Objectives: (i) Exploring how professionals in Marseille (France) conceptualise NBSPs; (ii) Identifying perceived facilitators and barriers to implementing NBSPs among residents facing social isolation and loneliness. Methods: Twelve semi-structured interviews were conducted with health, social-care, and urban–environment professionals selected via network mapping and snowball sampling. Verbatim transcripts underwent inductive thematic analysis informed by Social Representation Theory, with double coding to enhance reliability. Results: Five analytic themes emerged: (1) a holistic health paradigm linking nature, community, and well-being; (2) stark ecological inequities with limited green-space access in deprived districts; (3) work challenges due to the urgent needs of individuals facing significant socio-economic challenges in demanding contexts; (4) a key tension between a perceived top-down process and a preference for participatory approaches; (5) drivers and obstacles: strong professional endorsement of NBSPs meets significant systemic and institutional constraints. Conclusions: Professionals endorse NBSPs as a promising approach against loneliness, provided programmes tackle structural inequities and adopt participatory governance. Results inform the Marseille RECETAS pilot and contribute to global discussions on environmentally anchored health promotion.

Keywords: loneliness; social isolation; nature-based social prescription; social representations; qualitative research; urban inequalities; participatory approaches; health promotion; health inequalities

1. Introduction

Loneliness, defined as the perceived gap between desired and actual social relationships, has become a major public-health determinant [1]. In France, the proportion of adults who report feeling lonely "often or almost every day" rose from 19% in 2020 to 29% in 2022 [2]. This rise mirrors global trends driven by rapid urbanisation, fragmentation of family ties and, more recently, COVID-19 distancing measures. Chronic loneliness is linked to a 26% increase in all-cause mortality and is an established risk factor for cardiovascular disease, depression, and cognitive decline [3]. Despite substantial evidence, loneliness remains insufficiently acknowledged in public health and social policy and continues to be predominantly conceptualised as an individual deficit rather than as the outcome of structural social, economic, or environmental determinants [2,4–6].

Addressing loneliness, therefore, requires systemic, cross-sectoral interventions that tackle its social and environmental determinants. Social prescribing, as developed within the UK National Health Service, connects individuals to non-medical community activities, such as creative workshops, walking groups or volunteering, and has shown positive effects on well-being and social connectedness [7,8]. Among the different forms of social prescribing, Nature-Based Social Prescription (NBSP) offers unique potential by leveraging the restorative, socially connective, and health-promoting qualities of natural environments. Rooted in the framework of the social determinants of health (SDH), it seeks to address the combined effects of social isolation, socio-economic deprivation, limited access to healthcare, and territorial fragmentation in urban settings [9].

In Marseille, France's second-largest city, these challenges are concentrated in the northern districts, where most of the 38 Priority Neighbourhoods (Quartiers Prioritaires de la Ville, QPV) are located and poverty rates are more than double the national average [10,11]. These areas, shaped by successive migration waves, are home predominantly to residents of North African, sub-Saharan African and Comorian origin [12]. They experience intersecting forms of disadvantage, including economic hardship, territorial stigmatisation, language barriers and limited administrative literacy, which restrict social support networks and reinforce structural isolation [13]. Vulnerability is not evenly distributed: young people, low-income older adults, people with disabilities or chronic illness, and single-parent families in precarious situations are particularly overrepresented among socially isolated residents [14].

Mobility and environmental inequalities further compound these challenges. Although Marseille is five times larger than Lyon, its public transport network extends only 30 km compared to 73 km in Lyon. In the most deprived districts, 40% of households lack a private vehicle, limiting access to employment, services and social participation [15]. Green space provision is equally unequal: despite the Calanques National Park covering 20% of the city, Marseille offers only 5 m^2 per inhabitant, six times less than Lyon and far below the WHO minimum recommendation of 9 m^2 [16,17]. For many vulnerable residents in northern districts, these combined mobility and environmental constraints make nature both physically and symbolically distant, despite its well-documented benefits for health and social connection.

In this context, loneliness in Marseille reflects the combined impact of social, territorial, and environmental inequalities. This intersection is precisely where the European project RECETAS (Reimagining Environments for Connection and Engagement: Testing Actions for Social Prescribing in Natural Spaces) operates. Launched in 2021, RECETAS pilots NBSP interventions in six cities: Barcelona, Cuenca, Helsinki, Marseille, Melbourne, and Prague. The project's central aim is to reduce loneliness in urban settings by testing and evaluating an innovative intervention based on NBSP [18]. In Marseille, the focus is on residents of deprived neighbourhoods who face migration-related barriers and multiple, overlapping forms of exclusion, placing them at heightened risk of chronic loneliness [19]. To adapt the intervention to this local context, RECETAS designed a co-creative process with local actors, structured in the following three progressive phases: diagnosis, participatory diagnosis, and co-creation [19]. The initial diagnosis phase sought to build a foundational understanding of the local context, its challenges, and the network of actors able to propose nature-based solutions, before the intervention design was co-developed with beneficiaries in later phases.

As part of this initial diagnosis phase, NBSP was found to be largely unfamiliar: a 2021 mapping of local actors showed that 89% of professionals in Marseille did not know the term. Understanding how such an unfamiliar concept is interpreted requires an analytical framework that explains how new ideas are made meaningful. Social Representation Theory (SRT) provides such a framework, with the concept of anchoring describing how novel interventions are incorporated into pre-existing knowledge, values, and practices [20,21]. By situating the study within SRT, the analysis not only explores local perceptions of NBSPs but also aims to illuminate processes and dynamics that may inform its adoption in other urban contexts facing comparable socio-environmental challenges. The objective of this study is, therefore, to explore how professionals in health, social care, and urban–environment sectors conceptualise NBSP at the outset, and to identify perceived facilitators and barriers to its implementation.

2. Methods

2.1. Study Design

This study adopted an exploratory qualitative approach. The methodology was grounded in a constructivist and interpretivist epistemological stance, which holds that knowledge is co-constructed through interaction and shaped by social and professional contexts. In this perspective, reality is not considered fixed and objective, but rather the product of shared meanings emerging through dialogue between participants and researchers. The constructivist stance emphasises that these meanings are context-dependent, while the interpretivist stance focuses on understanding the subjective experiences and interpretations of individuals within their specific socio-professional environments.

This positioning aligns with the theoretical framework of Social Representation Theory, particularly the process of anchoring, through which a new social object, such as NBSP, is made meaningful based on pre-existing knowledge and shared understandings held by individuals, for instance, regarding conceptions of health and nature [22]. Based on the principle that this knowledge is mobilised by actors and accessible through individual discourse, an inductive approach using research interviews made it possible to explore the categories and meanings used to construct the concept of NBSPs [23]. Accordingly, the research design privileged open-ended, flexible questioning and reflexive analysis to capture the diversity of perspectives. This approach also allowed for the co-construction of meaning throughout the data collection process. The holistic nature of qualitative inquiry is especially well-suited to capturing the complexity involved in integrating an emerging concept such as NBSP across different professional domains, where disciplinary boundaries, limited institutional recognition, and unfamiliarity with the approach may challenge its implementation. The study is reported in accordance with the COREQ (Consolidated Criteria for Reporting Qualitative Research) checklist [24].

2.2. Participants and Recruitment

Participant recruitment was based on a 2021 mapping of local actors. This mapping took the form of a Social Network Analysis (SNA), conducted in collaboration with Visible Network Labs via the PARTNER platform. Its objective was to understand how organisations in the pilot cities addressed loneliness and well-being through social prescribing and nature-based activities. For the Marseille context, this analysis identified a network of 392 organisations, from which the 12 professionals were ultimately selected to participate in this study based on the inclusion criteria (see Table 1).

Table 1. Distribution of the sample according to professional affiliation.

Interview	Profession	Organisation	NBSP Domain
1	Educator (o)	Social support drop-in centre	S
2	Coordinator (o)	Local non-profit association	S
3	General practitioner (o)	Primary healthcare unit	H
4	Manager (dm)	Regional public health agency	H
5	Head of service (o)	Shelter and social reintegration centre	S
6	Project officer (dm)	Municipal urban agriculture initiative	UN
7	Project officer (o)	Municipal urban agriculture initiative	UN
8	Coordinator (dm)	Public health and urban health programme	H
9	General practitioner (o)	Hospital-based healthcare unit	H
10	Project officer (dm)	Regional public health agency	UN
11	Coordinator (dm)	Municipal environmental department	H
12	Volunteer, Association President (o)	Community gardening association	UN

NBSP domain: H = Health; S = Social action; UN = Urban nature. Role: (dm) = Decision-making; (o) = Operational. Participants were selected to ensure coverage of all three domains and representation of both decision-making and operational roles.

Drawing on the Marseille dataset, the sample was constructed using purposive sampling, supplemented by snowball sampling [25], where initial participants meeting the inclusion criteria were first identified from the SNA list and invited to participate. This extended recruitment to actors not captured in the original mapping and ensured sectoral diversity across fields such as health, social work, urban planning, and environmental NGOs. The inclusion criteria were twofold: (1) representing key NBSP domains (health, social action, urban nature) and (2) holding either a decision-making or operational role, to capture representations across different hierarchical levels. Recruitment and preliminary analysis were conducted iteratively, with interviews transcribed and coded in parallel to identify emerging themes. Thematic saturation was considered reached when two consecutive interviews yielded no new codes or substantial insights relevant to the research objectives. This point occurred after the tenth interview, with two additional interviews conducted to confirm it. This resulted in a total of twelve participants [26].

2.3. Data Collection

Twelve semi-structured interviews (SSIs) were conducted in person, each lasting between 45 and 75 min. The interviews took place at participants' workplaces or, in two cases, in neutral public spaces to ensure confidentiality and participant comfort. All professionals were informed of the study's objectives and the voluntary nature of their participation. They were also informed that no nominative data (direct or indirect) would be collected. Verbal informed consent was obtained prior to each interview, in accordance with ethical standards for minimal-risk qualitative research [27]. The NBSP intervention in Marseille was approved by the Ethics Committee of the University of Aix-Marseille (N/Ref: 2023-01-05-03). With participants' authorisation, all interviews were audio-recorded and transcribed verbatim for analysis. The interviews were conducted by a health psychologist trained in qualitative methods and discourse analysis, ensuring both methodological consistency and sensitivity to the personal and professional dimensions explored. The interviewer maintained a reflexive stance throughout the research process, acknowledging her professional background in health psychology and prior involvement in the RECETAS project, and considering how these might influence data collection and interpretation. The wider research team, which included public health specialists, social scientists, and environmental health experts, regularly discussed how their diverse disciplinary backgrounds, professional experiences, and positions within the project could shape the interpretation and emphasis of specific themes. A reflexive journal was kept to document potential biases and analytical decisions. Each interview began with a free-association task in which professionals were asked to spontaneously cite four words or ideas that came to mind upon hearing the term "Nature-Based Social Prescription". (prompt: "Please tell me the four words, expressions, or ideas that spontaneously come to mind when you hear 'Nature-Based Social Prescription'"). This technique, commonly used in research on social representations, is designed to elicit immediate associations and latent representations prior to engaging in a guided discussion [23]. Unlike some approaches that analyse these evocations in isolation, it was decided to incorporate them directly into the broader thematic analysis, consistent with a holistic interpretation of meaning construction on a new social object such as NBSP.

The remainder of the interview followed a semi-structured guide organised around five thematic areas: (1) professional role and positioning; (2) professional experiences with the target populations; (3) perceptions of loneliness and well-being; (4) the role of nature in health and social action; (5) conditions for the appropriation of NBSP and the involvement of target groups. The guide was developed collaboratively by the research team, piloted with two professionals from outside the study sample, and refined for clarity and relevance before data collection began.

2.4. Data Analysis

All interviews were transcribed verbatim in their original language (French) and analysed using an inductive thematic analysis following a six-step approach [28]. Data management and coding were facilitated using NVivo 12 software (QSR International, Melbourne, Australia), which allowed for the systematic organisation of codes and themes. After an initial immersion phase involving repeated readings of the transcripts, each interview was systematically coded into distinct units of meaning, which were then grouped to form potential initial themes. To ensure reliability, this initial coding was conducted independently by two health psychologists, who then met to compare their coding, resolve discrepancies, and establish a consensual coding scheme. This scheme was subsequently applied to the entire dataset, focusing on identifying commonalities and differences across interviews. A comparative matrix in NVivo mapped convergences and divergences in coding, allowing the naming and hierarchical organisation of final themes and sub-themes. The process also examined differences and similarities in representations according to professional sectors (health, social, urban/environment) and hierarchical roles (operational vs. decision-making).

This combined integration of spontaneous discourse from the free-association task and more developed reflections enabled a nuanced interpretation of the anchoring processes shaping professionals' emerging representations of NBSP. As an additional validation strategy, preliminary themes were discussed within the research team to ensure interpretive coherence and minimise individual bias. However, no formal member checking with participants was conducted, due to time constraints and the exploratory nature of the study, which prioritised timely thematic synthesis over iterative participant validation.

3. Results

Thematic content analysis revealed five major themes and thirteen sub-themes, as detailed in Table 2. These themes are: (I) a holistic conception of health, community, and nature; (II) structural inequalities in Marseille; (III) populations facing cumulative disadvantage; (IV) pathways toward participation and recognition; (V) barriers and facilitators to NBSP implementation.

Table 2. Thematic structure of the analysis: key themes and sub-themes regarding the implementation of NBSP.

	Theme		Sub-Themes
I.	A holistic conception of health, community, and nature	1	Health as a multidimensional and interconnected phenomenon
		2	The need for social belonging as a core human experience
		3	Perceived continuity between humans and nature
		4	Nature-based activities as catalysts for social connection
II.	Structural inequalities in Marseille	5	Urban living conditions as a barrier to well-being
		6	Reproduction of social inequalities through unequal access to nature
III.	Populations facing cumulative disadvantage	7	A focus on basic needs limiting long-term engagement
		8	Expressions of psychosocial distress among target groups
IV.	Pathways toward participation and recognition	9	Conditions for meaningful public participation
		10	Recognition of local knowledge and lived experience
V.	Barriers and facilitators to NBSP implementation	11	Difficulties in engaging structurally isolated populations
		12	Institutional constraints and top-down dynamics
		13	Enablers of NBSP implementation

3.1. A Holistic Conception of Health, Community, and Nature

This first theme comprises three sub-themes: an ecosystemic view of health, the fundamental role of social belonging, and nature as a vital and socially mediating entity, each with distinct yet interconnected dimensions.

Professionals consensually articulated an integrated vision of health, nature, and community. Health was unanimously described as a dynamic ecosystem involving multiple interacting factors. One professional explained that basic needs like eating and housing are often considered priorities, "without realizing that this is already part of global health" (SSI 9). In this ecosystemic view of health, the focus was on the interdependence between physical, social, and environmental conditions as structural determinants of well-being, rather than on isolated factors. This perspective primarily emphasised the systemic and environmental context in which health is maintained.

Following this, the social belonging dimension, raised by 11 out of 12 professionals across all sectors, referred specifically to the perceived need to feel part of a group or community. Whereas the ecosystemic view addresses macro-level interconnections between health, society, and the environment, social belonging was described at the micro- and meso-levels, focusing on interpersonal bonds, emotional support, and collective identity. Together, these two dimensions were presented as complementary components of an "interdependent well-being" framework. Most professionals (10 out of 12) stated that nature-based interventions foster strong social bonds. One professional highlighted the need to "feel surrounded, to feel like we belong to a community, even if it's just for the duration of a one-hour activity" (SSI 6), while another described interventions such as

NBSP as enabling a "social encounter between inhabitants of the same neighbourhood or building" (SSI 10).

Finally, nature was perceived as a foundational element, "what keeps us alive" (SSI 12), and as a means of connection, helping to "break symbolic barriers" (SSI 3). All but one professional (11 out of 12) described nature as both a vital need for humans and a socially mediating entity, often anchored in familiar and positively valued symbolic meanings. Within the Social Representation Theory framework, this symbolic anchoring positions nature as a universally recognisable and culturally shared reference point that facilitates inclusion, trust, and shared purpose in social interactions. A spiritual dimension to this ontological connection was mentioned by nine professionals across all sectors, and was described as an intrinsic part of the relationship with nature rather than a separate belief system. Nature was described as a superior and autonomous entity that surpasses us, is intrinsically beautiful, and universal across all cultures. One professional stated, "it seems to me that spirituality is completely part of the relationship with nature. We are part of a whole" (SSI 5). This shared vision was seen as favourable to the acceptance of NBSP, which was perceived as a logical extension of this interdependent and holistic perspective. While this shared holistic vision provides a strong conceptual basis for NBSP, professionals also emphasised that its translation into practice is shaped—and often constrained—by the structural inequalities specific to Marseille's urban environment.

3.2. Structural Inequalities in Marseille

This theme comprises two sub-themes: what 10 out of 12 professionals described as a "hostile environment", referring to disadvantaged neighbourhoods of Marseille, and the unequal distribution of natural spaces. Professionals described Marseille's urban context as a significant barrier to well-being, pointing to a stark imbalance between concrete and green areas. This is illustrated by comments such as, "In my neighbourhood, there's concrete everywhere, not even a single tree" (SSI 3). According to professionals, this perception of hostility was fuelled by the degraded state of the built environment, dense housing conditions, traffic congestion, and noise, which together contributed to an atmosphere they perceived as "difficult to live in, noisy, and tiring" (SSI 16). As one professional summarised, "living in Marseille is in itself a factor of stress, and when you add precarity on top of that, it's really hard to breathe" (SSI 7).

This challenging environment is marked by a starkly unequal distribution of natural resources. This point was highlighted by six professionals, specifically among field actors and institutional representatives from the health and social sectors, and was seen as a social divide. This is highlighted by observations like, "in the chic neighbourhoods there's greenery, and in the others much less" (SSI 11), framing nature access as a 'luxury'. Consequently, even major assets like the Calanques National Park, described as a "green lung", are considered difficult to access for certain populations. Access is limited not only by physical distance but also by a combination of social and symbolic barriers. The theme of symbolic barriers, identified by six professionals from nature institutions, health institutions, and local social actors, refers to situations where residents felt "out of place" in certain spaces or perceived them as "not meant for them." Past negative experiences sometimes reinforced this sense of exclusion. These structural and symbolic inequalities directly shape the lived realities of the target populations for NBSP, influencing not only their access to nature but also their capacity to participate in community-based health initiatives.

3.3. Populations Facing Cumulative Disadvantage

This theme is structured around three sub-themes: the effects of precarity on social isolation and loneliness, specific barriers to participation, and the potential of nature as a resource for social recognition.

Professionals from health institutions, local health actors, and local social actors described the target populations as facing multiple and intersecting forms of disadvantage. They referred to situations of "uprooting" (SSI 1), loss of reference points and social status, often intensified by stigma. One professional described them as a "politically easy target" (SSI 9). This demanding work context, professionals reported, is dominated by a "very short-term vision" (SSI 9), as their efforts are constantly focused on addressing target populations' primary concerns. Basic physiological needs, such as housing and food, were reported as dominant concerns: "finding housing, food, a roof over their heads" (SSI 6). Several specific obstacles to participation were highlighted, including "language barriers", "cultural practices" (SSI 9); institutional mistrust: "fear of being caught by the police on the way" (SSI 9); and significant symbolic barriers that confine individuals to their immediate surroundings: "outside of their housing estate they don't dare to go out, it's complicated for them… Even their knowledge of their own city…" (SSI 10). According to four professionals from health institutions, nature institutions, and local social actors, this last observation reflects not only practical constraints but also internalised forms of exclusion, illustrating the "symbolic barriers" theme. These descriptions may also reflect a degree of distance between service providers and beneficiaries, underscoring the importance of critically reflecting on professionals' own positionality to avoid reinforcing an us-versus-them perspective.

Nevertheless, five professionals identified nature as a potential vector for recovery of competence and personal recognition, especially for individuals with a rural background who could reconnect with past agricultural skills. It was seen as a way to restore self-esteem and competencies: "it shows them they haven't lost their skills" (SSI 1). Some individuals, particularly women, were reported to have explicitly asked professionals for access to natural spaces: "they ask to go out and ask for access to nature" (SSI 4). Addressing these cumulative disadvantages requires strategies that go beyond access, focusing on empowerment and co-construction of solutions with communities.

3.4. Pathways Toward Participation and Recognition

This theme comprises two sub-themes: the importance of participatory design and empowerment, and the tensions surrounding the term "prescription."

The first sub-theme, mentioned by a majority of professionals across all sectors, emphasised the need for a participatory approach, starting with a diagnosis of needs developed with the community itself. They expressed the desire to "start from [people's] experiences and the lessons they draw from them" (SSI 5), and to build on their internal resources, asking, "How to help the other find their own solutions… starting from their experiences, that's what's important" (SSI 5). Some suggested forming a "core group to drive the process" (SSI 12), often composed of both professionals and motivated community members, whose responsibilities could range from co-designing activities to participating in key decision-making steps. Others highlighted the value of "close, hands-on support" (SSI 10), such as accompanying participants during the first sessions, providing regular feedback, or facilitating peer support groups, with the ultimate goal of fostering autonomy. Assigning responsibilities was described as "highly empowering and ego-boosting" (SSI 1).

The second sub-theme, concerning the semantic tension surrounding the term "prescription," was raised by all actors except local health actors. The critique of the term mainly focused on its association with medical authority and an asymmetrical power dynamic. Some professionals argued, "Prescription sounds like a medical order. That's not what we want, we want to start from them" (SSI 6), highlighting a resistance to a top-down approach. At the same time, others perceived the prescription as a motivating element: "It provides structure, it's reassuring for patients, they know it's not just a walk" (SSI 10). Interestingly, local health actors did not explicitly comment on the term "prescription." For them, as healthcare professionals, the strength of the programme lies precisely in its capacity to function as supportive care, complementing medical treatment rather than imposing an external mandate. This professional perspective reflects an understanding of prescription not only as a formal directive but as a means to legitimise and integrate the intervention within the healthcare pathway. However, the very terminology used to describe NBSP emerged as a point of contention among professionals.

3.5. Barriers and Facilitators to NBSP Implementation

This final theme includes four sub-themes related to territorial constraints, limited institutional resources, identity-based levers, and a shared set of professional values.

Professionals from all sectors identified several structural barriers to the implementation of NBSP. For instance, a lack of nearby green spaces and difficulties accessing natural sites like the Calanques were mentioned by eight professionals. These territorial constraints, often linked to transportation issues, the spatial layout of urban areas, and, in some cases, perceived safety concerns, limit the ability of professionals to fully apply NBSP principles in practice, sometimes forcing adaptations or compromises. Operational constraints also emerged among local actors from health and social sectors, who reported workload saturation: "We're already overloaded, we can't do everything" (SSI 8). Furthermore, professionals highlighted the inherent difficulty of mobilising and sustaining involvement over time, noting that for multi-vulnerable individuals, "if you ask people to commit long-term, it's complicated" (SSI 11).

At the same time, several facilitators were identified. First, the alignment of NBSP principles with existing professional values was perceived as a key lever, noted by most professionals across sectors. This process can be understood as the anchoring of a new social representation (NBSP) within pre-existing professional knowledge, as one professional noted: "We're not inventing anything new, we're just putting a framework around what we already do" (SSI 11). This anchoring helped professionals persevere despite external constraints and bridged the semantic and institutional practice levels. Second, nature was unanimously seen as a powerful vehicle for restoring self-esteem: "It helps them regain confidence because it's not medical, it's alive" (SSI 1). This motivating factor supports engagement, even when structural barriers exist. Furthermore, NBSP was considered replicable for other populations by professionals from health and nature sectors, as one professional noted: "these people are participating in a pilot project that could later serve other publics" (SSI 7). Finally, a strong sense of social urgency in response to growing loneliness and social isolation reinforced the perceived necessity of the NBSP intervention. Together, these barriers and facilitators illustrate both the structural challenges and the professional commitment that shape the current and future implementation of NBSP, paving the way for a discussion on its scalability and transferability.

Ultimately, results showed that conceptualisations of NBSPs are shaped by two intersecting dimensions: sectoral affiliation (health, social action, urban nature) and hierarchical role (operational vs. decision-making). Operational actors, across all sectors, tended to anchor NBSP in their day-to-day realities, emphasising logistical feasibility, immediate participant needs, and the value of relational proximity. Decision-makers, by contrast, often framed NBSP within strategic and programmatic narratives, focusing on alignment with policy frameworks, institutional mandates, and long-term scalability. Sectoral perspectives further refined these patterns: health professionals tended to interpret NBSP through integrated care and public health paradigms; social action professionals foregrounded empowerment and community development; and urban nature actors emphasised ecological accessibility and environmental justice. These cross-cutting patterns enrich the understanding of how NBSP is anchored across different professional contexts and set the stage for the discussion of its broader implications.

4. Discussion

Thematic analysis, interpreted through the lens of Social Representation Theory, highlighted the dynamics through which NBSP is appropriated by mobilising pre-existing knowledge related to nature and health, and social and territorial inequalities. Within this framework, the process of anchoring unfolds along three main axes: (1) a consensual anchoring of NBSP in a holistic vision of health and nature, connected to established health promotion and environmental psychology frameworks; (2) its perceived relevance for addressing Marseille's pronounced territorial inequalities; and (3) a paradox between participatory ideals and practical barriers to implementation, crystallised around the term "prescription", which reflects tensions between empowerment and medicalisation.

4.1. Anchoring NBSP in a Representation of Nature as a Lever for Biopsychosocial Health Promotion

Receptiveness to the concept of NBSP is closely linked to its anchoring in a widespread social representation of nature as a fundamental pillar of health. This anchoring operates through multiple theoretical traditions: health promotion, which offers a systemic, equity-oriented approach linking social and environmental determinants; environmental psychology, which emphasises nature's restorative and relational benefits; and the One Health approach, situating these benefits within the broader interdependence of human, animal, and ecosystem health.

In this perspective, nature connection is framed as a determinant of well-being that goes beyond the biomedical model, supporting individual autonomy and social belonging through interaction with natural environments. This understanding aligns with the Ottawa Charter [29] and subsequent health promotion models, which conceptualise health as a complex, intersectoral and multi-level framework involving diverse actors, participation, and empowerment [30]. The benefits of nature align with key theories in environmental psychology, particularly Ulrich's stress reduction theory and Wohlwill's characterisation of the qualities of nature-based experiences. Ulrich posits an innate biophilia, whereby nature constitutes an intrinsically soothing and aesthetic environment capable of alleviating the anxiety associated with loneliness [31]. Wohlwill further identifies four experiential qualities of nature: its autonomous character, whose organic growth and transformations inspire wonder; its visual properties, perceived as more ordered and predictable than urban spaces, which foster a sense of safety; its capacity to slow down vigilance mechanisms; and its profound symbolic meanings [32]. For some, the connection between nature and health extends beyond well-being to encompass identity formation, reflecting the principle that nature and the self are closely intertwined across individual life trajectories [33].

The anchoring of NBSP is thus both collective and individual, resonating with deeply personal experiences. In SRT terms, this anchoring not only shapes how nature is understood but also legitimises its use as a lever for health promotion. By acting on both individuals (through emotional relief) and environments (through the creation of opportunities for social interaction), nature addresses loneliness on two levels. Immersion in nature can reduce both emotional and social loneliness by fostering community integration [34]. From this perspective, loneliness is framed as a rupture in the relationship between human well-being and the surrounding social–natural environment. This view resonates with broader contemporary approaches, such as the One Health concept, which emphasises the interdependence of human, animal and ecosystem health [35]. It also foreshadows the perspective of Planetary Health, in which loneliness may be interpreted as a symptom of a fractured relationship between human civilisation and global natural systems [36]. In Marseille, NBSP's positive reception among professionals reflects not only interest in an innovative intervention, but also a deeper need to repair these human–nature connections. Future research should assess the robustness of this anchoring across sectors and analyse how it is operationalised within institutional constraints.

4.2. Territorial Disparities in Marseille as Drivers of Health and Loneliness Inequalities

While the idea of nature as a source of well-being is broadly universal, its application through NBSP is anchored in the specific context of Marseille. NBSP is seen as a targeted response to territorial fractures, which, as shown by the analysis of social determinants of health in the city, directly contribute to residents' social vulnerability and experiences of loneliness.

The city exhibits marked contrasts between the dense, under-resourced northern districts and the more affluent southern neighbourhoods. This reflects the concept of the social gradient in health, showing how differences in income and living conditions translate into observable disparities in health outcomes [37]. Such a context constitutes a form of environmental injustice, where those most exposed to loneliness due to economic precarity also face limited opportunities for informal social encounters as a result of poor-quality public spaces. From an SRT perspective, these challenges can be understood as symbolic barriers anchored in representations of certain urban areas as inaccessible or socially inappropriate. Past negative experiences may reinforce these perceptions, fostering exclusion and self-stigmatisation, which in turn encourage avoidance behaviours and intensify social isolation. This process creates a second, territorially based determinant of social isolation.

Structural barriers, such as mobility constraints, further exacerbate this dynamic. In Priority Neighbourhoods, limited public transport and the absence of private vehicles for many households reinforce geographic confinement and limit access to larger natural areas [15]. These constraints are perceived not only as practical obstacles but also as disincentives to participation, resulting in avoidance of long or unfamiliar trips, reduced activity participation, and reliance on poor-quality local spaces. From a Social Representation Theory perspective, such constraints anchor NBSP in a representation of Marseille as fragmented, influencing which solutions are deemed legitimate, and favouring proximity-based, culturally adapted interventions. This interpretive lens also shapes which forms of "nature" are perceived as accessible, acceptable, and meaningful for target populations. This territorial dimension of loneliness is inseparable from its psychosocial consequences. As the literature highlights, loneliness is closely associated with stigma and is often experienced through shame and self-deprecation, leading to social avoidance [2,4–6]. The relevance of NBSP lies precisely in its potential to address these psychological barriers by reducing fear of judgement, restoring self-esteem, enhancing recognition of individual strengths, and deconstructing internalised obstacles to social connection.

4.3. The Tension Between an Empowerment Ideal and a Perceived Top-Down Intervention Model

The implementation of NBSPs among vulnerable populations reveals a central paradox, oscillating between a philosophy grounded in empowerment and a form of pragmatism shaped by structural determinism.

On the one hand, professionals express an intervention ideal strongly aligned with humanistic approaches. Starting from lived experiences and supporting the search for self-defined solutions directly echoes Rogers' person-centred approach [38]. This ideal corresponds to what is referred to as praxis: an action aimed at recognising the other as the main agent of their own autonomy, particularly in their effort to overcome loneliness [39]. However, this ideal of doing with comes into sharp contrast with an analysis of beneficiaries' living conditions. To justify the difficulty, or even the impossibility, of fostering participation, frequent reference is made to Maslow's hierarchy of needs [40]. In their view, it is unrealistic to expect engagement in needs for belonging or self-actualisation, even though these needs are central to alleviating loneliness, when basic physiological and safety needs remain unmet. This reasoning, which attributes vulnerability to external structural factors, aligns with Strauss's perspective, in which vulnerability is understood as the product of social processes embedded in everyday life [41].

This is where the paradox emerges. While professionals are clearly attuned to the structural determinants of loneliness, some accounts suggest a tendency to reassign responsibility back onto individuals. Within the framework of Social Representation Theory, such categorisation reflects one of the core social functions of representations, namely the classification of individuals and groups in ways that can legitimise existing power relations. In this case, the implicit distinction between participants and non-participants risks reinforcing social boundaries instead of dismantling them. This dynamic risks legitimising exclusion rather than dismantling it, thereby constraining the transformative potential of community-based interventions such as NBSPs. This tension reflects an ambivalent framing of the problem, situated somewhere between structural approaches and individualising models. As suggested by Abric, such a stance may also reflect a representation of the social worker's role as primarily assisting individuals in difficulty, rather than engaging in complex efforts to dismantle mechanisms of social exclusion [42]. This ambivalence underscores the need for a paradigm shift in health promotion, favouring community-based and systemic action, such as that proposed by NBSP.

The paradox between participatory ideals and pragmatic constraints is clearly illustrated by the semantic debate surrounding the term "prescription". The term is far from neutral. It crystallises tensions between two models of intervention and reveals competing professional cultures. In the nature and social sectors, it is anchored in a representation of medical authority that is hierarchical and potentially exclusionary, often perceived as paternalistic and incompatible with empowerment logics. In the health sector, by contrast, "prescription" fits more easily into care pathways, conveying legitimacy and structured support. In SRT terms, these contrasting interpretations reflect two anchoring processes: one embedding the term in integrated care pathway representations, the other in representations of medical authority. In line with previous work in health promotion, practitioners have suggested replacing the term "prescription" with alternative expressions such as "referral" or "well-being pathway," which could better align with participatory and empowerment-oriented approaches by reducing the imprint of medical authority. Considering such terminology shifts could help broaden NBSP's legitimacy and acceptability across both professional sectors and community stakeholders.

These divergences show how terminological choices can reproduce sectoral boundaries and power relations. They also illustrate how language can be used strategically to align

NBSP with participatory health promotion principles. Ultimately, this tension risks shifting NBSP from a collective, structural intervention towards an individualising model. Yet loneliness is linked not only to individual experiences but also to social networks, civic participation, and social recognition. By mobilising nature as a non-stigmatising third space that fosters collective narratives and strengthens cohesion, NBSP can reduce emotional loneliness, restore self-worth, and reactivate local social dynamics.

Despite the paradoxes observed, NBSP retains the potential to repair social bonds, transforming loneliness into an experience that can be shared, tolerated, and even used as a foundation for mental well-being.

5. Limits

This study presents several contextual, methodological, and epistemological limitations. First, the specific context of Marseille, marked by significant territorial disparities, a particular urban geography, and high levels of social precarity, constitutes both a source of analytical richness and a limiting factor for the transferability of the findings to other settings.

From a methodological perspective, the sample size, although aligned with qualitative standards in terms of thematic saturation [26], does not allow for generalisation of the results, particularly regarding the relationship between professional affiliation and social representations and the specific context of the study, conducted in Marseille. Furthermore, the absence of interviewee feedback (member checking), although justified by the intention to preserve the spontaneity of responses, limits the external validation of the interpretations.

A further limitation is the absence of direct perspectives from beneficiaries in this phase of the study. However, the participatory diagnostic phase of the RECETAS project involved co-constructing a menu of NBSP activities through participatory methods, thereby including beneficiaries. This process allowed for a more refined understanding of the needs of those directly concerned, while the present study specifically focused on understanding how NBSP is integrated into professional practices.

Regarding the analysis, although conducted with rigour, it inevitably involves a degree of subjectivity inherent in qualitative approaches. The complementary use of textual analysis software could have further enriched the interpretation. Likewise, while the decision to integrate free associations into the overall thematic analysis is consistent with an interpretative stance, some readers might question the absence of a distinct structural or prototypical analysis, which could have shed additional light on the underlying socio-cognitive dimensions.

Practical Implications for NBSP Implementation

This study led to the formulation of a set of operational recommendations that subsequently guided the implementation of NBSP in Marseille. Rooted in both the specific territorial context and the principles of health promotion, these actions aimed to strengthen the relevance, effectiveness, and equity of NBSP as a strategy to address loneliness.

To enhance accessibility, NBSP was primarily implemented in priority neighbourhoods, in partnership with locally embedded professionals. A set of progressive and adaptable activities, such as nature walks and gardening workshops, was co-designed with professionals and the target populations during the second and third phases of the co-creation process of RECETAS. These included a participatory diagnostic phase and the collective definition of a panel of NBSP activities. Five focus groups supported this process, which aimed not only to foster empowerment by valuing individuals' own resources but also to build a shared culture around care, social connection, and nature. Professional reflexivity was also supported through interprofessional exchange sessions designed to foster a common culture. Finally, a mixed-methods evaluation was implemented to assess lived experience, changes in perceived loneliness, well-being and quality of life outcomes. By integrating environmental, social, cultural, and psychological dimensions, NBSP emerges as a systemic response to the multidimensional determinants of loneliness. This study highlights that this approach is positively received by professionals due to its grounding in a holistic view of health and in shared representations of nature as a source of well-being and social connection. In relation to the semantic discussions raised earlier, at this stage of the project, and in coherence with the other pilot teams involved in RECETAS, no change in terminology has been implemented locally. The decision to retain or adapt the term "prescription" will be revisited collectively at the end of the project, once all pilot sites have gathered empirical evidence on its acceptability and impact. This staged approach allows for cross-context learning while maintaining a consistent vocabulary during the initial implementation phase.

6. Conclusions

In the Marseille context, marked by significant territorial inequalities, NBSP is perceived as an innovative lever for disrupting mechanisms of social exclusion. The uniqueness of this territory lies in the coexistence of diverse natural environments, offering a distinctive potential to create spaces for social encounters where nature can function as a relational third place, safe and non-stigmatising. It is precisely this collective dimension that NBSP aims to strengthen by facilitating the emergence of new shared narratives and reinforcing psychosocial cohesion at the local level. Its anticipated effects include a reduction in emotional loneliness (by alleviating the feeling of facing difficulties alone), subjective enhancement (through a renewed sense of belonging and social usefulness), and reconnection with others through the reactivation of localised social dynamics (renewed contacts, integration into other activities). Thus, despite the paradoxes identified and supported by other works that have studied the representation of nature in Marseille and shown both the richness of its peripheral natural spaces and a fragmented urban nature, ref. [43] NBSP may act as a genuine mechanism for repairing social bonds, contributing to a transformation of loneliness into a shareable, more tolerable experience, and even a potential foundation for the restoration of mental well-being. However, this dynamic encounters structural tensions. Although professionals advocate for participatory ideals, they are confronted with the material and psychological constraints of the target populations, which may lead to more top-down forms of intervention than initially envisioned. These findings invite us to consider NBSP not merely as a sector-specific innovation but as an opportunity to renew public health paradigms.

Firstly, it suggests the need to explicitly frame the reduction in emotional loneliness and the strengthening of social belonging as central objectives. To achieve its full potential, NBSP must move beyond the boundaries of individual interventions and be embedded within a collective and contextualised strategy, supported by ambitious public policies and training programmes that promote professional reflexivity and active beneficiary involvement. Secondly, NBSP, as a new social object and intervention in France, derives its meaning from a deep interdependence between health, natural spaces, and social relations. The recognition of this interdependence implies an integration of human and ecosystem health, a concept known as Planetary Health [36]. This holistic and integrative representation of health, through which the interviewed professionals understand NBSP, also reflects a shift towards an ecological model of public health [44]. This new ecological public health transcends individualistic preventive and curative approaches and, much like the field of health promotion, calls for a consideration of social determinants of health at the macro level and an expanded responsibility for health across disciplines beyond traditional healthcare boundaries.

A further significant finding is the profoundly relational character of NBSP, where nature is conceptualised as a resource for developing social bonds. This characteristic suggests reframing ecology itself (and by extension, the ecological public health model previously cited) in a resolutely relational orientation, thinking of ecology as the possibility of forging connections between humans, and between humans and natural spaces [45]. This notion is supported by previous research on the social representations of nature, which has highlighted the importance of introducing relational values (between people and between people and nature) to develop systemic strategies around nature and human well-being [46].

Author Contributions: L.C. and A.D. contributed to the development of the methodology and the analysis of the results. L.C. and S.G. co-wrote the manuscript in English. S.G. also supervised the overall research process and validated the final version of the article. G.G.V. co-wrote and reviewed the consistency of the contextualisation with the RECETAS project framework. All authors have read and agreed to the published version of the manuscript.

Funding: This research was funded by the European Union's Horizon 2020 research and innovation programme under the RECETAS project, grant agreement No. 945095. The APC was funded by the RECETAS project.

Institutional Review Board Statement: The NBSP intervention in Marseille was approved by the Ethics committee of the University of Aix-Marseille (N/Ref: 2023-01-05-03).

Informed Consent Statement: Oral informed consent was obtained from all subjects involved in the study. Professionals were informed that anonymized quotes from the interviews might be used in publications, and none expressed opposition to this.

Data Availability Statement: The data presented in this study are available on request from the corresponding author due to privacy and ethical considerations.

Acknowledgments: We would like to thank all the professionals who kindly agreed to participate in our study.

Conflicts of Interest: The funders had no role in the design of the study; in the collection, analyses, or interpretation of data; in the writing of the manuscript; or in the decision to publish the results.

References

1. Reinhardt, G.; Vidovic, D.; Hammerton, C. Understanding loneliness: A systematic review of the impact of social prescribing initiatives on loneliness. *Perspect. Public Health* **2021**, *141*, 204–213. [CrossRef]
2. Fondation de France. *Solitudes 2022: Regards sur les Fragilités Relationnelles*; CREDOC & CERLIS: Paris, France, 2022. Available online: https://www.fondationdefrance.org/images/pdf/2023/solitudes-2022.pdf?trk=public_post_comment-text (accessed on 14 June 2025).
3. Holt-Lunstad, J.; Smith, T.B.; Baker, M.; Harris, T.; Stephenson, D. Loneliness and social isolation as risk factors for mortality: A meta-analytic review. *Perspect. Psychol. Sci.* **2015**, *10*, 227–237. [CrossRef] [PubMed]
4. Kerr, N.A.; Stanley, T.B. Revisiting the social stigma of loneliness. *Personal. Individ. Differ.* **2021**, *171*, 110482. [CrossRef]
5. Barreto, M.; Van Breen, J.; Victor, C.; Hammond, C.; Eccles, A.; Richins, M.T.; Qualter, P. Exploring the nature and variation of the stigma associated with loneliness. *J. Soc. Pers. Relatsh.* **2022**, *39*, 2658–2679. [CrossRef]
6. Rotenberg, K.J. Stigmatization of transitions in loneliness. *J. Soc. Pers. Relatsh.* **1998**, *15*, 565–576. [CrossRef]
7. NHS England. Social Prescribing. Available online: https://www.england.nhs.uk/personalisedcare/social-prescribing/ (accessed on 14 June 2025).
8. Liebmann, M.; Pitman, A.; Hsueh, Y.C.; Bertotti, M.; Pearce, E. Do people perceive benefits in the use of social prescribing to address loneliness and/or social isolation? A qualitative meta-synthesis of the literature. *BMC Health Serv. Res.* **2022**, *22*, 1297. [CrossRef]

9. Leavell, M.A.; Leiferman, J.A.; Gascon, M.; Braddick, F.; Gonzalez, J.C.; Litt, J.S. Nature-based social prescribing in urban settings to improve social connectedness and mental well-being: A review. *Curr. Environ. Health Rep.* **2019**, *6*, 297–308. [CrossRef] [PubMed]
10. INSEE. Dossier Complet—Commune de Marseille (13055). Available online: https://www.insee.fr/fr/statistiques/2011101?geo=COM-13055#tableau-REV_G1 (accessed on 14 June 2025).
11. Commission Exigence Sociale, Prévention, Santé. *Pauvreté(s): Eléments de Diagnostic*; Délégation Générale du Conseil de Provence: Marseille, France, 2021. Available online: https://www.departement13.fr/mon-departement/les-instances-consultatives/le-conseil-de-provence/nos-travaux/rapports-avis (accessed on 20 June 2025).
12. Beauchemin, C.; Hamel, C.; Simon, P. *Trajectoires et Origines: Enquête sur la Diversité des Populations en France*; INED: Paris, France, 2016.
13. Baby-Collin, V.; Dahdah, A. Miroir de la précarité sociale et (carrefour) des dynamiques migratoires. Les hôtels dits meublés du centre-ville marseillais. *Faire Savoirs Sci. Hum. Soc. Rég. PACA* **2017**, *13*, 65–74.
14. Dorier, E.; Dario, J. *Marseille 2018–2019: De la Crise du Logement à la Crise Humanitaire*; Haut Comité au Logement pour les Personnes Défavorisées (HCLPD): Paris, France, 2020.
15. INSEE. La Mobilité Résidentielle et Ses Impacts Dans Les Quartiers de la Politique de la Ville (QPV)—Provence-Alpes-Côte d'Azur. Available online: https://www.insee.fr/fr/statistiques/5650474?sommaire=5650644 (accessed on 20 June 2025).
16. INSEE. Un Accès Inégal Aux Espaces Verts Dans Les Grands Centres Urbains—Insee Première—2049. Available online: https://www.insee.fr/fr/statistiques/8558420 (accessed on 14 June 2025).
17. World Health Organization, Regional Office for Europe. *Urban Green Spaces and Health*; WHO Regional Office for Europe: Copenhagen, Denmark, 2016. Available online: https://iris.who.int/handle/10665/345751 (accessed on 20 June 2025).
18. Litt, J.S.; Coll-Planas, L.; Sachs, A.L.; Rochau, U.; Jansson, A.; Dostálová, V.; Daher, C.; Beacom, A.; Bachinski, K.; Garcia Velez, G.E.; et al. Nature-based social interventions for people experiencing loneliness: The rationale and overview of the RECETAS project. *Cities Health* **2024**, *8*, 418–431. [CrossRef]
19. Yáñez, P.P.; Vélez, G.G.; Pesántez, K.V.; Páez, D.A. Hacia la prescripción social basada en la naturaleza para aliviar la soledad: Una experiencia co-creativa desde Ecuador. *Ciênc. Saúde Coletiva* **2025**, *30*, 3–6. [CrossRef]
20. Jodelet, D. Représentation sociale: Phénomènes, concepts et théories. In *Psychologie Sociale*; Moscovici, S., Ed.; Presses Universitaires de France: Paris, France, 1984.
21. Moscovici, S. *La Psychanalyse, Son Image et Son Public*; Presses Universitaires de France: Paris, France, 1976. Available online: https://www.persee.fr/doc/bupsy_0007-4403_1977_num_31_332_11441_t1_0028_0000_2 (accessed on 20 June 2025).
22. Apostolidis, T. Représentations sociales et triangulation: Une application en Psychologie Sociale de la Santé. *Psicol. Teor. Pesqui.* **2006**, *22*, 211–226. [CrossRef]
23. Dany, L. Analyse qualitative du contenu des représentations sociales. In *Les Représentations Sociales*; Lo Monaco, G., Delouvée, S., Rateau, P., Eds.; Les Représentations Sociales; de Boeck: Bruxelles, Belgium, 2016; pp. 85–102.
24. Tong, A.; Sainsbury, P.; Craig, J. Consolidated criteria for reporting qualitative research (COREQ): A 32-item checklist for interviews and focus groups. *Int. J. Qual. Health Care* **2007**, *19*, 349–357. [CrossRef] [PubMed]
25. Goodman, L.A. Snowball sampling. *Ann. Math. Stat.* **1961**, *32*, 148–170. [CrossRef]
26. Paillé, P.; Mucchielli, A. *L'analyse Qualitative en Sciences Humaines et Sociales*; Armand Colin: Paris, France, 2016.
27. Painter, S. La recherche du consentement: Enjeux et méthode dans une enquête qualitative auprès de personnes en fragilité psychique. *Carnets Géogr.* **2020**, *14*, 4–6. [CrossRef]
28. Braun, V.; Clarke, V. Using thematic analysis in psychology. *Qual. Res. Psychol.* **2006**, *3*, 77–101. [CrossRef]
29. World Health Organization. *The Ottawa Charter for Health Promotion*; First International Conference on Health Promotion: Ottawa, ON, Canada, 1986. Available online: https://www.who.int/teams/health-promotion/enhanced-wellbeing/first-global-conference (accessed on 20 June 2025).
30. Trickett, E.J.; Beehler, S.; Deutsch, C.; Green, L.W.; Hawe, P.; McLeroy, K.; Miller, R.L.; Rapkin, B.D.; Schensul, J.J.; Schulz, A.J.; et al. Advancing the science of Community-Level interventions. *Am. J. Public Health* **2011**, *101*, 1410–1419. [CrossRef]
31. Ulrich, R.S. View Through a Window May Influence Recovery from Surgery. *Science* **1984**, *224*, 420–421. [CrossRef]
32. Wohlwill, J.F. The concept of nature: A psychologist's view. *Hum. Behav. Environ.* **1983**, *6*, 5–37.
33. Olivos, P.; Clayton, S. Self, Nature and Well-Being: Sense of connectedness and environmental identity for quality of life. In *Handbook of Environmental Psychology and Quality of Life Research*; Fleury-Bahi, G., Pol, E., Navarro, O., Eds.; International Handbooks of Quality-of-Life; Springer: Cham, Switzerland, 2017; pp. 107–126. [CrossRef]
34. Paquet, C.; Whitehead, J.; Shah, R.; Adams, A.M.; Dooley, D.; Spreng, R.N.; Aunio, A.-L.; Dubé, L. Social Prescription Interventions Addressing Social Isolation and Loneliness in Older Adults: Meta-Review Integrating On-the-Ground Resources. *J. Med. Internet Res.* **2023**, *25*, e40213. [CrossRef]

35. Pitt, S.J.; Gunn, A. The one health concept. *Br. J. Biomed. Sci.* **2024**, *81*, 1–2. [CrossRef] [PubMed]
36. Whitmee, S.; Haines, A.; Beyrer, C.; Boltz, F.; Capon, A.G.; de Souza Dias, B.F.; Ezeh, A.; Frumkin, H.; Gong, P.; Head, P.; et al. Safeguarding human health in the Anthropocene epoch: Report of The Rockefeller Foundation–Lancet Commission on planetary health. *Lancet* **2015**, *386*, 1973–2028. [CrossRef]
37. Mackenbach, J.P.; Bakker, M.J.; European Network on Interventions and Policies to Reduce Inequalities in Health. Tackling socioeconomic inequalities in health: Analysis of European experiences. *Lancet* **2003**, *362*, 1409–1414. [CrossRef]
38. Rogers, C.R. *The Carl Rogers Reader*; Kirschenbaum, H., Henderson, V.L., Eds.; Houghton, Mifflin and Company: Boston, MA, USA, 1989.
39. Fablet, D. Les groupes d'analyse des pratiques professionnelles: Une visée avant tout formative. *Connexions* **2004**, *82*, 105–117. [CrossRef]
40. Maslow, A.H. A theory of human motivation. *Psychol. Rev.* **1943**, *50*, 370–396. [CrossRef]
41. Bungener, M. La Trame de la Négociation, Sociologie Qualitative et Interactionnisme, Anselm L Strauss, Textes Réunis et Présentés par Isabelle Baszanger. *Persée*. Available online: https://www.persee.fr/doc/sosan_0294-0337_1992_num_10_4_1742 (accessed on 20 June 2025).
42. Abric, J.-C. *Les Représentations Sociales: Aspects Théoriques et Pratiques Sociales de L'insertion et de la Prévention*; Communication au Séminaire sur les Représentations Sociales, un Outil au Service de l'Insertion et de la Prévention, Barcelone, Espagne; Presses Universitaires de France (PUF): Paris, France, 1996.
43. Mouad, B. Les Trames Vertes Urbaines: Analyse des Représentations Sociales de la «Nature en Ville» à Marseille et à Strasbourg. Doctoral Dissertation, Université de Nanterre-Paris X, Nanterre, France, 2018.
44. Lang, T.; Rayner, G. Ecological public health: The 21st century's big idea? An essay by Tim Lang and Geof Rayner. *BMJ* **2012**, *345*, e5466. [CrossRef] [PubMed]
45. Gervais, M. Quel travail social et quelle écologie? Revenir sur la division nature/culture pour une écologie comme capacité à nouer des liens. *Le Sociographe* **2024**, *86*, XVII–XXXII. [CrossRef]
46. De Vreese, R.; Van Herzele, A.; Dendoncker, N.; Fontaine, C.; Leys, M. Are stakeholders' social representations of nature and landscape compatible with the ecosystem service concept? *Ecosyst. Serv.* **2019**, *37*, 100911. [CrossRef]

International Journal of
Environmental Research and Public Health

MDPI

Review

Loneliness by Design: The Structural Logic of Isolation in Engagement-Driven Systems

Lauren Dwyer

School of Communication Studies, Faculty of Business, Communication Studies, and Aviation, Mount Royal University, Calgary, AB T3E 6K6, Canada; ldwyer@mtroyal.ca

Abstract

As the prevalence of public discourse pertaining to loneliness increases, digital interventions, such as artificial intelligence companions, are being introduced as methods for fostering connection and mitigating individual negative experiences of loneliness. These tools, while increasing in volume and popularity, operate within and are shaped by the same engagement-driven systems that have been found to contribute to loneliness. This meta-narrative review examines how algorithmic infrastructures, which are optimized for retention, emotional predictability, and behavioural nudging, not only mediate responses to loneliness but participate in its ongoing production. Flattening complex social dynamics into curated, low-friction interactions, these systems gradually displace relational agency and erode users' capacity for autonomous social decision making. Drawing on frameworks from communication studies and behavioural information design, this review finds that loneliness is understood both as an emotional or interpersonal state and as a logical consequence of hegemonic digital and technological design paradigms. Without addressing the structural logics of platform capitalism and algorithmic control, digital public health interventions risk treating loneliness as an individual deficit rather than a systemic outcome. Finally, a model is proposed for evaluating and designing digital public health interventions that resist behavioural enclosure and support autonomy, relational depth, systemic accountability, and structural transparency.

Keywords: loneliness; digital technologies; artificial intelligence; design; public health; digital public health

1. Introduction

Reports of loneliness have surged since the onset of the COVID-19 pandemic, drawing renewed attention to what public health officials now describe as a global crisis [1]. Recent policy analyses underscore that loneliness is increasingly framed not only as a personal health issue but also as a policy concern, with clear technological dimensions [2,3]. Goldman and colleagues [2] provide a cross-national review of loneliness and social isolation policies, noting that many governments now explicitly include technology-based interventions in their strategic plans. In the UK, additional studies by Jentoft and colleagues show how political discourse around loneliness often situates older adults within narratives of digital inclusion, even as these narratives risk oversimplifying structural inequities [3,4]. In 2020, 54% of Canadians and 36% of Americans reported heightened feelings of isolation, a marked increase from previous years [5,6]. Hawkley [7] similarly emphasizes that public policy must grapple with both the social determinants of loneliness and the role of emerging technologies in shaping them. Although loneliness is not formally classified as a mental illness in the Diagnostic and Statistical Manual of Mental Disorders (DSM-5-TR) [8], it is deeply entangled with mental health outcomes, including depression [9], and is linked to significant physical health risks such as cardiovascular disease and early mortality [10]. Developmental perspectives add further nuance, as Hang et al. [11] highlight how chronic loneliness can take root early in life, with digital environments playing a formative role in either buffering or exacerbating social disconnection. Now described as a "parallel pandemic," the crisis of disconnection has persisted even as the stigma surrounding loneliness has shifted in its cultural weight [12,13]. In response, digital intervention (i.e., artificial intelligence companions, chatbots, and social wellness apps) have emerged as scalable, accessible tools that have shown promise in fostering emotional support and facilitating connection, particularly for older adults and geographically or socially isolated individuals [13–19].

Despite these advantages, the literature on human–computer interaction (HCI) and design studies suggest the same digital infrastructures designed to alleviate loneliness are implicated in its ongoing production [20–26]. This paradox highlights a deeper tension at the intersection of public health, design, and algorithmic media: while AI systems may mediate individual experiences of disconnection, they are also structurally embedded within platform logics that prioritize engagement, predictability, and behavioural nudging over relational depth. In other words, the systems offering therapeutic solutions are often architected around the same imperatives that displace meaningful social interaction in the first place.

The roots of this contradiction lie, in part, in transformations to how information is filtered, circulated, and experienced in digital life. Gatekeeping theory, once central to media and communication studies, described the editorial decisions made by individuals, journalists, broadcasters, editors about what entered the public sphere [27]. The gate was visible and accountable, albeit imperfectly. Today, as algorithmic systems increasingly determine what we see, believe, and engage with, gatekeeping has become computational. It is no longer a social negotiation but a proprietary operation encoded into the infrastructure of digital platforms. As Tarleton Gillespie notes [28,29], choices made by designers working within commercial ecosystems embed algorithmic systems with values like frictionless navigation to minimize frustration and challenges in the digital sphere. These values are not neutral; they shape what rises to visibility and what disappears into algorithmic oblivion. In this sense, platforms do not merely mediate attention, as they actively structure epistemological and emotional life.

The result is a digital media environment where visibility becomes synonymous with legitimacy [30], and emotional salience rather than informational value determines what circulates. Zuboff's concept of surveillance capitalism [31] and Casas-Cortés and colleagues' concept of platform capitalism [32] explain how these systems move beyond the passive prediction of behaviour toward its active shaping. In this environment, reality itself becomes what is most clickable, most shareable, and most emotionally intense. Tufekci [33] illustrates how attention is redirected by rewarding engagement over accuracy, pulling users toward more polarizing or addictive experiences. In this context, scholars have argued that loneliness may be more than a byproduct of digital life, suggesting that it is shaped and, in some cases, reinforced by dominant design logics embedded in platform capitalism [34–36]. The same algorithmic infrastructures that provide social recommendation, affirmation, or simulated empathy are often optimized to fragment user attention [33], narrow emotional range [31], and displace complexity in favour of simplified, coherent narratives [29,37]. Where earlier generations encountered propaganda as deliberate and centralized, today it is ambient, embedded in interface design, emotional profiling, and the algorithmic ordering of experience. Targeting is no longer demographic but psychographic, functioning through predictive emotional calibration.

This review examines the research surrounding loneliness not only as an emotional or interpersonal state but as a structural consequence of the technologies designed to treat it. Drawing on the fields of communication and media studies, HCI, design, and public health, the analysis examines how algorithmic infrastructures mediate, perpetuate, and produce loneliness within the logics of platform capitalism. It explores how personalization, artificial intimacy, and engagement-maximizing design displace agency and relationality, while simultaneously offering interventions that treat loneliness as an individual pathology. Finally, we propose a human-centered, ethically grounded framework for designing AI and digital public health tools that resist behavioural enclosure, support relational autonomy, and center human flourishing in an age of algorithmic control.

2. Methodology

This study follows a meta-narrative review methodology, guided by the Realist and Meta-narrative Evidence Synthesis (RAMESES) framework [38,39]. The meta-narrative approach was selected for its suitability in examining how different research traditions (public health, communication studies, behavioural design, and human–computer interaction (HCI)) and their respective epistemic cultures conceptualize loneliness in the context of digital and technological design [40]. This method prioritizes pluralism, reflexivity and historicity over a single standard of evidence, enabling insights to be considered from diverse epistemic traditions that rarely intersect in conventional systematic reviews [40].

2.1. Research Questions

This review is guided by two central questions:

1. How is loneliness framed in the fields of digital and technological design (including HCI and communication studies), compared to its clinical and public health representations?
2. How can these perspectives inform the design of ethical digital public health interventions?

2.2. Rationale for Review Type

The meta-narrative review methodology was chosen for its comparative mapping of concepts, theories, and evidence across distinct epistemic traditions. The RAMESES framework provides guidance for integrating differing perspectives to identify conceptual convergences and divergences, ultimately informing a new evaluative framework for digital public health designs [38,39].

2.3. Search Strategy

An exploratory scoping phase was undertaken during April and May of 2025 to familiarize the researcher with the breadth of the literature and terminology used across the relevant fields. This initial review consisted of informal browsing of electronic databases, citation chasing of seminal works, and informal consultations with experts in public health, communication studies, and human–computer interaction. This stage identified and helped to draw connections and distinctions between the key epistemic traditions being explored in this review: public health/clinical research, behavioural science, communication and media studies, and design/technology studies. This work informed the iterative development of search terms and inclusion/exclusion criteria.

The formal search strategy combined electronic database searches, hand-searching of reference lists from selected articles for additional relevant publications, and a grey literature review of policy reports, white papers, and industry documentation from organizations such as the WHO, OECD, and various national public health agencies. The following databases were searched using university access: PubMed, APA PsycInfo, Communication & Mass Media, ACM Digital Library. Additional searches were run through Google Scholar. These databases were chosen to ensure coverage across the health, psychology, social science, and technology literature.

Search terms were combined using Boolean operators and adapted for each database. Initial terms and concepts included the following: *Loneliness* OR *social isolation* AND *Digital public health* OR *digital intervention* OR *AI companion* OR *social robot* OR *mental health app* OR *wellness app; Design paradigm* OR *algorithmic infrastructure* OR *platform capitalism* OR *engagement-driven* OR *behavioural nudging* OR *artificial intimacy.*

Boolean operators and truncations were adapted for each database. Searches were limited to works published between January 2010 and May 2025, in English, to capture the literature reflecting the rise of algorithmically mediated social environments and the proliferation of digital health interventions. Where available on database searches, the peer reviewed and references available filters were applied.

Initial results yielded a combined 7786 articles, books, and grey literature. Searches were re-run at key points in the review to incorporate newly published studies and with considerations given to the evolving nature of new technologies. Citation trails were followed from influential works to better understand the narratives of each field.

2.4. Inclusion/Exclusion, Screening and Selection Processes

Inclusion criteria: Articles consisted of empirical studies, theoretical papers, systematic reviews, policy analyses, or critical essays engaging with loneliness in the context of digital or technological mediation. Works examining the design logic, algorithmic mediation, or infrastructural dynamics of digital platforms relevant to loneliness were included. Studies contributing conception or empirical insights into public health, communication, or design implications were also included.

Exclusion criteria: Studies on loneliness with no reference to digital or technological systems were not included; however, seminal texts that define loneliness were initially referenced to define the field. Interventions limited to traditional telehealth without algorithmic or engagement-driven features were not included. Opinion pieces lacking substantive engagement with the existing literature were not included.

Selection was guided by pragmatism, with sources being retained only if they were likely to inform cross-disciplinary sense making. Quality appraisal was tradition-specific: public heath articles were assessed for methodological rigour using health sciences standards; design and communication studies were judged according to qualitative and theoretical scholarship criteria; and human–computer interaction research was considered under quantitative methodological standards.

All retrieved records were imported into reference management software (Zotero 7.0.24), where duplicates were removed. Titles and abstracts were screened for relevance, and potentially relevant records proceeded to full-text review, during which inclusion and exclusion decisions were documented alongside justifications. Iterative searching occurred throughout to refine search terms to those discovered in included works and cross-citation mapping between traditions. Figure 1 summarizes the search, screening, and selection process, including database searching, grey literature, and citation chasing.

Data extraction was designed to support meta-narrative cross-disciplinary sense making rather than mechanical coding. Synthesis followed the RAMESES principles by prioritizing sources most useful for building cross-disciplinary understanding; evaluating each tradition's sources based on their own quality criteria and epistemic assumptions, considering the traditions' evolutions over time; informal peer review through discussions with colleagues with relevant expertise but outside of the researcher's primary discipline and maintaining awareness of the researcher's own positionality as a communications and design scholar with a background in artificial intelligence and social robotics.

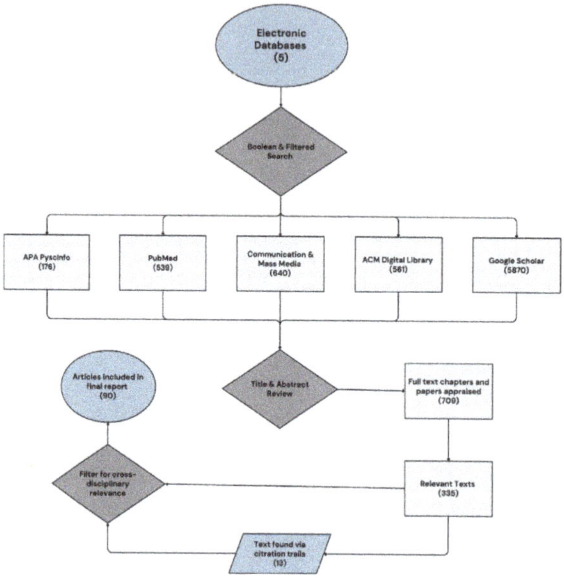

Figure 1. RAMESES search criteria and screening process.

3. Analysis and Results

Cross-disciplinary analysis of the literature identified four principal research traditions that engage with loneliness in the context of digital and technological design: (1) Public Health and Clinical Epidemiology, (2) Behavioural Science and Psychology, (3) Human–computer Interaction (HCI) and Design Research, and (4) Communication and Media Studies. Within these traditions, the meaning of loneliness and the factors deemed most salient to its emergence and the perceived role of digital interventions varied substantially. The following synthesis outlines the prevailing conceptualizations, with comparisons made to identify commonalities, divergences, and opportunities for cross-disciplinary integration. Table 1 below outlines these findings. A systems thinking approach was applied to bridge these gaps, treating technological design, social practices, and policy environments as interlinked components of a single dynamic system. This perspective was used to consider the feedback loops between technological affordances, user behaviours, and psychosocial outcomes as well as account for multi-level determinants of loneliness such as interface features and community infrastructure. Potential unintended consequences of engagement-driven designs offering short-term relief but deepening long-term disconnection formed the basis for this article's proposed discussion between these traditions.

The following discussions build on this synthesis by unpacking four thematic domains that cut across traditions: (1) the hegemony of digital design paradigms, (2) the role of algorithmic infrastructures as mediators and producers of loneliness, (3) structural logics of platform capitalism and algorithmic control, (4) the convergence and tensions between public health and design perspectives. A fifth theme emerged in the readings, suggesting a framework for priorities for (5) a digital public health design framework. This progression moves from critical examination of underlying structures to the development of an integrative framework that preserves the conceptual integrity of each tradition while offering a coherent, ethically grounded approach to digital public health design. A table noting the selected articles, their tradition, and thematic domains can be found in the Supplemental Materials, Table S1.

Table 1. Ethical design priorities for digital interventions addressing loneliness.

Research Tradition	Framing of Loneliness + Technology	Methodological Orientation	Design Implications
Public Health	Technology positioned as a scalable mechanism to address loneliness, primarily treated as a modifiable health risk.	Epidemiological surveys, longitudinal studies, validated psychometric scales, intervention trials.	Integrate structural critiques into intervention design to avoid treating loneliness solely as an individual pathology.
Behavioural Science & Psychology	Technology as a medium for behaviour change, social skills training, and cognitive reframing to reduce loneliness.	Behaviour change theory, CBT, nudge theory, experimental and quasi-experimental studies.	Ensure long-term relational outcomes by combining behavioural strategies with safeguards against dependency and over-reliance
HCI/Design	Technology as a sociotechnical system whose affordances shape relational depth, agency, and connection quality.	User-centered and participatory design, affordance theory, systems thinking, usability studies.	Prioritizes hybrid online-offline connections, design "positive friction" and preserve user agency in relational contexts.
Communication & Media	Technology as embedded in political-economic systems that commodify connection and influence emotional life.	Political economy of media, gatekeeping theory, critical discourse analysis.	Address platform logics and governance structures to design interventions that resist commodification and structural disconnection.

4. The Hegemony of Digital Design Paradigms

4.1. Hegemonic Digital Infrastructures and the Structuring of Loneliness

The influence of structural logics as infrastructures on social experience reflects deeper questions about agency in the digital age [30,35]. Ågerfalk [41] describes AI as a form of digital agency, mediating and even substituting human decision making in ways that reconfigure relational autonomy, which Ho [42] defines as the ability to act meaningfully within relationships while retaining independence from coercive digital mediation. Extending this, Kuss and Meske [43] and Dattathrani and De' [44] consider how AI shifts agency from individuals to sociotechnical systems, while Burkitt's [45] relational sociology frames agency itself as emerging from networks of human and non-human actors. Loneliness, far from being solely an emotional or psychological phenomenon, emerges systematically in the literature as having a reciprocal relationship to prevailing hegemonic paradigms in digital and technological design [13–19,46]. Contemporary digital infrastructures, shaped by commercial imperatives and optimization strategies, are found to embed structural logics that significantly contribute to the persistence and exacerbation of loneliness [2,7,46].

While this review focuses on shared structural logics, it is important to distinguish between the design approaches and relational impacts of three overlapping but distinct categories of digital intervention that appear in the literature: (1) AI companions and conversational agents, such as Replika, ChatGPT, or ElliQ, designed to simulate relational presence and provide emotional support; (2) digital wellness and mental health apps, which use behavioural nudges, gamified CBT, or journaling to manage mood and stress; and (3) social media platforms, which are not explicitly therapeutic but significantly shape users' affective and social landscapes through algorithmic curation. While each of the above differs in function and intent, they operate within a shared infrastructure of platform capitalism and engagement-driven design. Despite their functional differences, each of these systems operates within infrastructures that reward predictability, data extraction, and continuous engagement. Chen et al.'s [47] work documents how adolescents encounter algorithmic features (such as infinite scroll and autoplay) that intentionally extend usage sessions while narrowing the diversity of social interaction. Studies like Chen et al. [47] demonstrate how large-scale empirical work on engagement-prolonging designs confirms these tendencies. As a result, they may contribute to a common relational outcome: digitally saturated environments that amplify disconnection, emotional flattening, and the erosion of relational autonomy [47].

Central to these paradigms is the prioritization of superficial interactions over meaningful relational depth [13,15,17]. Social media platforms, driven by commercial imperatives for maximum engagement, favour quantifiable metrics such as follower counts, likes, and frequent yet brief interactions [15,31]. This logic results in social experiences that are abundant in volume but lacking in emotional authenticity, leaving individuals digitally connected yet emotionally alienated [48,49]. The subsequent sense of disconnection illustrates a paradox central to contemporary digital design, wherein increased connectivity fails to correspond to genuine relational satisfaction or emotional fulfillment.

Digital design paradigms that subscribe to hegemonic practices are also frequently found to result in the displacement of meaningful face-to-face interactions [13,48,49]. Technologies engineered for continual user engagement inherently encourage increased screen time, inadvertently reducing opportunities for more enriching, embodied interpersonal encounters [50,51]. This displacement not only impoverishes the social experience but also diminishes users' opportunities to engage in complex, nuanced interactions, interactions that provide emotional nourishment and relational depth not readily replicated through digital channels [48,51].

4.2. *Simulated Intimacy and the Erosion of Relational Depth*

The dominance of algorithmically driven artificial intimacy further compounds this isolation. AI companions and conversational agents, designed to provide consistently empathetic and conflict-free (i.e., frictionless) interactions, promote dependency by offering emotionally predictable relationships [15,17,50,52]. The design ethos of frictionless interactions, although comforting, can inhibit users from engaging with the complexities and emotional messiness of authentic human relationships [53–55]. While "frictionless" interfaces are often celebrated in commercial design, Kemper [53] critiques this as an aesthetic and philosophical orientation that erases opportunities for meaningful pause or reflection. Chen and Schmidt [56] similarly propose "positive friction" as a countermeasure, in which small, intentional points of resistance are introduced to preserve user agency and promote deeper and more critical engagement. Over-reliance on these predictable forms of artificial intimacy undermines the intrinsic relational growth that arises through genuine human friction, negotiation, and compromise, thereby intensifying users' underlying loneliness [50,52,56].

Algorithmic designs often create an "illusion of recognition," providing users with simulations of empathy and understanding without the reciprocal depth fundamental to authentic relationships [50]. Empirical studies of AI companions confirm the risks of these relationships; Jacobs [50] shows that reliance on AI-mediated "recognition" can shift patterns of social validation, while George et al. [52] interrogate the ethics of simulated intimacy in generative AI, warning that such systems may offer comfort at the expense of authentic reciprocity. Rather than genuinely alleviating loneliness, such monologic interactions result in what scholars' term "digitized loneliness," wherein individuals are effectively conversing with reflections of their own emotional states within algorithmically curated echo chambers [50,52,55,57]. Illusory intimacy, while compelling, is fundamentally incomplete and reinforces rather than resolves users' emotional isolation [48,57].

4.3. Design Affordances, Sensory Deficits, and Affective Disconnection

Hegemonic digital paradigms are likewise characterized by their commercial incentives, frequently producing addictive designs intended to maximize continuous user engagement [31,32,34]. Platforms intentionally incorporate social metrics and reward mechanisms that encourage persistent social comparison through continuous presence online and an emotional dependency on digital approval [47,58–60]. Such designs are as commercially advantageous as they are relationally detrimental, exacerbating experiences of loneliness by discouraging users from pursuing meaningful offline connections and creating cycles of compulsive digital interaction. Concurrently, digital communication systems suffer from inherent sensory impoverishment [25,51]. Designed primarily for textual and visual communication, they lack critical relational cues such as tone of voice, body language, and nuanced emotional expressions, all of which are fundamental to deep emotional resonance [51]. This sensory deficit inevitably diminishes the emotional quality of digital interactions, rendering them less fulfilling and leaving users feeling emotionally detached despite apparent digital connectivity.

The reproduction and reinforcement of societal biases within algorithmic systems additionally contribute to loneliness [13,46,61]. AI models trained on inadequately diverse datasets risk perpetuating discriminatory views, inadvertently amplifying prejudices and contributing to the social isolation of already-marginalized groups [61]. This bias-driven amplification further entrenches social divisions, reducing opportunities for inclusive integration and meaningful cross-group social engagement [61].

4.4. Individualisation, Medicalization, and the Obfuscation of Structural Causes

Digital technology interventions, whether they be AI companions, chatbots, digital wellness and mental health apps, or social media platforms, may provide short-term relief; however, they fail to sustainably address chronic loneliness, as they inherently lack the reciprocal emotional intimacy central to long-term relational satisfaction [16]. This design misalignment fosters cycles of temporary relief followed by enduring dissatisfaction and emotional isolation. When dominant digital paradigms frequently individualize and medicalize loneliness, the hegemonic framing becomes one of individual deficit or medical condition [62]. The pervasive emphasis on individualized technological solutions for self-management, reflecting broader neoliberal ideologies, can deflect attention from underlying systemic and socioeconomic drivers of loneliness. By framing loneliness as primarily an individual responsibility, digital designs obscure necessary discussions of community structures, socioeconomic inequities, and broader collective conditions that systematically produce relational disconnection [62]. When technologies prioritize immediacy, constant connectivity, and sustained engagement, over the users' deeper emotional needs for meaningful connection and relational authenticity [25,61], loneliness becomes a predictable outcome. The experience then reflects the logic of hegemonic digital design, driven by commercial engagement metrics, algorithmic optimization, and individualizing narratives [32,61]. Addressing loneliness effectively must require systemic reorientations in technological design, moving beyond short-term emotional validation and toward fostering relational depth, equitable access, authentic interpersonal reciprocity, and structural accountability.

5. Algorithmic Infrastructures as Mediator and Producer

Algorithmic infrastructures, by design, mediate contemporary social interaction by shaping both the nature and availability of interpersonal engagements [13,24,48–50]. These systems, encompassing AI, digital technologies, and social media platforms, play a dual role in both alleviating and intensifying loneliness, depending on the design and usage context [50,63,64].

5.1. Technology as Mediator

On the alleviating side, digital technologies provide meaningful pathways to social connection, which is particularly beneficial for those geographically isolated, socially marginalized, or experiencing situational loneliness [7,50,63,64]. Platforms such as online forums, social networking sites, and digital wellness apps can effectively bridge physical and metaphorical distances, creating virtual spaces where users connect over shared experiences, interests, or identities [23]. This capacity became critically evident during the COVID-19 pandemic, when telehealth platforms, virtual support groups, and social media networks offered indispensable social support amid widespread physical isolation [65]. Additionally, algorithmic personalization enhances the emotional resonance and relevance of these digital interactions [23,52]. Emotionally intelligent AI technologies, such as the social robot ElliQ, use behavioural analytics to infer emotional states, adapting their interactions to subtly encourage social engagement among older adults [23]. Likewise, AI-powered companions like Replika and even later versions of ChatGPT offer synthetic yet responsive conversational partners, designed explicitly to make users feel understood, recognized, and supported, which are crucial psychological elements identified in loneliness interventions [17,55].

5.2. Technology as Producer

Despite these advantages, algorithmic mediation, like all algorithmic interventions, is not inherently benign. The same technologies that enable personalized interactions also structure environments characterized by censorship in the form of computational enclosure, a narrowing of informational experience through automated affirmation and selective exposure [66–68]. Milli et al. [58] demonstrate how engagement algorithms amplify divisive or emotionally charged content, while Ibrahim et al. [59] identify the specific design patterns that lead to harm, including narrowing emotional range and reinforcing dependency. Building on Tufekci's [69] account of computational agency as a narrowing of informational experience, Grabher's Enclosure 4.0 [70] analysis of how platforms capture data and scale predictive logics, and Couldry and Mejias's [71] framing of datafication as a form of digital enclosure, I use the term "behavioural enclosure" to describe how predictive systems quietly constrain users' affective and behavioural horizons. Rather than explicitly forbidding certain content, platforms gradually reduce friction, ambiguity, and contradiction to preserve emotional continuity and platform retention [53,56,64]. Personalization algorithms, learning continuously from users' behavioural data and emotional cues, systematically reinforce existing beliefs and emotional preferences, filtering out contradictory or challenging content [37,69,72]. Rather than enabling true social agency, this personalization constrains informational autonomy, creating an experience of algorithmically facilitated frictionlessness that prioritizes comfort over genuine relational growth. These dynamics raise questions of relational autonomy [42]. Unlike traditional forms of censorship that restrict content by explicit force, algorithmic enclosure subtly removes complexity, contradiction, and discomfort by rendering them less visible or less accessible [66]. Such algorithmically driven filtering risks entrenching a narrowed worldview, diminishing users' tolerance for ambiguity, and ultimately weakening relational depth in favour of superficial engagement [61]. By prioritizing ease of interaction and emotional predictability, platforms inadvertently encourage interactions that are frequent but emotionally shallow, exacerbating rather than alleviating loneliness over time.

The dynamics of algorithmic mediation have significant implications for democratic social engagement. Personalized realities, individually curated by algorithms, undermine a collective baseline of shared information, weakening capacities for collective decision making [31–33]. Users no longer merely disagree; they inhabit fundamentally different informational ecosystems, constructed by distinct algorithmic logics, each sustained by their own self-reinforcing truths [27–29]. In this way, algorithmic infrastructures not only shape individual experiences of loneliness but influence broader social cohesion, potentially deepening feelings of alienation and disconnection.

Critical perspectives highlight that reliance on digital solutions such as AI companions can lead to dependence on the appeasement of the system, potentially eroding users' motivation and ability to engage authentically in offline human relationships [50]. The risk here lies in digital relationships supplanting rather than supplementing genuine human connections, potentially leaving users feeling superficially connected yet fundamentally isolated [52,68].

Algorithmic mediation also raises critical issues of access and equity. Socioeconomic status, age, cultural context, and digital literacy significantly affect individuals' ability to benefit from digital interventions [49]. The result is an ambivalent landscape in which, as Cahyono and Adiawaty [49] observe, the same technologies that promise to connect us often operate in ways that entrench isolation. Without careful attention to these structural barriers, algorithmic infrastructures may inadvertently reinforce existing inequalities, marginalizing those who stand to gain the most from meaningful digital connections.

6. Structural Logics of Platform Capitalism and Algorithmic Control

6.1. Platform Capitalism and the Infrastructure of Loneliness

The structural logics that make up the scaffold of what Casas-Cortés et al. [32] define as "platform capitalism," are a mode of economic organization where value is extracted from social interactions themselves, and in what Nowotny [26] terms the "illusion of control" in predictive algorithms, which obscures the asymmetry between user agency and platform power. Platform capitalism and algorithmic control fundamentally shape both the lived experience of loneliness and the dominant technological responses proposed to address it. These algorithms are characterized by imperatives of scalability, engagement maximization, and data extraction that prioritize profit over well-being by embodying the specific values and priorities that often conflict with the conditions necessary for meaningful social connection [18,62]. In the context of digital loneliness interventions, such logics offer the appearance of connection and care, while frequently reproducing or exacerbating the very forms of isolation they claim to remedy.

At the center of platform capitalism lies the pursuit of profit through engagement [31]. Commercial platforms are incentivized to design technologies that prioritize user retention and behavioural predictability, often through the use of engagement-prolonging features (EPFs) such as infinite scroll, autoplay, and social nudging mechanisms [20,52,61,73]. These mechanisms range from profile view alerts to interaction streaks and leverage social anxieties and cognitive biases to maintain user presence rather than to foster relational depth. Within this model, attention is a commodity, and loneliness becomes an opportunity for monetization, giving rise to what has been described as a "billion-dollar loneliness industry" [62,74]. As Ruckenstein [24] argues, algorithmic systems are not neutral mediators but active producers of affect, shaping how users feel and act in order to sustain engagement [36]. This builds on Pariser's [37] "filter bubble" and Couldry and Mejas's [71] "costs of connection," both of which describe how datafication transforms social life into a resource for extraction. Emotional vulnerability, far from being addressed, is instrumentalized as a means of generating value.

6.2. *Affective AI and the Commodification of Emotional Vulnerability*

The logic of personalization further entrenches this profit-through-engagement dynamic. Algorithms that simulate empathy or tailor content to user affective states are framed as therapeutic tools, offering frictionless, always-available companionship [75]. AI-based chatbots and digital humans are explicitly designed to make users feel heard and supported, traits widely identified as effective in reducing the perception of loneliness [75]. While some studies show digital interventions can provide temporary relief, their effects are often "short-lived" [16]. Quantitative evidence from Maples et al. [76] and Magid et al. [63] suggests that while such tools may temporarily improve mood or reduce distress, they often fail to sustain long-term social connection, echoing the paradox described above. They are noted for not providing "real human interaction" and, thus, "cannot replace human contact," failing to reduce social disconnectedness on a long-term basis [16]. This suggests that current digital treatments act as surface-level rather than long-term solutions. Yet these interactions often constitute the above-mentioned "illusion of recognition": a simulation of social reciprocity without true mutuality or intersubjectivity [50]. Qualitative studies such as Meadows and Hine [57] and Fullam [55] show how users of mental health chatbots experience these systems not simply as tools but as affective environments that reshape expectations of intimacy and care. Rather than disrupting isolation, they reorganize it and transform loneliness from a felt absence of connection into a perpetual state of digitally mediated pseudo-connection. This is the paradox of affective AI within capitalist infrastructures: it relieves symptoms while sustaining the underlying condition.

6.3. *Algorithmic Affordances and the Redefinition of Connection*

Algorithmic infrastructures displace the role of embodied, face-to-face communication by offering convenient, scalable substitutes [77]. Digital platforms are often positioned as solutions to access barriers by providing support to users in remote regions, with limited mobility, or lacking traditional mental health resources; however, their increasing integration into daily life risks supplanting, rather than supplementing, high-quality human relationships [25,48,77,78]. The very affordances that make digital interventions scalable (i.e., predictability, availability, and affective responsiveness) can also produce dependency, flatten emotional complexity, and disincentivize engagement with the "inherent messiness" of real-world relationality [48,57,61,68]. What emerges is not just the erosion of social skill or opportunity but the redefinition of connection itself according to the logics of responsiveness, efficiency, and user retention.

6.4. *Extraction, Bias, and the Medicalized Reframing of Loneliness*

These background actors are also mechanisms of classification and control. Through digital phenotyping and the collection of granular behavioural data, platforms actively structure users' engagement with emotional experiences [18]. Data become a currency that is harvested, analyzed, and often commodified to predict user states, automate interventions, and refine engagement strategies [79]. This orientation positions the user simultaneously as a subject in distress and a data source to be mined, rendering the affective experience of loneliness legible primarily as a behavioural variable within a feedback system. While such models purport to offer care, they do so within architectures that are fundamentally extractive, opaque, and profit driven [79].

Trained on narrow datasets and optimized for broad-market appeal, these systems are also embedded with epistemic and representational limitations. AI systems risk reinforcing dominant cultural norms, societal biases, and normative assumptions about intimacy and relational need [61,79]. If left unexamined, these biases can reproduce exclusionary dynamics, marginalizing users whose identities, values, or communication styles fall outside those anticipated by the system. What results is not a universal tool for connection but a highly contingent intervention shaped by the market's image of loneliness and the individual it imagines as its subject.

Finally, the structural logics of platform capitalism encourage the previously described medicalized and individualized framing of loneliness. Digital loneliness interventions often locate the "problem" within the individual that positions users as deficient or dysregulated subjects in need of affective optimization [62]. This responsibility aligns with broader neoliberal discourses of self-management, in which structural determinants of disconnection (e.g., precarious labour, urban alienation, racialized exclusion, or defunded public infrastructure) are rendered invisible. In treating loneliness as a symptom to be managed through personalized digital solutions, such systems deflect attention from the social, political, and economic conditions that produce it [62]. Public health becomes reframed as a technological marketplace while systemic reform is replaced by therapeutic interface.

7. Public Health and Technological Design

7.1. *The Systemic Framing of Loneliness in Public Health and Design*

The convergence of public health and technology by way of design reflects a growing recognition that loneliness is not only a psychological state but also a systemic and technologically mediated phenomenon [9,15,49]. Policy analyses increasingly highlight that digital tools are being positioned as a part of national strategies to address loneliness, embedding technological interventions within broader public health frameworks [2–4,7]. While both public health and design fields acknowledge AI's potential to mediate social connection, empirical studies also show that algorithmic systems can perpetuate or even produce loneliness through their underlying logics, reshaping relational norms and displacing authentic human interaction [17,50].

Public health institutions have increasingly identified loneliness as a pervasive and urgent public health concern, particularity following the COVID-19 pandemic, associated with heightened risks of depression, anxiety, cardiovascular disease, cognitive decline, and premature mortality [1,6,8,10,12–16]. Recent epidemiological studies extend this picture: Fahy and Barry [65] show how online social capital interacts with loneliness, while Infurna et al. [80] find that loneliness levels in midlife have risen over decades, especially in digitally saturated contexts. Leading bodies such as the World Health Organization and the U.S. Surgeon General have positioned loneliness as a global crisis, calling for systemic responses and explicitly recommending the development of "pro-connection technology" and the exploration of digital interventions [61,62,81,82]. These imperatives, situated within a broader framework of the social determinants of health, have catalyzed the design field to develop responsive technologies aimed at connection, care, and accessibility.

7.2. *Digital Interventions and Conditional Promises of Connection*

Despite this review's already-significant critiques of technology-based public health interventions, both fields also recognize the potential of AI to mediate connection under specific conditions. Digital technologies can address access barriers to traditional mental health care, offering support to those facing geographic, financial, or mobility constraints [83,84]. Virtual meetups, telehealth, and digital peer support networks have proven particularly valuable during moments of crisis, such as the COVID-19 pandemic [48]. Some AI companions and platforms incorporate therapeutic frameworks like Cognitive Behavioural Therapy (CBT) or narrative coaching, providing structured support that may alleviate subjective feelings of loneliness in the short term [54,76]. Certain interventions have been designed with transitional intent such as helping users develop communicative competencies or encouraging re-engagement with real-world social environments through hybrid tools such as location-based games or social prompts [67].

7.3. Designing for Relational Justice: Toward Ethical and Inclusive Systems

What emerges from this intersection is a call for ethically grounded, human-centered design [13,48]. Ethical analyses such as Jecker et al. [61] argue for policy safeguards when deploying digital solutions for social support, noting that the capacity for simulated empathy demands corresponding protections against misuse. Public health perspectives insist that loneliness must be understood as a socially patterned and structurally produced phenomenon, not merely a symptom to be managed through individual digital use [49,52,54,61]. This orientation challenges the design field to develop interventions that resist individualization, foreground user autonomy, and account for social, economic, and cultural inequities. Design responses should be informed by participatory methods, community-based research, and ethical foresight, with particular interest to those that center accessibility, transparency, and inclusivity, which can help mitigate some of the harms introduced by commercial and algorithmic systems [52,54,61,65].

At the policy level, both fields advocate for increased regulation, interdisciplinary oversight, and long-term evaluation of digital mental health interventions [2,4,14,85]. There is growing consensus that ethical and technical governance must be instituted to protect vulnerable populations from manipulation, surveillance, or further marginalization [54,57,79,86]. This is further coupled with an urgent need to move beyond short-term assessments of efficacy to examine the long-term psychosocial effects of digital interactions on loneliness, relational depth, and communal cohesion [57,79,82].

The connection between public health and design is not simply one of task delegation, where health systems define problems and designers generate solutions, but one of epistemological and ethical entanglement. Both fields must engage in ongoing dialogue to interrogate how digital infrastructures are conceptualized, deployed, and experienced. From a design justice perspective, Pendse et al. [79] call for decolonial approaches that challenge dominant narratives and ensure technologies are shaped by, and accountable to, the communities they serve. Addressing loneliness in the context of AI requires not only technological innovation but also a collective commitment to reimagining relationality, accountability, and care in an era shaped by algorithmic systems.

8. Digital Public Health Design Framework

The preceding sections traced how the four interconnected domains of hegemonic digital design paradigms, algorithmic mediation, and public health framing shape the experience of loneliness and the interventions proposed to address it. The structural critiques outlined in Section 5 identify the commercial and algorithmic logics that undermine relational depth, pointing to the need for relational personalization and digital well-being by design. Section 6's analysis of algorithmic mediation highlights the narrowing of informational and emotional experience, underscoring the importance of hybrid and real-world connection and adaptive, non-coercive support. Behavioural science offers several design strategies to support adaptive, non-coercive interventions: Mele et al. [23] describe "smart nudging" as a way to co-create value with users, Joachim et al. [87] apply nudge theory to AI-driven health platforms, and Chiam et al. [88] demonstrate how algorithmic nudging can be personalized to health outcomes while maintaining transparency. Section 7's integration of public health perspectives calls for participatory, equitable and accountable approaches. Together, these thematic insights directly inform the ethical design priorities that follow.

To address loneliness as both a public health crisis and a technologically mediated condition, this review proposes a human-centered and ethically grounded framework for the design of AI and digital interventions. Rather than reproducing the logic of behavioural enclosure, this framework supports relational autonomy, structural responsiveness, and ethical accountability. Rooted in public health imperatives, human-centered design principles, and critical analyses of platform capitalism, it offers an alternative to engagement-driven models that often exacerbate the very issues they seek to resolve [49]. Instead of managing the symptoms of loneliness, it foregrounds the structural and systemic conditions that produce and perpetuate it.

The framework begins with a philosophical reorientation. Loneliness should not be treated solely as a pathological deficit to be remedied through technological substitution. Instead, it must be understood as a relational signal, an embodied, affective form of attunement that indicates unmet needs for social connection [11–13]. In this reframing, digital tools are positioned as facilitators of social repair rather than surrogates for social life. This shift is rooted in a model of relational autonomy, which is the understanding that autonomy is not the absence of dependence but the ability to act meaningfully within a network of social, cultural, and structural relationships [41,42,45]. Unlike individualistic models of choice, relational autonomy recognises that agency is shaped by context, care, and reciprocity [42]. This demands recognition of the structural determinants shaping experiences of loneliness, including economic precarity, housing insecurity, systemic discrimination, and unequal access to care [13,15,61,62]. Technology, in this context, should be designed to support human flourishing in culturally and materially specific ways. It requires an ethical shift away from replacement logics toward the augmentation of human relationships. AI systems must scaffold, prompt, and gently encourage connection, not reroute relational energy into synthetic stand-ins. A decolonial, context-sensitive approach is essential, one that centers lived experience, acknowledges cultural specificity, and actively disrupts power asymmetries in how technologies are imagined, designed, and accessed [79].

At the heart of this framework lies a set of ethical principles, adapted from Löchner et al.'s TEQUILA model (Trust, Evidence, Quality, Usability, Interests, Liability, Accreditation) [18], and revised to address the specific challenges of AI in public health. Trust must be earned through transparent data governance, continuous and informed consent, and clear communication of the capacities and limitations of artificial agents. Users should retain full control over their emotional, behavioural, and biometric data, and transparency must include explicit disclosures about AI-generated content and simulated empathy.

High standards of evidence and quality are also critical. Interventions must be rigorously evaluated through long-term, methodologically robust studies across diverse populations [18,61,82]. Success should be measured not by engagement metrics but by their capacity to foster emotional resilience, deepen social ties, and promote community integration [61]. Clinical accreditation and regulatory oversight are essential for systems with therapeutic claims, alongside meaningful human oversight for any AI making interpretive judgments about users' mental health [82].

Equally vital is a participatory design process grounded in human-centered values. End users, mental health practitioners, and public health experts must be involved throughout development, from needs assessment to outcome evaluation [14,48,79,87]. Systems should empower users by promoting autonomy and discouraging dependency, avoiding manipulative design patterns that exploit vulnerability [25,48,73]. Algorithmic systems must be audited for bias and actively corrected to avoid reproducing structural inequities related to race, gender, disability, or class [61,79]. Equity must be embedded in the design logic from the outset.

Clear lines of accountability must be maintained throughout the entire lifecycle of digital interventions. Responsibility for outcomes, from data handling to harm mitigation, cannot be diffused through technical abstraction [18,54,89]. The myth of algorithmic neutrality must be replaced with governance structures that acknowledge the political and material stakes of AI systems. Certification protocols are particularly important for platforms and agents performing quasi-clinical functions in mental health.

While all digital interventions must be evaluated for bias and equitable access, AI companions require safeguards around emotional simulation and user dependency. To operationalize these ethical commitments, Figure 2 identifies the following key functional priorities:

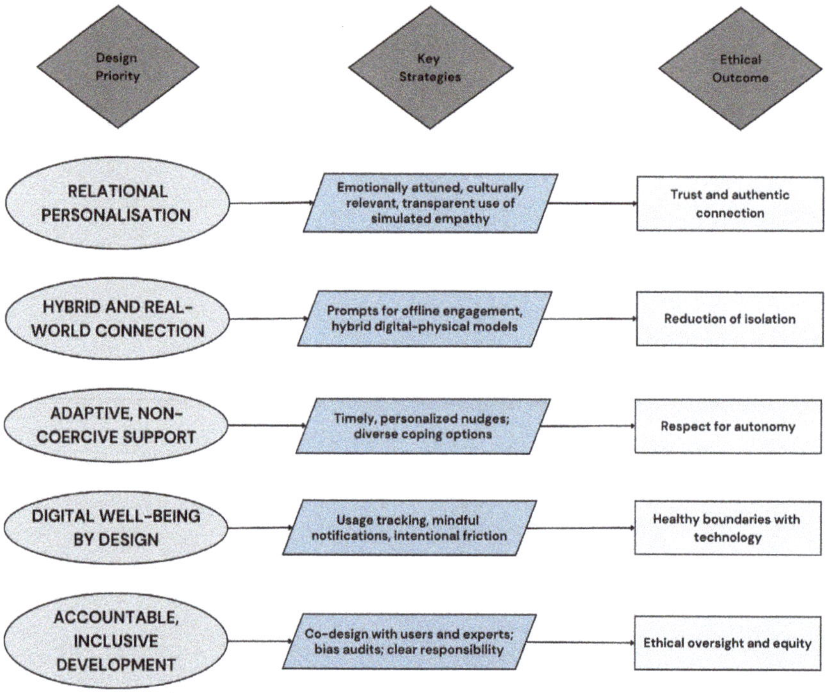

Figure 2. Ethical outcomes of design priorities for digital interventions addressing loneliness.

Personalization should be used not to increase retention but to ensure relevance, emotional recognition, and cultural sensitivity [14,48,82,87]. While emotionally intelligent responses and simulated empathy can help users feel recognized, these functions must remain transparent to avoid misidentification or confusion. In the case of social robots, nonverbal cues such as gaze or gesture may enhance interaction but must be carefully calibrated to avoid the phenomenon commonly known as the uncanny valley, which can disrupt trust and emotional resonance.

Digital systems should also reinforce real-world connection. Features such as prompts to connect with friends, community event suggestions, and referrals to local resources help bridge online engagement with embodied sociality [14,48,82,90]. Hybrid models that integrate online tools with offline support can mitigate the risk of relational displacement. Adaptive systems, such as Just-in-Time Adaptive Interventions (JITAIs), can offer timely and context-sensitive nudges that promote well-being without coercion [21,23,25]. These should encourage, not compel, social activity, movement, and emotional regulation. A practical illustration of the "hybrid and real-world connection" priority is the +*Connect* smartphone application, a positive psychology-based program co-designed with young people who self-identified as experiencing loneliness [14]. The intervention delivered daily digital content over six weeks, including short videos, reflective exercises, and "real-world" missions, which prompt users to initiate or deepen social interactions offline [14]. In a pilot randomized controlled trial involving young adults both with and without social anxiety disorder, +*Connect* achieved high rates of engagement and yielded measurable improvements in self-reported social connectedness and reductions in loneliness [14]. Qualitative feedback highlighted the value of combining asynchronous, self-paced digital learning with structured encouragement to practice skills in everyday life, supporting the idea that digital public health interventions can be designed to bridge online engagement with offline relationship building in ways that are perceived as supportive rather than intrusive [14].

Rather than promoting a universalized vision of healthy behaviour, interventions must recognize and support the diverse coping strategies users already employ. From creative expression and distraction to introspection and social withdrawal, digital tools must be flexible enough to accommodate varied paths through loneliness [25,48]. Systems should also help prevent overdependence: tools such as usage dashboards, mindful notification settings, and intentional design friction can support digital well-being and more reflective engagement [48,73]. Pretolesi et al. [91] explore user preferences for customization, Janković et al. [92] show how adaptive notifications can improve engagement in behaviour-change apps, and Auf et al. [60] examine gamification techniques that balance motivation with user autonomy. Crucially, interventions must maintain a clear boundary between technological support and relational replacement while maintaining trust through empathy [48,73,93,94].

Meaningful solutions to loneliness require sustained and interdisciplinary collaboration between fields, humans, and machines [48,95,96]. Designers, engineers, social scientists, ethicists, clinicians, and policymakers must work together from ideation to implementation. Feedback loops must be built into these systems, allowing for iterative refinement based on lived experience and emergent harms. Longitudinal studies are needed to assess not only clinical efficacy but also the social and political consequences of intervention. Policy frameworks must promote equitable access, mandate accountability, and protect vulnerable users from exploitation.

Addressing loneliness through AI and digital public health tools requires a multidimensional approach, philosophical, ethical, functional, and political. By resisting reductive engagement metrics and centering relational integrity, this framework offers a path toward technologies that support connection, compassion, and human flourishing in complex and context-specific ways.

9. Conclusions

As loneliness emerges as a defining public health challenge of the digital age, it becomes increasingly urgent to examine not only the individual experiences of disconnection but also the technological, economic, and epistemological systems that shape them. This review has argued that loneliness must be understood as both a socially embedded condition and a logical outcome of hegemonic design paradigms, particularly those structured by the logics of platform capitalism and algorithmic control. The very infrastructures that promise to alleviate loneliness, such as AI companions, wellness apps, and digital health tools, are embedded in the logics of platform capitalism and engagement-driven design, monetizing attention [26,32]. The intimacy through simulated empathy replaces genuine social connection with commercially mediated interactions [15,42,63].

By tracing the evolution of gatekeeping from a human editorial process to an opaque, computational logic embedded in algorithmic infrastructures, the analysis has shown how visibility, emotion, and legitimacy are increasingly governed by profitability and predictive accuracy. Within this paradigm, loneliness is not merely mediated; it is produced. In this new algorithmic epistemology, emotional profiling replaces public discourse, and behavioral nudging becomes a quiet, ambient form of governance [20]. This review proposes that loneliness is not only framed and mediated but produced through what might be called "algorithmic epistemology," a logic of knowing grounded in engagement-generated, affect-oriented, and predictive algorithms [89,95]. As Maalsen [89] shows, algorithmic systems reconfigure epistemic landscapes by actively shaping how we come to know and interpret social and spatial realities. This epistemological shift is further underscored by Loosen and Scholl [95], who argue that algorithms function as observing systems that construct meaning rather than passively reflect it, and by Milano et al. [96], who demonstrate how algorithmic profiling can fragment individuals' interpretive capacities, limiting their ability to share experiences and resist system-driven sense making. These systems do not just reflect user reality; they recalibrate it. What is most seen becomes what is most real.

This review recognizes that digital interventions vary widely in function and design; however, the shared infrastructure of algorithmic governance and behavioural design necessitates a critical lens across domains. Digital interventions are not inherently harmful, but when embedded in systems optimized for surveillance, scalability, and retention, they risk becoming part of the problem they seek to solve. If designed without critical reflection, they may individualize systemic issues, reinforce existing inequities, and offer only superficial comfort in place of sustained, structural solutions. Addressing loneliness, therefore, demands more than innovation; it requires transformation of design priorities, business models, regulatory structures, and public imaginaries.

The framework proposed in this review offers a path forward, one grounded in public health ethics, human-centered design, and political accountability. By reframing loneliness as a relational signal rather than a personal failure, and by designing AI tools to augment rather than replace human connection, it is possible to develop digital interventions that respect autonomy, enable genuine engagement, and resist exploitative logics. Such tools must be transparent, context-sensitive, and continually evaluated for their long-term impacts, not just on individuals but on the social fabrics they inhabit.

Designing for loneliness is not only a technological challenge; it is a moral and cultural one. It calls for interdisciplinary collaboration, policy reform, and, above all, a renewed commitment to human dignity in an age of machine mediation. In reimagining how we relate to both each other and the systems we build, we are not simply addressing loneliness; we are redefining the terms of connection itself.

10. Limitations and Future Directions

A meta-narrative review, by design, does not aim for exhaustive inclusion of all possible studies, nor does it provide a quantitative meta-analysis. Instead, it prioritizes conceptual depth and cross-disciplinary dialogue. As such, some relevant empirical studies may not have been captured, particularly outside the time frame or language searched. The focus on English-language sources and the reliance on available database indexing may also introduce selection bias. All conclusions and the framework presented here should be read as integrative, rather than definitive, offering a foundation for further empirical testing and refinement.

The growing integration of AI-driven systems into loneliness interventions presents a critical area for future research at the intersection of technology, public health, and relational design. One area of note is social robotics and digital humans. As these fields evolve beyond assistive functions toward roles as emotionally responsive companions, they raise important questions about the reconfiguration of care, connection, and intimacy in technologically mediated contexts. Future research should expand Freitas et al.'s [17] work, which provides evidence that AI companions can reduce loneliness in controlled settings, as well as the work of Mahajan [54], who explores their potential for integration into family-like roles, and Lynch et al. [90], who cautions that such automation can displace human affective labour.

Future studies should investigate how affective AI systems simulate empathy, personalize interaction, and offer scalable support for structurally underserved populations. Equally important is the need to assess the long-term psychosocial impacts of such systems, including risks of dependency, emotional flattening, and the commodification of human relationships. Work by Sharma et al. [93] and Pralat et al. [94] demonstrates that human–AI collaboration can foster more empathetic, trust-building interactions, findings which could inform ethical frameworks and technical implantation.

This research agenda must also address ethical and governance concerns, including consent, bias mitigation, and accountability, in the collection and use of affective data. Frameworks such as TEQUILA [12] offer starting points for evaluating responsible deployment but require empirical testing and contextual adaptation.

As AI companions increasingly blur the boundaries between care, commerce, and relationality, interdisciplinary research is needed to ensure these systems enhance rather than erode the conditions for meaningful social connection. The challenge lies not only in developing technically sophisticated tools but in reimagining digital interventions that prioritize human dignity, autonomy, and structural equity.

Supplementary Materials: The following supporting information can be downloaded at: https://www.mdpi.com/article/10.3390/ijerph22091394/s1, Table S1: Classification of articles for analysis.

Funding: This research received no external funding.

Institutional Review Board Statement: Not applicable.

Informed Consent Statement: Not applicable.

Data Availability Statement: No new data were created or analyzed in this study. Data sharing is not applicable to this article.

Conflicts of Interest: The author declares no conflicts of interest.

References

1. Petersen, A. Pandemics as Socio-Political Phenomena. In *Pandemic Societies a Critical Public Health Perspective*; Bristol University Press: Bristol, UK, 2024; pp. 1–24. [CrossRef]
2. Goldman, N.; Khanna, D.; El Asmar, M.L.; Qualter, P.; El-Osta, A. Addressing loneliness and social isolation in 52 countries: A scoping review of National policies. *BMC Public Health* **2024**, *24*, 1207. [CrossRef]
3. Jentoft, E.E. Technology and older adults in British loneliness policy and political discourse. *Front. Digit. Health* **2023**, *5*, 1168413. [CrossRef]
4. Jentoft, E.E.; Sandset, T.; Haldar, M. Problematizing loneliness as a public health issue: An analysis of policy in the United Kingdom. *Crit. Policy Stud.* **2025**, *19*, 1–18. [CrossRef]
5. Isolation, Loneliness, and COVID-19: Pandemic Leads to Sharp Increase in Mental Health Challenges, Social Woes. Available online: http://angusreid.org/isolation-and-loneliness-covid19/ (accessed on 10 June 2025).
6. Weissbourd, R.; Batanova, M.; Lovison, V.; Torres, E. Loneliness in America: How the Pandemic Has Deepened an Epidemic of Loneliness and What We Can Do About It. Report by the Making Caring Common Project in Harvard Graduate School of Education 2021. Available online: https://mcc.gse.harvard.edu/reports/loneliness-in-america (accessed on 2 June 2025).
7. Hawkley, L. Public policy and the reduction and prevention of loneliness and social isolation. In *Loneliness and Social Isolation in Old Age, Correlates and Implications*; Routeledge: New York, NY, USA, 2023; pp. 181–190.
8. American Psychiatric Association. *Diagnostic and Statistical Manual of Mental Disorders: DSM-5-TR (5th Edition Text Revision)*; American Psychiatric Association Publishing: Washington, DC, USA, 2013.
9. von Känel, R.; Weilenmann, S.; Spiller, T.R. Loneliness Is Associated with Depressive Affect, But Not with Most Other Symptoms of Depression in Community-Dwelling Individuals: A Network Analysis. *Int. J. Environ. Res. Public Health* **2021**, *18*, 2408. [CrossRef]
10. Caciopo, S.; Grippo, A.J.; London, S.; Cacioppo, J.T. Loneliness: Clinical Import and Interventions. *Perspect. Psychol. Sci. A J. Assoc. Psychol. Sci.* **2015**, *10*, 238–249. [CrossRef]
11. Hang, S.; Jost, G.M.; Guyer, A.E.; Robins, R.W.; Hastings, P.D.; Hostinar, C.E. Understanding the development of chronic loneliness in youth. *Child Dev. Perspect.* **2024**, *18*, 44–53. [CrossRef]
12. Rokach, A.; Boulazreg, S. Loneliness or Solitude: Which will we experience? *Ruch Filoz.* **2023**, *79*, 95–139. [CrossRef]
13. Dwyer, L. Canadian perspectives on loneliness; digital communication as meaningful connection. *Front. Public Health* **2024**, *12*, 1389099. [CrossRef] [PubMed]
14. Lim, M.H.; Rodebaugh, T.L.; Eres, R.; Long, K.M.; Penn, D.L.; Gleeson, J.F.M. A Pilot Digital Intervention Targeting Loneliness in Youth Mental Health. *Front. Psychiatry* **2019**, *10*, 604. [CrossRef] [PubMed]
15. Nieves, J.C.; Osorio, M.; Rojas-Velazquez, D.; Magallanes, Y.; Brännström, A. Digital Companions for Well-being: Challenges and Opportunities. *J. Intell. Fuzzy Syst.* **2024**, 219336. [CrossRef]
16. Shah, S.G.S.; Nogueras, D.; van Woerden, H.C.; Kiparoglou, V. Evaluation of the Effectiveness of Digital Technology Interventions to Reduce Loneliness in Older Adults: Systematic Review and Meta-analysis. *J. Med. Internet Res.* **2021**, *23*, e24712. [CrossRef] [PubMed]
17. Freitas, J.D.; Uguralp, A.K.; Uguralp, Z.O.; Stefano, P. AI Companions Reduce Loneliness. *arXiv* **2024**. [CrossRef]
18. Löchner, J.; Carlbring, P.; Schuller, B.; Torous, J.; Sander, L.B. Digital interventions in mental health: An overview and future perspectives. *Internet Interv.* **2025**, *40*, 100824. [CrossRef]
19. Alqahtani, F.; Al Khalifah, G.; Oyebode, O.; Orji, R. Apps for Mental Health: An Evaluation of Behavior Change Strategies and Recommendations for Future Development. *Front. Artif. Intell.* **2019**, *2*, 30. [CrossRef] [PubMed]
20. Matias, J. Nudging Algorithms by Influencing Human Behavior: Effects of Encouraging Fact-Checking on News Rankings. Open Science Framework. 2020. Available online: https://osf.io/m98b6/ (accessed on 2 June 2025).
21. Toner, J.; Allen-Collinson, J.; Jones, L. 'I guess I was surprised by an app telling an adult they had to go to bed before half ten': A phenomenological exploration of behavioural 'nudges'. *Qual. Res. Sport Exerc.* **2024**, *14*, 413–427. [CrossRef]
22. Torous, J.; Bucci, S.; Bell, I.H.; Kessing, L.V.; Faurholt-Jepsen, M.; Whelan, P.; Carvalho, A.F.; Keshavan, M.; Linardon, J.; Firth, J. The growing field of digital psychiatry: Current evidence and the future of apps, social media, chatbots, and virtual reality. *World Psychiatry* **2021**, *20*, 318–335. [CrossRef]
23. Mele, C.; Russo Spena, T.; Kaartemo, V.; Marzullo, M.L. Smart nudging: How cognitive technologies enable choice architectures for value co-creation. *J. Bus. Res.* **2021**, *129*, 949–960. [CrossRef]
24. Ruckenstein, M. *The Feel of Algorithms*; University of California Press: Oakland, CA, USA, 2023.
25. Salamida, M. Designing Meaningful Future Digital Interactions: Fostering Wellbeing to Reduce Techno-Induced Stress. 2024. Available online: https://www.politesi.polimi.it/handle/10589/227729 (accessed on 2 June 2025).
26. Nowotny, H. *In AI We Trust: Power, Illusion and Control of Predictive Algorithms*; John Wiley & Sons: Hoboken, NJ, USA, 2021.

27. Shoemaker, P.J.; Vos, T. *Gatekeeping Theory*; Taylor & Francis: Oxfordshire, UK, 2009.
28. Gillespie, T. The Politics of 'Platforms. *New Media Soc.* **2010**, *12*, 347–364. [CrossRef]
29. Gillespie, T. Do Not Recommend? Reduction as a Form of Content Moderation. *Soc. Media Soc.* **2022**, *8*, 20563051221117552. [CrossRef]
30. Couldry, N. Media in Modernity: A Nice Derangement of Institutions. *Rev. Int. Philos.* **2017**, *281*, 259–279. Available online: https://shs.cairn.info/journal-revue-internationale-de-philosophie-2017-3-page-259?lang=en (accessed on 26 May 2025). [CrossRef]
31. Zuboff, S. *The Age of Surveillance Capitalism: The Fight for a Human Future at the New Frontier of Power*; Public Affairs: New York, NY, USA, 2019.
32. Casas-Cortés, M.; Cañedo, M.; Diz, C. *Platform Capitalism*; Oxford Research Encyclopedias, Anthropology: Oxford, UK, 2023. [CrossRef]
33. Tufecki, Z. "Not This One": Social Movements, the Attention Economy, and Microcelebrity Networked Activism. *Am. Behav. Sci.* **2013**, *57*, 848–870. [CrossRef]
34. Srnicek, N. The Challenges of Platform Capitalism: Understanding the Logic of a New Business Model. *Juncture* **2017**, *23*, 254–257. [CrossRef]
35. Turkle, S. *Alone Together: Why We Expect More from Technology and Less from Each Other*; Basic Books Inc.: New York, NY, USA, 2011.
36. Illouz, E. *Cold Intimacies: The Making of Emotional Capitalism*; Polity: New York, NY, USA, 2007.
37. Pariser, E. *The Filter Bubble: What The Internet Is Hiding from You*; Penguin Books Limited: London, UK, 2011.
38. Greenhalgh, T.; Wong, G.; Jagosh, J.; Greenhalgh, J.; Manzano, A.; Westhorp, G.; Pawson, R. Protocol—The RAMESES II Study: Developing Guidance and Reporting Standards for Realist Evaluation. *BMJ Open* **2015**, *5*, e008567. [CrossRef]
39. Wong, G.; Greenhalgh, T.; Westhorp, G.; Buckingham, J.; Pawson, R. RAMESES Publication Standards: Meta-Narrative Reviews. *BMC Med.* **2013**, *11*, 20. [CrossRef] [PubMed]
40. Sukhera, J. Narrative Reviews: Flexible, Rigorous, and Practical. *J. Grad. Med. Educ.* **2022**, *14*, 414–417. [CrossRef]
41. Ågerfalk, P.J. Artificial Intelligence as Digital Agency. *Eur. J. Inf. Syst.* **2020**, *29*, 1–8. [CrossRef]
42. Ho, A. *Live Like Nobody Is Watching: Relational Autonomy in the Age of Artificial Intelligence Health Monitoring*; Oxford University Press: New York, NY, USA, 2023.
43. Kuss, P.; Meske, C. *From Entity to Relation? Agency in the Era of Artificial Intelligence*; Social Science Research Network: Rochester, NY, USA, 2025. [CrossRef]
44. Dattathrani, S.; De', R. The Concept of Agency in the Era of Artificial Intelligence: Dimensions and Degrees. *Inf. Syst. Front.* **2023**, *25*, 29–54. [CrossRef]
45. Burkitt, I. Relational Agency: Relational Sociology, Agency and Interaction. *Eur. J. Soc. Theory* **2016**, *19*, 322–339. [CrossRef]
46. Hughes, G.; Moore, L.; Hennessy, M.; Sandset, T.; Jentoft, E.E.; Haldar, M. What kind of a problem is loneliness? Representations of connectedness and participation from a study of telepresence technologies in the UK. *Front. Digit. Health* **2024**, *6*, 1304085. [CrossRef] [PubMed]
47. Chen, Y.; Fu, Y.; Chen, Z.; Radesky, J.; Hiniker, A. The Engagement-Prolonging Designs Teens Encounter on Very Large Online Platforms. *arXiv* **2025**. [CrossRef]
48. Dwyer, L. Isolated Circuits: Human Experience and Robot Design for the Future of Loneliness. Ph.D. Thesis, Toronto Metropolitan University, Toronto, ON, Canada, 2023.
49. Cahyono, M.Y.M.; Adiawaty, S. The Ambivalent Impact of Digital Technology on Loneliness: Navigating Connection and Isolation in the Digital Age. *Sinergi Int. J. Psychol.* **2024**, *2*, 181–197. [CrossRef]
50. Jacobs, K.A. Digital loneliness—Changes of social recognition through AI companions. *Front. Digit. Health* **2024**, *6*, 1281037. [CrossRef]
51. Comment, T.D. The Impact of Social Media Use on Loneliness Through an Interpersonal-Connection-Behavior Framework. Master's Thesis, Kent State University, Kent, OH, USA, 2024.
52. George, A.S.; George, A.S.H.; Baskar, T.; Pandey, D. The Allure of Artificial Intimacy: Examining the Appeal and Ethics of Using Generative AI for Simulated Relationships. *Partn. Univers. Int. Innov. J.* **2023**, *1*, 132–147. [CrossRef]
53. Kemper, J. *Frictionlesssness: The Silicon Valley Philosophy of Seamless Technology and the Aesthetic Value of Imperfection*; Bloomsbury Publishing: Santa Barbara, CA, USA, 2023.
54. Mahajan, P. Beyond Biology: AI as Family and the Future of Human Bonds and Relationships. HAL Archives Ouvertes. Available online: https://hal.science/hal-04987496 (accessed on 2 June 2025).
55. Fullam, E. The Social Life of Mental Health Chatbots. Ph.D. Thesis, Birbeck, University of London, London, UK, 2024.
56. Chen, Z.; Schmidt, R. Exploring a Behavioral Model of "Positive Friction" in Human-AI Interaction. In *Design, User Experience, and Usability*; Marcus, A., Rosenzweig, E., Soares, M.M., Eds.; Springer Nature: Cham, Switzerland, 2024; pp. 3–22. [CrossRef]

57. Meadows, R.; Hine, C. Entanglements of Technologies, Agency and Selfhood: Exploring the Complexity in Attitudes Toward Mental Health Chatbots. *Cult. Med. Pyschiatry* **2024**, *48*, 840–857. [CrossRef] [PubMed]
58. Milli, S.; Carroll, M.; Wang, Y.; Pandey, S.; Zhao, S.; Dragan, A.D. Engagement, User Satisfaction and the Amplification of Divisive Content on Social Media. *PNAS Nexus* **2025**, *4*, pgaf062. [CrossRef]
59. Ibrahim, L.; Rocher, L.; Valdivia, A. Characterizing and Modeling Harms from Interactions with Design Patterns in AI interfaces. *arXiv* **2024**. [CrossRef]
60. Auf, H.; Dagman, J.; Renström, S.; Chaplin, J. Gamification and Nudging Techniques for Improving User Engagement in Mental Health and Well-being Apps. *Proc. Des. Soc.* **2021**, *1*, 1647–1656. [CrossRef]
61. Jecker, N.S.; Sparrow, R.; Lederman, Z.; Ho, A. Digital Humans to Combat Loneliness and Social Isolation: Ethics Concerns and Policy Recommendations. *Hastings Cent. Rep.* **2024**, *54*, 7–12. [CrossRef]
62. Sagan, O. Organized loneliness and its discontents. *Divers. Incl. Res.* **2024**, *1*, e12008. [CrossRef]
63. Magid, K.; Sagui-Henson, S.J.; Sweet, C.C.; Smith, B.J.; Chamberlain, C.E.W.; Levens, S.M. The Impact of Digital Mental Health Services on Loneliness and Mental Health: Results from a Prospective, Observational Study. *Int. J. Behav. Med.* **2024**, *31*, 468. [CrossRef]
64. Primack, B.A.; Shensa, A.; Sidani, J.E.; Whaite, E.O.; Lin, L.Y.; Rosen, D.; Colditz, J.B.; Radovic, A.M.; Miller, E. Social Media Use and Perceived Social Isolation Among Young Adults in the U.S. *Am. J. Prev. Med.* **2017**, *53*, 1–8. [CrossRef] [PubMed]
65. Fahy, M.; Barry, M. Investigating the interplay of loneliness, computer-mediated communication, online social capital, and well-being: Insights from a COVID-19 lockdown study. *Front. Digit. Health* **2024**, *6*, 1289451. [CrossRef] [PubMed]
66. Woolley, S. *Computational Propaganda: Political Parties, Politicians, and Political Manipulation on Social Media*; Oxford University Press: Oxford, UK, 2018.
67. Kitchen, N.; Curtis, S. "If you Build It, They Will Come." Infrastructure, Hegemonic Transition, and Peaceful Change. *Glob. Stud. Q.* **2025**, *5*, ksaf021. [CrossRef]
68. Ghantous, D. Between the Self and Signal the Dead Internet & A Crisis of Perception. Master's Thesis, OCAD University, Toronto, ON, Canada, 2025.
69. Tufekci, Z. Algorithmic Harms Beyond Facebook and Google; Emergent Challenges of Computational Agency. *Colo. Technol. Law J.* **2015**, *13*, 203.
70. Grabher, G. Enclosure 4.0: Seizing Data, Selling Predictions, Scaling Platforms. *Sociologica* **2020**, *14*, 241–265. [CrossRef]
71. Couldry, N.; Mejias, U.A. Data Colonialism: Rethinkking Big Data's Relation to the Contemporary Subject. *Telev. New Media* **2019**, *20*, 336–349. [CrossRef]
72. Bozdag, E.; van den Hoven, J. Breaking the Filter Bubble: Democracy and Design. *Ethics Inf. Technol.* **2015**, *17*, 249–265. [CrossRef]
73. Zaheer, S. Designing for Digital Well-Being: Applying Behavioral Science to Reduce Tech Addiction. *Int. J. Res. Lead. Publ.* **2023**, *4*, 1–12. [CrossRef]
74. Rosenzwig, M. Boyfriends for Rent, Robots, Camming: How the Business of Loneliness Is Booming. In *The Guardian*. 1 November 2020. Available online: https://www.theguardian.com/society/2020/nov/01/loneliness-business-booming-pandemic (accessed on 1 June 2025).
75. Li, H.; Zhang, R.; Lee, Y.C.; Kraut, R.E.; Mohr, D.C. Systematic review and meta-analysis of AI-based conversational agents for promoting mental health and well-being. *npj Digit. Med.* **2023**, *6*, 1–14. [CrossRef]
76. Maples, B.; Cerit, M.; Vishwanath, A.; Pea, R. Loneliness and suicide mitigation for students using GPT3-enabled chatbots. *npj Ment. Health Res.* **2024**, *3*, 1–6. [CrossRef]
77. Duradoni, M.; Serritella, E.; Severino, F.P.; Guazzini, A. Exploring the Relationships Between Digital Life Balance and Internet Social Capital, Loneliness, Fear of Missing Out, and Anxiety. *Hum. Behav. Emerg. Technol.* **2024**, *2024*, 1–9. [CrossRef]
78. Jokić, B.; Ristić Dedić, Z.; Šimon, J. Time Spent Using Digital Technology, Loneliness, and Well-Being Among Three Cohorts of Adolescent Girls and Boys—A Moderated Mediation Analysis. *Psihol. Teme* **2024**, *33*, 25–46. [CrossRef]
79. Pendse, S.R.; Nkemelu, D.; Bidwell, N.J.; Jadhav, S.; Pathare, S.; De Choudhury, M.; Kumar, N. From Treatment to Healing: Envisioning a Decolonial Digital Mental Health. In Proceedings of the 2022 CHI Conference on Human Factors in Computing Systems, New Orleans, LA, USA, 29 April–5 May 2022; Association for Computing Machinery: New York, NY, USA, 2022; pp. 1–23. [CrossRef]
80. Infurna, F.J.; Dey, N.E.Y.; Gonzalez Avilès, T.; Grimm, K.J.; Lachman, M.E.; Gerstorf, D. Loneliness in Midlife: Historical Increases and Elevated Levels in the United States Compared with Europe. *Am. Psychol.* **2024**, *80*, 744–756. [CrossRef] [PubMed]
81. WHO Launches Commission to Foster Social Connection. Available online: https://www.who.int/news/item/15-11-2023-who-launches-commission-to-foster-social-connection (accessed on 2 June 2025).
82. Yang, Y.; Wang, C.; Xiang, X.; An, R. AI Applications to Reduce Loneliness Among Older Adults: A Systematic Review of Effectiveness and Technologies. *Healthcare* **2025**, *13*, 446. [CrossRef] [PubMed]

83. Andersson, G.; Titov, N. Advantages and Limitations of Internet-Based Interventions for Common Mental Disorders. *World Psychiatry* **2014**, *13*, 4–11. [CrossRef]
84. Naslund, J.A.; Aschbrenner, K.A.; Araya, R.; Marsch, L.A.; Unützer, J.; Patel, V.; Bartels, S.J. Digital Technology for Treating and Preventing Mental Disorders in Low-Income and Middle-Income Countries: A Narrative Review of the Literature. *Lancet Psychiatry* **2017**, *4*, 486–500. [CrossRef]
85. Danieli, M.; Ciulli, T.; Mousavi, S.M.; Riccardi, G. A Conversational Artificial Intelligence Agent for a Mental Health Care App: Evaluation Study of Its Participatory Design. *JMIR Form. Res.* **2021**, *5*, e30053. [CrossRef]
86. Thieme, A.; Hanratty, M.; Lyone, M.; Palacios, J.; Marques, R.F.; Morrison, C.; Doherty, G. Designing Human-centered AI for Mental Health: Developing Clinically Relevant Applications for Online CBT Treatment. *ACM Trans. Comput.-Hum. Interact.* **2023**, *30*, 1–50. [CrossRef]
87. Joachim, S.; Forkan, A.R.M.; Jayaraman, P.P.; Morshed, A.; Wickramsinghe, N. A Nudge-Inspired AI-Driven Health Platform for Self-Management of Diabetes. *Sensors* **2022**, *22*, 4620. [CrossRef]
88. Chiam, J.; Lim, A.; Teredesai, A. NudgeRank: Digital Algorithmic Nudging for Personalized Health. In Proceedings of the KKD '24: The 30th ACM SIGKDD Conference on Knowledge Discovery and Data Mining, Barcelona, Spain, 25–29 August 2024; Association for Computing Machinery: New York, NY, USA, 2024; pp. 4873–4884. [CrossRef]
89. Pretolesi, D.; Motnikar, L.; Bieg, T.; Gafert, M.; Uhl, J. Exploring User Preferences: Customisation and Attitudes towards Notification in Mobile Health and Well-Being Applications. *Behav. Inf. Technol.* **2025**, *44*, 2–18. [CrossRef]
90. Jankovič, A.; Kolenik, T.; Pejović, V. Can Personalization Persuade? Study of Notification Adaptation in Mobile Behavior Change Intervention Application. *Behav. Sci.* **2022**, *12*, 116. [CrossRef]
91. Maalsen, S. Algorithmic Epistemologies and Methodologies: Algorithmic Harm, Algorithmic Care and Situated Algorithmic Knowledges. *Prog. Hum. Geogr.* **2023**, *47*, 197–214. [CrossRef]
92. Loosen, W.; Scholl, A. The Epistemological Dimension of Algorithms. *Constr. Found.* **2021**, *16*, 369–371.
93. Milano, S.; Prunkl, C. Algorithmic Profiling as a Source of Hermeneutical Injustice. *Philos. Stud.* **2025**, *182*, 185–203. [CrossRef] [PubMed]
94. Lynch, C.R.; Bissell, D.; House-Peters, L.A.; Del Casino, V.J., Jr. Robotics, Affective Displacement, and the Automation of Care. *Ann. Am. Assoc. Geogr.* **2022**, *112*, 684–691. [CrossRef]
95. Sharma, A.; Lin, I.W.; Miner, A.S.; Atkins, D.C.; Althoff, T. Human-AI Collaboration Enables More Empathetic Conversations in Text-Based Peer-to Peer Mental Health Support. *Nat. Mach. Intell.* **2023**, *5*, 46–57. [CrossRef]
96. Pralat, N.; Ischen, C.; Voorveld, H. Feeling Understood by AI: How Empathy Shapes Trust and Influences Patronage Intentions in Conversational AI. In *Chatbots and Human-Centered AI*; Følstad, A., Papadopoulos, S., Araujo, T., Law, E.L.-C., Luger, E., Hobert, S., Brandtzaeg, P.B., Eds.; Springer Nature: Cham, Switzerland, 2025; pp. 234–259. [CrossRef]

MDPI AG
Grosspeteranlage 5
4052 Basel
Switzerland
Tel.: +41 61 683 77 34

International Journal of Environmental Research and Public Health Editorial Office
E-mail: ijerph@mdpi.com
www.mdpi.com/journal/ijerph

www.ingramcontent.com/pod-product-compliance
Lightning Source LLC
Chambersburg PA
CBHW040313270926
51850CB00007BC/1211
* 9 7 8 3 7 2 5 8 5 8 5 9 0 *